Mindfulness and Yoga
for Self-Regulation

Catherine P. Cook-Cottone, PhD, is a licensed psychologist, registered yoga teacher, and associate professor at the University at Buffalo, The State University of New York. She is also a researcher specializing in embodied self-regulation (i.e., yoga, mindfulness, and self-care) and psychosocial disorders (e.g., eating disorders). She has written four books and over 50 peer-reviewed articles and book chapters. Presenting nationally and internationally, Catherine uses her model of embodied self-regulation to structure discussions on empirical work and practical applications. She teaches classes on mindfulness therapy, yoga for health and healing, the history of psychology, and counseling with children and adolescents. She also maintains a private practice specializing in the treatment of anxiety-based disorders (e.g., posttraumatic stress disorder and generalized anxiety disorder), eating disorders (including other disorders of self-care), and development of emotional regulation skills.

Mindfulness and Yoga for Self-Regulation

A Primer for Mental Health Professionals

CATHERINE P. COOK-COTTONE, PhD

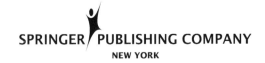
SPRINGER PUBLISHING COMPANY
NEW YORK

Springer Publishing Company, LLC
11 West 42nd Street
New York, NY 10036
www.springerpub.com

Acquisitions Editor: Nancy S. Hale
Composition: S4Carlisle Publishing Services

ISBN: 978-0-8261-9861-7
e-book ISBN: 978-0-8261-9863-1

15 16 17 18 19 / 5 4 3 2 1

The author and the publisher of this Work have made every effort to use sources believed to be reliable to provide information that is accurate and compatible with the standards generally accepted at the time of publication. The author and publisher shall not be liable for any special, consequential, or exemplary damages resulting, in whole or in part, from the readers' use of, or reliance on, the information contained in this book. The publisher has no responsibility for the persistence or accuracy of URLs for external or third-party Internet websites referred to in this publication and does not guarantee that any content on such websites is, or will remain, accurate or appropriate.

Library of Congress Cataloging-in-Publication Data

Cook-Cottone, Catherine P.
 Mindfulness and yoga for self-regulation : a primer for mental health professionals/Catherine P. Cook-Cottone, PhD.
    pages cm
 Includes bibliographical references and index.
 ISBN 978-0-8261-9861-7—ISBN 978-0-8261-9863-1 1. Mind and body. 2. Self. 3. Yoga—Psychological aspects. I. Title.
 BF161.C696 2015
 158.1—dc23
                                                                                                       2015004056

Special discounts on bulk quantities of our books are available to corporations, professional associations, pharmaceutical companies, health care organizations, and other qualifying groups. If you are interested in a custom book, including chapters from more than one of our titles, we can provide that service as well.

For details, please contact:
Special Sales Department, Springer Publishing Company, LLC
11 West 42nd Street, 15th Floor, New York, NY 10036-8002
Phone: 877-687-7476 or 212-431-4370; Fax: 212-941-7842
E-mail: sales@springerpub.com

Printed in the United States of America by McNaughton & Gunn.

This book is dedicated to
Jerry W. Cottone,
my husband, partner, and love.

Contents

Foreword

Yoga and mindfulness programs have grown in popularity at an unprecedented rate over the past few decades. Both are now frequently offered at medical centers, mental health clinics, schools, and elderly care facilities around the world. People of every age and stage of life are turning to yoga and mindfulness-based approaches as therapy for physical and mental health issues.

Although the scientific evidence for the effectiveness of these programs for myriad health concerns is rapidly emerging, medical and mental health professionals rarely receive formal graduate training in these practices. Consequently, interested practitioners receive yoga and mindfulness instruction outside the context of their professional sphere, and integration of these approaches is left to the individual. What's more, in most cases, training is not comprehensive enough to address the vast complexity of biopsychosocial issues that practitioners face. Clearly, an evidence-based road map for navigating the synthesis of Eastern and Western healing traditions is needed.

Emerging scientific evidence suggests that regular yoga and mindfulness practice have positive mental health outcomes. For example, yoga has been found to reduce the stress response and may be useful in alleviating symptoms of mood disorders, including anxiety and depression. Although encouraging, the field of yoga research is still nascent, with an overwhelming majority of the studies lacking sufficient empirical rigor to paint a convincing picture. At best we can conclude that the data are promising, and at worst we can point to methodological inconsistencies, weak research designs, and a plethora of other issues that render many of these findings speculative at best.

The dynamic interplay of mind and body and its role in the emergence, persistence, and treatment of physical and psychological problems remain a multifaceted mystery. Although psychobiological theories of mental illness and the yogic, mindfulness, and Ayurvedic traditions concur that the *issues are in our tissues*, treatment is not a simple, linear proposition. Rather, it is a dance of the physical body releasing its storehouse of repressed experience and the mind searching for meaning. It is akin to opening Pandora's Box while providing the crucible for discovery. This undertaking is remarkable to behold, yet it requires tremendous skill, flexibility, and wisdom for clinicians to navigate. The consequences of failing to understand, appreciate, or respect this mind–body interface can be dire, causing more harm than good.

Mindfulness and Yoga for Self-Regulation: A Primer for Mental Health Professionals is oriented around the premise that the *hungry self* is a driving force behind cognitive and behavioral dysregulation. This dysregulation sets the stage for mood disorders, anxiety, and the craving and desire that fuel self-defeating cycles and behavioral addictions. Catherine Cook-Cottone skillfully weaves the threads of Western and Eastern healing traditions into a framework for embodied self-regulation. This framework offers a model for holistic healing that emphasizes the synergy of mind and body and the embodiment of illness and recovery.

Unlike many of the existing philosophical and scientific texts on this topic, Dr. Cook-Cottone provides an accessible entrée into the philosophical underpinnings of yoga and mindfulness and the evidence supporting these practices that sets the stage for an embodied framework for clinical work. The framework is distilled into 12 embodied practices, which are interwoven throughout the chapters that follow. Yoga and mindfulness practice are presented in pragmatic, on- and off-the-cushion formats that support the idea of life as practice, honoring the conviction that we are all fellow travelers on the path to wellness.

This elegantly clear and accessible book is a timely and necessary offering for health professionals wishing to incorporate yogic and mindfulness principles and practices into their work. It offers a model for engaging clients that is scientifically grounded, pragmatic, and informed by time-honored yogic, Buddhist, and contemporary mindfulness traditions. Infused with illustrative accounts of the author's clinical work, this primer offers a much-needed blend of theory, practice, and tools to support therapists and clients in their integration of modern medicine with contemplative practice.

B. Grace Bullock, PhD
Founding Director
International Science & Education Alliance
Former Editor in Chief
International Journal of Yoga Therapy

Preface

Aim Namah Shivaya:
I bow to the infinite within and without, who is the bringer of
harmony, beauty, wisdom, and inner peace.
SANSKRIT YOGA MANTRA; AUTHOR UNKNOWN

THE HUNGRY SELF

Mindfulness and Yoga for Self-Regulation: A Primer for Mental Health Professionals presents an introduction to mindfulness-based and yoga approaches within the context of the dysregulating, culture-wide battle involving consumption and the struggle for identity. This clinician-oriented, introductory text explores the influences that lead to the externally oriented, idealized, and ultimately self-defeating construction of self adopted by many within Westernized culture—*the hungry self.* Over my years of work as a researcher, practicing psychologist, and certified yoga instructor trained in both traditional hatha and vinyasa flow methodologies, a persistent pattern became clear: Many individuals have become convinced that the antidote to their woes is found outside of themselves. Driven by an unrelenting media culture that correlates consumption with happiness, individuals eat, diet, shop, drink, gamble, medicate, and otherwise search for oft-promised satiety and peace of mind. For many, this externalized search results in a self-perpetuating cycle of longing, perceived failure, and dysregulation. In the absence of an internal sense of the self, a focus on consumption for happiness can exacerbate struggles with mood, anxiety, eating, and substance use, as well as a variety of additional addictive and compulsive behaviors.

This text provides the structure and practical applications for clinicians to help their clients find an internal sense of satiety and peace of mind. The body of research supporting mindfulness and yoga as wellness and preventive practices, as supplemental treatments, and integrated into treatment protocols is there. Mindfulness and yoga-based approaches have been found to be effective in helping individuals find a steady, regulated experience of self. Further, researchers are beginning to understand and document the mechanisms of action. Through mindful and yogic practice, the self (i.e., body and mind) is experienced as a living entity that can be responded to and learned from. The result of this embodied practice is physiological, psychological, and even neuropsychological change.

Illustrating the success of the field, there is a growing body of disorder-specific empirical work explicating mindfulness and yoga approaches for mood regulation, eating issues, depression, anxiety, and substance use. There are several manualized programs (e.g., dialectic behavioral therapy, acceptance and commitment therapy, and mindfulness-based stress reduction). Currently, there are a variety of texts that more generally address mindfulness and emotional regulation, the manualized programs, and mindfulness and yoga within the context of specific disorders (e.g., depression, anxiety). Currently, no text presents mindfulness and yoga as practices that help clients manage the psychosocial epidemic of dysregulation manifest in Western culture. Accordingly, this text defines the *dysregulated self* within the consumer context and presents mindfulness and yoga approaches as an alternative pathway toward a contented, regulated experience of self. Written for clinicians interested in learning more about why and how to integrate mindfulness and yoga techniques into their practice, this text introduces basic theoretical foundations, articulates key practices, and provides a brief overview of comprehensive protocols. Mindful self-care is reviewed, and the Mindful Self-Care Scale is introduced to facilitate patient and therapist self-evaluation and goal setting.

Background

In 1985, Kim Chernin's book *The Hungry Self: Women, Eating, and Identity* captured the struggle of women as they searched for a modern female identity and the corresponding epidemic of disordered eating. She was one of a pioneering group of researchers, theorists, and practitioners who had come to see that the struggle with consumption had something to do with the struggle for identity. Today, the struggle not only endures, it manifests in our overall approach to self and affects both men and women. Perhaps even more potent now than ever, the external influences integral to our consumer culture continue to create a tendency for self-identity to evolve from the outside in. Guided by media, many individuals turn to what can be consumed in order to feel whole, regulated, and content. However, as quickly realized, this approach does not satisfy. The development of individual identity moves away from an interactive and attuned unfolding of internal needs and external demands and resources. The authentic experience of self is lost. An externally driven, consumptive approach to well-being leaves one perpetually hungry as actual physiological, emotional, and intellectual needs are unmet.

Documentation of this struggle between consumption and identity dates back to biblical references, when Adam and Eve eat from the tree of knowledge and immediately become self-aware (Chernin, 1987). To be sure, hunger is a real and basic drive. Individuals need to consume to survive and ultimately to thrive. However, many confuse physiological hunger and needs with other hungers. They reach to consume (i.e., externally regulate) because they are afraid, alone, bored, excited, happy, and a whole variety of other feelings and states. Many also suffer from the delusion that all of these hungers or drives can be satisfied like real hunger, or worse yet, that they should be. These individuals come to see all of their drives as hungers that must be immediately met with food or a satisfaction of some kind (e.g., a purchase, a drink, or an accomplishment). If they crave security, they seek a relationship. If they crave status or acceptance, they seek material goods. Many believe that they are constantly hungry, and the media has created a science out of agreeing with them: *You are hungry and we have just the thing for you.*

The consequence of the consumption culture is that the prevalence of mood, anxiety, substance, and eating disorders continues to rise. Within many individuals, there is a neglected inner self that is in need of healthy attunement and care. Enter mindfulness and yoga. These traditions span thousands of years and have been passed down through sacred texts and practices. Yoga, by definition, is the yoking or integration of the mind and body in search of the true self. More recently, Western science has integrated these approaches as complementary and alternative mental health practices showing efficacy in a variety of areas (e.g., depression, anxiety, eating disorders). This text focuses specifically on the aspects of the hungry self as manifest in compulsive, externalized drives and behaviors and the basics of the integration of mindful and yogic practices that can help address these issues.

General Organization of the Text

The book is structured in four parts. Part I provides the conceptual, empirical, and theoretical foundations of embodied self-regulation. The chapters in this section address the various aspects of embodied self-regulation, introduce the dysregulated self, briefly define the disorders associated with poor self-regulation (e.g., disordered eating, mood disorders, compulsive shopping, and gambling), and present the mindful and yogic self. Parts II, III, and IV comprise the bulk of the text, as they hold the most utility for the practicing mental health professional. In Part II, the conceptual and philosophical aspects of mindfulness are explained in order to serve as a cognitive framework for a healthier, regulated self. Two chapters follow explicating the formal (i.e., on-the-cushion) and informal (i.e., off-the-cushion) mindful practices. In Part III, the conceptual and philosophical aspects of yoga are explained. As in the coverage of mindfulness, three chapters follow explicating formal yoga practices (i.e., on the mat), guidelines for developing a personal yoga practice, and informal yoga practices (i.e., off the mat). Part IV reviews evolving mindful and yogic applications as they are utilized within various empirically supported mindfulness and yoga-based protocols and in self-care.

Part I: Embodied Self-Regulation: A Conceptual Model

Part I is an introduction to the problem and the pathway to change. First, in Chapter 1, Embodied Self-Regulation: A Conceptual Model of the Role of Embodied Practices in Self-Regulation, the conceptual model of the text is presented. Using the self-representational model (Cook-Cottone, 2006), this chapter reviews the theoretical underpinnings and empirical support underlying the development of a consumptive approach to well-being. Chapter 2, The Dysregulated Self: From Craving, to Consumption, to Disorder, reviews a model of the dysregulated self and details disorders of dysregulation. Subclinical- and clinical-level disorders of mood, anxiety, and behavioral regulation are defined. In this chapter, the transition from risk to disorder is detailed. Specifically, the roles of genetic and internal variables that place individuals at risk are briefly reviewed. Finally, the role of the dynamic interface between individual vulnerability and family, community, and cultural influences is explicated. In Chapter 3, The Mindful and Yogic Self: Embodied Practices, the model of the mindful and yogic self is presented along with the 12 embodied mindful and yogic practices. This chapter explains the role of mindfulness and yoga in the search for self. With this brief chapter, the context will serve to transition the reader toward the review of mindfulness and yogic philosophy and practice. The conceptual aspects of mindfulness and yoga are presented as a framework for a healthier experience of self.

Part II: The Mindful Self

In Part II, the philosophy and conceptualization of self as presented in mindfulness philosophy are reviewed. Applied directly to clinical practice, each chapter addresses specific aspects of the mindful philosophical traditions that can serve as a new empowering cognitive and embodied self-regulation framework for clients. Chapter 4, Mindfulness: The Basic Principles, reviews the three basic principles of mindfulness approaches: impermanence, suffering, and not-self. Further, newer conceptualizations such as Siegel's *Mindsight* (Siegel, 2010) are reviewed. The principles are examined within the context of the literature on consumption and the utility of these concepts in shifting the client's perspectives and cognitions. Specific difficulties and disorders are used to demonstrate the role of mindful cognitive structures in well-being and recovery. Chapter 5, On the Cushion: Formal Mindfulness Practices, defines and describes formal practices within the mindfulness tradition (e.g., meditations). Finally, Chapter 6, Off the Cushion: Informal Mindfulness Practices, defines and describes the informal practices that are easily integrated into our daily lives, such as single-mindedness, the distinction between pain and suffering in all activities, and mindful being (e.g., mindful eating).

Part III: The Yogic Self

As a primer for clinicians, this section is grounded in the basic yoga practices as described in the Yoga Sutras and the Bhagavad Gita. Chapter 7, Yoga: The Basic Principles, defines the eight limbs, or steps, of yoga: yama (commitments), niyama (personal practices), asanas (body postures), pranayama (breath control), pratyahara (sense moderation), dharana (concentration and perceptual awareness), dhyana (meditation), and samadhi (the realization of self). The basic principles of yoga are presented as an integrated pathway to structure cognitions and support behavioral change. Chapter 8, On the Mat: Formal Yoga Practices, details formal yoga practices. These are the postures, posture sequences, breathing exercises, and meditations.

In Chapter 9, Creating a Regulating Practice: Yoga Teachers, Styles, Risks, and Tools, the types of yoga are described as well as the postures and sequences thought to be effective in addressing craving and consumption. Risks and contraindications are also covered. Please note that although the review of the practice of yoga is relatively comprehensive, this text does not include detailed guidance on specific poses. There are many guides for instruction in asana practice (see Chapter 9 for a guide to asana texts). For example, *Yoga Journal* (www.yogajournal.com) and the Himalayan Institute's *Yoga International* (yogainternational.com) offer free access to asana, yoga, classes, and boundless information on yoga. Each offers descriptions of asana, including step-by-step instructions, tips, and contraindications for each pose.

Chapter 10, Off the Mat: Informal Yoga Practices, details informal yoga practices. Similar to the informal mindfulness practices, these yoga techniques are used during an individual's daily life. These include the yamas (e.g., practicing nonviolence, demonstrating a commitment to truthfulness, sense control, and moderation) and niyamas (e.g., practices such as acceptance, contentment, and self-study). The practices are described within the context of their utility in self-regulation and the cultivation of the healthy self. Utility in specific areas of disorder is also integrated.

Part IV: Evolving Mindful and Yogic Approaches

Part IV addresses new directions in mindfulness and yoga. Chapter 11, Comprehensive Treatment Protocols and Empirical Support, reviews various prevention and treatment protocols that integrate mindfulness and yoga techniques. These include but are not limited to mindfulness-based stress reduction, dialectic behavioral therapy, acceptance and commitment therapy, mindfulness-based eating awareness training, and yoga protocols. Limitations in the research as well as cautions and contraindications are highlighted. Clinicians will be able to use this section as a resource and a road map for how to continue to build their expertise beyond the scope of this text.

Chapter 12, Mindful Self-Care, is a critical chapter and unique in its approach to effective remediation of an externally focused, dysregulated self. Chapter 12 addresses the balance between the care of the emotional and physiological self within the context of an individual's commitments outside of self. Often, those who struggle with self-regulation have great difficulty balancing service to others and external drives with the routine practice of self-care. This chapter details the cultivation of such a practice. Mindful self-care is presented as appropriate for both therapists and patients. Mindful self-care is defined, and a domain-by-domain description and assessment are provided. Each domain and each item can be easily translated into prescriptive goals.

THE MINDFUL AND YOGIC SELF
AS A PATHWAY TO SELF-REGULATION

You are about to begin a transformative process. This text was designed to inform clinicians in an easily accessible manner with use of case studies, practice scripts, tables, and figures to illustrate key concepts and practices. I encourage you to begin, or continue, practicing mindfulness and yoga as you enter into the reading of this text. Throughout the text, I refer to you and your patients, or clients, inclusively. Mindful and yogic practices are meant to be your practices as well as those of your clients. In Chapter 3, the journey and commitment of the therapist are detailed. As a therapist, you can guide patients on the path because you are a fellow traveler. Practice. Your active, embodied practice will bring the words to life as you have a felt sense of the meaning in your body. It is my hope that the love and gratitude that I have for these practices shine through the pages as you read. Mindfulness and yoga have changed my life. I hope the same for you and your patients. Welcome to a new way of being.

REFERENCES

Chernin, K. (1985). *The hungry self: Women, eating, and identity.* New York, NY: Harper & Row.

Chernin, K. (1987). *Reinventing Eve: Modern woman in search of herself.* New York, NY: Harper & Row.

Cook-Cottone, C. P. (2006). The attuned representation model for the primary prevention of eating disorders: An overview for school psychologists. *Psychology in the Schools, 43,* 223–230.

Siegel, D. (2010). *The mindful therapist. A clinician's guide to mindsight and neural integration.* New York, NY: W. W. Norton.

Acknowledgments

Be who God meant you to be and you will set the world on fire.
ST. CATHERINE OF SIENA[1]

Writing a book is a work of love. Given the right conditions, love can do amazing things. This book began as a seed, the emergence of an authentic expression of my self. It was born from my heart, my own personal growth, and the life-affirming process of personal inquiry. I have an ever-idle pinecone sitting in my office that reminds me that seeds cannot grow alone. Ease comes to authentic self-expression when those around you validate and support. That is, they see your light, the seed, and wholeheartedly help it grow. Seeds need a container, nourishing soil, water, sun, and tending.

I am the container. To make sure I am strong, healthy, and able to write I engage in self-care (see Chapter 12), which includes running with a wonderful group of people at Fleet Feet in Buffalo, New York, and the Snyder Running Club, as well as a soul-nourishing yoga practice at Power Yoga Buffalo. Thank you! Also, a big thank you to lululemon Buffalo (Walden Galleria) for all of your support of the athletes and yogis in the Buffalo area, including me. You brought the music and the strobe light to the party, and we have been rocking it. Thank you, Nancy S. Hale, for seeing this text to fruition—from idea to print—with encouragement and support. Thank you to Erga Lemish, who painstakingly read each letter of this text in preparation for submission. I am grateful to Christopher Hollister, associate librarian, who happily and effectively joined me in my quest to find obscure sources and citations. Thank you to my research team at the University at Buffalo, The State University of New York (SUNY). You are the light of the future. Thank you to all of my friends who laugh with me, for me, and sometimes at me—because sometimes you either laugh or cry, and although I like a good cry from time to time, I love to laugh. Yes, I am so thankful for the powerful communities and people who helped me take care of myself and stay inspired so that I could be the container for all of the concepts and ideas presented in this text.

A seed alone, in a container, is nothing without soil. A big thank you to my family: Oren and Elizabeth (Tink) Cook, Anne Cook, Patrick Cook, Cynthia Cook, and Stephen Cook. Growing up in our family provided endless motivation, creativity, and inspiration—I grew up in some great soil! I thank Utica College of Syracuse University, where I got a nurtured start in the field of psychology. Next, a big thank you to SUNY Oswego, where I secured my master's degree in school psychology. Finally, I have considerable gratitude for all I learned during my doctoral work at the University at Buffalo, SUNY, where I earned my degree in Combined Counseling and School Psychology.

The soil was not quite at the right mix for this particular seed to grow without my yoga training. Thank you to the Himalayan Institute (HI) for providing a pathway to knowledge, spirituality, and love of yoga. I am forever grateful for all I learned while earning my 200-hour yoga teacher certification through the HI at Buffalo. Also, thank you to Baptiste Power Vinyasa Yoga (BPVY). The Baptiste community has provided the tapas, the fire, that moved me from contemplating what I would like to contribute to the world to making it happen. I am forever grateful for all I have learned while receiving both the 200- and 500-hour yoga teacher certifications through BPVY.

All of this abundance and still more are needed. Without water, sun, and someone tending the process (the gardener), there can be no growth. Certainly, there is absolutely no way I could have written this book without the love and support of Chloe, Maya, and Jerry Cottone. You let me take over the kitchen table for months at a time, texted me the updates from lacrosse tournaments, and told me how proud you were of me when I wasn't sure about things or myself. You ate sushi, takeout, lots of pizza, turkey sandwiches, Annie's mac and cheese, and crockpot chili, all while—mostly—pretending that you did not mind. Chloe and Maya, you are my water and my sun. You nourish and inspire me. Chloe, ily∞ever. Maya, I love you more.

Jerry, you are the gardener. You always make sure that it all works. You noticed when I needed more support and when I needed less. You knew when to text and ask me to send you a grocery list and when to tell me to take a break and watch a movie. You drove all over the East Coast taking Chloe and Maya to lacrosse tournaments so that I could write. You taped games, made snacks, and texted updates. I am a very lucky wife. You believe in me, support me, and love me. And because of that, seeds like this book can grow.

I want you *all* to know that whenever a therapist, client, or anyone else reads this book and makes gains, puts down a drink, decides not to binge and purge, chooses to be present, or in any way uses these practices to improve his or her life situation, it will be because of all of you. You gave me everything I needed to grow this seed. Because of you, this seed can, in turn, plant seeds of hope and possibility in others. Love is generative like that.

NOTE

[1] "Be who God meant you to be," said Anglican Bishop of London Bishop Richard Chartres citing Saint Catherine of Siena in his address to the royal wedding couple Prince William and Kate Middleton at Westminster Abbey on April 29, 2011 (Bishop of London's amazing speech to William and Kate, Johannes1721/YouTube, retrieved from https://www.youtube.com/watch?v=l1vh-zWt9h8).

Embodied Self-Regulation
A Conceptual Model

Embodied Self-Regulation
A Conceptual Model of the Role
of Embodied Practices in Self-Regulation

However it may be of the stream of real life, of the mental river the saying
of Herakleitos is probably literally true: we never bathe twice in the same
water there.—WILLIAM JAMES (1884, p. 11)

THE SELF

Any discussion of self-regulation must begin with a discussion of the
self. The self: an entity or a process? Self as entity is a body, a thing,
an object. Self as process is a route, a journey, a practice, a river of
ever-changing experience. Within which way of seeing the self are we
most empowered as both conscious beings and as therapists? Since the
beginning of modern psychology there has been an ongoing inquiry
regarding the nature of the self. Great psychologists have tried to define it (e.g., William James, Sigmund Freud), whereas others minimize or ignore its existence (e.g., John B. Watson). Using empirical
tools, researchers have tried to measure, quantify, and study it. Yet, the
difficult-to-objectify *self* has remained elusive (Karoly, 1993). More recently, researchers have moved to understand the regulation of the self,
or self-regulation, as a comparatively more accessible construct to understand, measure, and modify.

This begs the question: Is *self-regulation* who we are? Are we the sum
total of our efforts to both regulate the inner workings of our physiology,

cognitions, and emotions and negotiate the outer influences of friends, family, community, and culture? In part, yes. The self—your self, my self, our clients' selves—is the sum total of three subsystems: the inner, outer, and integrative systems. Each of us has a self, or a sense of self, that is constructed from the roots of our internal, physiologically based predispositions, needs, and drives as well as from the demands and influences manifest in our environments. Accordingly, knowing who we are and functioning effectively requires mindfulness of each of the aspects of self-regulation. This includes a set of daily practices that cultivates and supports self-regulation.

In this chapter, the theoretical underpinnings of embodied self-regulation are explored and the empirical support is integrated. First, the construct of embodied self-regulation is described. Then, the first of several case studies is introduced. Finally, the Attuned Representation Model of Self (ARMS; Cook-Cottone, 2006) is reviewed.

The Self and Self-Regulation

Research indicates that mastery of self-regulation bears great fruits. For example, self-regulation is required to form and maintain close relationships with others (Molden & Dweck, 2006). Also, selfregulation is integral to the ability to immediately respond to setbacks and failures (Molden & Dweck, 2006). Many views of self-regulation (e.g., self-determination theory, or SDT) incorporate a focus on goals and one's regulation on the pathway toward achievement. Accordingly, when viewed in this way, interventions that enhance self-regulation can help clients achieve their goals. In fact, how self-regulation is studied and measured depends a great deal on how it is defined. It is important to clarify this point, as embodied self-regulation, as defined in this text, differs in key ways from Western views of self-regulation.

Self-regulation has many different definitions, or content emphases, depending on the perspectives of those seeking to define it. In 1993, Karoly defined self-regulation, in his often-cited paper, as voluntary action management. More specifically, according to Karoly (1993), self-regulation refers to:

- internal and/or transactional processes that enable individuals to guide their goal-directed activities over both time and changing circumstances or contexts;
- management of thought, affect, behavior, or attention through deliberate and/or automatized use of specific mechanisms and supportive meta-skills;

- processes that are initiated when routine activity is obstructed or when goal-directedness is otherwise made relevant (e.g., the appearance of a challenge, the failure of habitual or typical action patterns); and
- five interrelated and iterative component phases: (a) goal selection, (b) goal cognition, (c) directional maintenance, (d) directional change or reprioritization, and (e) goal termination.

Karoly's (1993) definition of self-regulation begins with a reference to goal-directed activities. Management of thoughts, feelings, and behaviors is conducted in order to maintain a trajectory toward goals. Self-regulatory processes are activated when a client notices an obstruction to, or deviation from, his or her goal-directed activity. At its core, this form of self-regulation begins with goals (i.e., goal selection) and ends with goals (i.e., goal termination), and between goal selection and goal termination regulation is engaged to serve the goals. I argue that this definition of self-regulation holds a prerequisite: a solid, felt sense of self. Without it, pursuit of goals can be a pathway to further loss of self, and with that your clients run the risk of challenges with self-regulation that go beyond failure to achieve goals and extend to challenges to the maintenance of mental health.

A key inspiration for this text is a book published in 1985, *The Hungry Self: Women, Eating and Identity* (Chernin, 1985). In her book, Chernin describes a process she observed in her work as a therapist. She noticed that as women lost their sense of self, a sense of who they are within their worlds, they had a corresponding struggle with food. She describes the loss of self as "There is no I" (Chernin, 1985, p. 20). Chernin's descriptions and analysis had a tremendous influence on how I came to understand "I" or "self" and the loss of self-regulation as well as the emergence of self-destructive behaviors such as eating disorders, shopping addictions, and substance abuse problems that manifest within the context of the triggers and demands present in the world. Clinical practice, research, and personal observations have convinced me that as the felt, embodied sense of self is lost, there is a corresponding increased risk for troubles with self-regulation. Considered another way, a hardy, effective self must be embodied to be known. In this way, self-regulation is a practice, an embodied practice.

Embodied Self-Regulation, Yoga, and Mindfulness

Embodied self-regulation differs from traditional self-regulation in four key ways: the target of the intervention, the emphasis, the endpoint or outcome, and the ecological scope (Table 1.1).

TABLE 1.1   A Comparison of Traditional Self-Regulation and Embodied Self-Regulation

Theoretical Facet	Traditional Self-Regulation	Embodied Self-Regulation
Target of intervention	Cognition-driven emotional and behavioral regulation	Mind and body integration within active practice
Emphasis	Motives, drives, and achievement	Honoring the process or the journey
Endpoint/outcome	Achievement of goals	Balanced and sustainable self-mastery
Ecological scope	Individual context	Attunement within self and among others

Distinct from more cognitive approaches to self-regulation, embodied self-regulation begins with the view of the body as a container of the self. With no physical entity, there is no manifest self. Accordingly, any self-work or self-regulation must integrate active practices that involve the body. Although cognitive approaches can be effective, often efficacy is enhanced through an integration of a behavioral component or embodied actions. In the same way, solely behavioral interventions for cognitively capable adolescents and adults prove more effective with an integration of cognitive components. This was illustrated by the emergence of cognitive behavioral therapy in the later part of the last century. Essentially, the birth of cognitive behavioral therapies was founded on the need for integration of the mind and body. The innovation continues as researchers and practitioners continue to seek increasingly more effective interventions.

As we have moved into the 21st century, many new therapies have emerged and the terms *emotional regulation* and *self-regulation* have become integral treatment targets in the latest wave of therapies (e.g., SDT). To various degrees, many of these therapies have integrated mindful and yogic approaches. Yogic approaches work. They have for thousands of years. The alignment of mindful and yogic practice and mental health is nearly seamless. The self, the whole self, craves and thrives on the integration of each of its aspects and functions best when well integrated (Siegel, 2010). Specifically, mindfulness and yoga help practitioners cultivate a receptive state of mind within which attention is informed by a sensitive awareness of what is occurring at the moment, both internally (e.g., psychological and somatic experiences) and externally (Brown & Ryan, 2003; Cook-Cottone, 2006; Schultz & Ryan, 2013).

The mindful and yogic path to self-regulation provides an embodied (i.e., lived experience) and cognitive framework for both knowing and regulating the whole, integrated self within the context of life experiences. Distinct from traditionally Western approaches to self-regulation, the mindful and yogic approach to self-regulation embraces the journey, perhaps more so than the goal. For example, in his yoga text, Patanjali (the original author of the Yoga Sutras) refers to the eight-limb path of yoga (Bryant, 2009). This pathway, formed of embodied practices, does in fact lead to a destination. However, it is not the completion of a marathon, earning of your first million dollars, or recovery. The destination is the realization of one's own true nature.

Embodied Self-Regulation Illustrated

Throughout this text, case studies are offered to further explicate and illustrate how self-regulation struggles might appear in practice. Self-regulation can look very different from person to person. People can vary substantially in how they process information, regulate emotions, and represent themselves within their social worlds (Molden & Dweck, 2006). These variables can lead them down substantially different developmental pathways (Molden & Dweck, 2006). We are whole beings. At our healthiest, we are the integration of our external and our internal selves. From an integrated, embodied self, we make decisions and regulate our emotions based on what we know to be true in our hearts (or emotional selves), our gut (our intuitive, sensing self), and our thoughts (the cognitive, neuropsychological self). Over the years, some of the most gifted therapists have made reference to this type of integration: Kim Chernin (1985), Marsha Linehan (1993), Niva Piran (Piran, Levine, & Steiner-Adair, 1999), and Daniel Siegel (2010). When an integrated, well-developed knowing of the self is embodied, there is an ability to live both intuitively and within the context of the knowledge we have accumulated from others over the years. Marsha Linehan (1993) calls this integration of the emotional and reasonable self *wise mind*. In her words, "wise mind adds intuitive knowing to emotional experience and logical analysis" (Linehan, 1993, p. 215).

To illustrate, Mathilde is happy and healthy. She is walking from the yoga studio to her apartment a few blocks away in Buffalo, New York. She thinks, "That was an awesome yoga practice. I feel alive." It's late spring and she smells the intermingled scents of the bakery up the street, the bouquet of fresh-cut grass, and the aroma of the coffee that she's holding in her hand. The sun is warm on her cheeks. It's a Saturday. Notably, a lot of things in her life are not quite on track. She is going out later to sit by a close friend who is terminally ill. Her boyfriend recently left for a new job in New York City and there is no knowing, for sure, if they are going to make it. She's 24 and in the second year of a career-path position with a not-so-great boss. She knows it is important to put in your time, make a commitment, and then move on. She has lots of reasons to be ruminating, sad, overeating, drinking, and even shopping for her happiness. Yet, she is not doing any of those things. As she walks today, she embodies happiness, strength, and self-love.

Danielle (Danny) is distracted and feeling lonely, anxious, and a little bit hung-over as she rushes to work, late again. She is a beautiful young lady, although a bit underweight. She is in her first 6 months of her third job as a legal aide. She is thinking about law school but never gets the deadlines right for the tests and applications. Her boyfriend Jared did not come home last night, again. He is a good-looking guy and she knows, "He can get whomever he wants." She is hoping once they get engaged, he will settle down. She starts feeling too full from her breakfast and wonders if the single bathroom at the entrance of the office will be open so she can make herself throw up before going upstairs. She had hoped it was going to be a "good day"—that is, no purging. She decides that she will make things right by skipping lunch. "It's okay for today," she rationalizes. This Jared thing has thrown her off. She walks in the door and the doorman asks her how she is. She smiles brightly and says "Great," knowing that she is not doing great at all. In fact, she now feels huge, horrible, and discouraged. She even hates her purse. Another decision made: This is a perfect day to drop by the mall on the way home. She has her mom's credit card from last weekend. Ah, that will perk her up—retail therapy.

Zuri is 13 years old and lives on the East Side in Buffalo, New York. Her mom is an alcoholic and she hasn't seen her dad in a long time. She is the middle child. Her older brother, Eric, is in and out of trouble. He has a lot of potential. He's bright and funny. Still, he hangs with a crowd that is up to dangerous dealings. Zuri worries for him and her younger brother Rashan. Rashan is still in elementary school and Zuri is essentially his caretaker. Funded by a wellness grant, Miss Amanda began working at Zuri's school as an after-school yoga teacher. Every day after school, Zuri practically runs from her locker to yoga class. Miss Amanda has no idea how important she is to Zuri. Miss Amanda's class is the one place Zuri is able to access her breath and, interestingly, her hope.

Mathilde, Danny, and Zuri are experiencing the world in very different ways. Circumstances challenge each of them. They each have a lot to negotiate. Yet, Mathilde and Zuri notice the sun and when they smile it is from the heart, a genuine experience. Conversely, Danny has learned to put on a good face. There is little attunement between her inner and outer experience. These seemingly subtle differences in ways of being can be nearly imperceptible to an outside observer. However, the inner experience of mis-attunement, dysregulation, and a false or lost sense of self can be intense and destructive.

From an integrated self, we are mindful of the effects our choices will have on the people whom we love and care for, as well as the community within which we live. We consider the cultural implications and social guidance (e.g., community values and moirés) for our choices. You see this in Mathilde as she allocates time to be with her friend who is sick and sticks with an entry-level position to aggregate experience and references. As you will see in this text, cultivating an integrated and embodied way of being takes some doing. For some, this is the natural unfolding of the self. The sense of attunement between the inner self (i.e., thoughts, feelings, and physiological needs) and outer self (i.e., the familial, community, and cultural self) is embodied within the context of love, support, and challenge. However, for a lot of our clients, like Danny, the experiences of attunement and integration are elusive and when present, fleeting. She experiences this cognitively, emotionally, and physically. She is hungry for a sense that things are okay. There are substantial forces pulling her in external directions: media culture, consumerism, idealization of financial wealth and beauty, and an emphasis on image and looking good (Thompson, Heinberg, Altabe, & Tantleff-Dunn, 1999). There has been a disruption in her relationship with her body (Piran, 2001). Accordingly, Danny looks outside of her-*self* for the cure (e.g., food, image, changing jobs, shopping)—a place she is not likely to find it, not for the long term.

Attuned Representational Model of Self: Embodied Self-Regulation

The Attuned Representational Model of Self (ARMS) was first conceptualized as a model for the development of a healthy, well-regulated self as well as to illustrate the factors that create risk for disordered eating (Cook-Cottone, 2006). ARMS is a comprehensive model that addresses cultural, community, and familial influences on individual development and individual behavior (Cook-Cottone, 2006; Cook-Cottone, Tribole, & Tylka, 2013; Cook-Cottone, Kane, Keddie, & Haugli, 2013a; Figure 1.1). According to the ARMS perspective, the self is a representation, or embodiment, of an integrated internal self (i.e., thoughts, feelings, and body/physiology) and the external experience, or social construction, of self (i.e., self within family, community, and culture; Cook-Cottone, 2006; Piran, 2001; Piran & Cormier, 2005). Risk and resiliency can arise from any one aspect of the self, internal or external. Further, risk and resilience

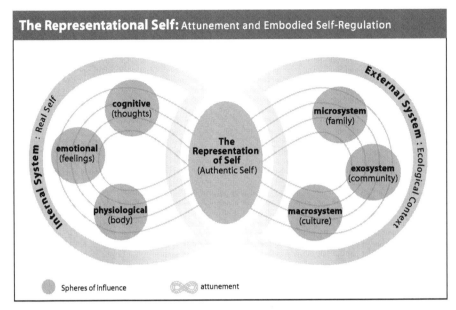

FIGURE 1.1 Attuned Representational Model of Self (ARMS).

are also created in the overall functioning of the system as the internal and external aspects of the self function with attunement or discordance. Specifically, internal and external attunement promote resiliency, and systemic discordance can lead to dysregulation and risk for disorder. Accordingly, there are both internal and external influences associated with self-regulation (Schultz & Ryan, 2013).

The healthy self is conceptualized as an authentic representation of an individual's thoughts (cognitive experience), feelings (emotional experience), and body (physiological experience). In order for the self to be a healthy, authentic representation of an individual's thoughts, feelings, and physiological needs, there must be an attunement among the coexisting components of the self, both internal and external. Similar to the SDT (Ryan & Deci, 2000), it is posited that individuals are growth oriented, naturally striving toward a coherent, unified sense of self, as well as integration of the self within a broader social network (Heatherton, 2011). Distinct from SDT, the ARMS model sees *attunement* and/or lack of *attunement* within the self and between the self and broader social systems as critical in the development of health and risk (Cook-Cottone, 2006; Heatherton, 2011). Specifically, attunement is defined as a reciprocal process of mutual influence and coregulation of thoughts, feelings, and physiological needs within the context of family, community, and culture (Cook-Cottone, 2006; Siegel, 1999). As an individual is mindful and responsive to his or her own needs, emotions, and thoughts, there can be an accompanying acceptance and validation of the individual within his or her social world (Piran, 2001).

Embodiment and embodied practice are critical elements in the development of a healthy self. In order for an individual to be resistant to or protected from externalized, dysregulated behaviors (e.g., disordered eating, shopping addictions, substance abuse, excessive exercise), he or she must *embody* a set of practices and ways of being that allow for and support regulation and attunement of cognitions, emotions, and physiological experiences. To *embody* is to give tangible form to something. In this way, an individual must be in action and practice to give form to attunement and health. Mindfulness and yoga are two pathways to embodied well-being. To be mindful is to embody and embodiment is the practice of yoga. In Gandhi's (2009) interpretation of the *Bhagavad Gita* he states that in order for the self to lead there must be complete harmony among thought, speech, and action. That is, to be in harmony with one's self, there must be embodied attunement. In an extension of the previous ARMS model (Cook-Cottone, Tribole, & Tylka, 2013b), the representation self (see Figure 1.1) manifests the embodied attunement and regulation of the internal self.

Embodiment and practice can also serve to be critical elements in the development of an unhealthy, dysregulated self. We see this as Danny struggles with her eating, changes jobs, drinks alcohol in excess, and shops. Danny experiences conflict between her own physiological needs for nourishment and the thinness and attractiveness messages she receives from her boyfriend and the media. At this point in her development, she is without tools and a health-promoting cognitive framework within which to process and reject these messages. Danny presents without an internal, embodied sense of direction or regulation and looks outside of herself (to her boyfriend, alcohol, and the mall) to feel okay.

Internal Aspects of Self

The internal self comprises an individual's cognitions (i.e., thoughts), emotions (i.e., feelings), and physiology (i.e., the body). Each aspect of the internal self represents an area that has been implicated in research as contributing to health and well-being or risk and disorder (Cook-Cottone, 2006; Cook-Cottone et al., 2013b). As presented in neurobiological theories (Siegel, 1999) and by Zen masters (Osho, 2003), the aspects of the self function best when they are in attunement or harmony. Osho (2003) described attunement as a deep, rhythmic harmony, a togetherness, in which the aspects of the self function in cooperation. He says that in this attunement you are "an orchestra of all your energies" (p. 153). At the core of self-regulation lies an individual's capacity to reflect upon and consider his or her own behavior and its congruency with the needs and drives of all the aspects of the internal self (Schultz & Ryan, 2013).

Physiological Self

The physiological, sensing self serves as the framework for self-regulation. It is in the physical experience that we exist. That is, we embody our lives (Herbert & Pollatos, 2012). It seems funny to feel compelled to write this. Yet, we have become so intellectualized, commoditized, and technology focused that we must be reminded of our bodies (Greenwood & Delgado, 2013; Siadat, Hasandokht, Farajzadegan, & Paknahad, 2013). Accordingly, there are schools of thought in the area of cognitive science that give the body a central role in shaping the mind (Herbert & Pollatos, 2012; Wilson, 2002). Piaget and Inhelder (1969) demonstrated that it is movement through the sensory motor stages that forms the framework for cognitive development, with roots in object permanence and understanding of basic concepts. In 1982, Kopp casted the antecedents of self-regulation within the critical transition from sensorimotor levels of functioning to reflective thought, task-oriented behaviors, and social interactions. Kopp (1982) posits that these early roots provide the ontogenetic framework for movements from neurophysiological modulation (birth to 2 to 3 months of age), to sensorimotor modulation (3 months to 9 months), to control (12 to 18 months), to self-control (24 months), and finally to the emergence of self-regulation (3 years and older).

Herbert and Pollatos (2012) describe the bodily sensations that are associated with endogenous homeostatic control mechanisms as intrinsically tied to life. These experiences represent relevant signals for survival and well-being and underlie the other two aspects of the internal self—emotional experience and cognitive processes (Herbert & Pollatos, 2012). Similarly, in her articles on embodied cognition, Margaret Wilson (2002) provides a theoretical rationale for understanding embodied cognition. From the perspective of embodied cognition, the starting point is not the mind working on abstract problems, but a body that compels the mind to make it function (Wilson, 2002). The term *embodied cognition* necessitates that the mind must be understood within the context of its relationship to a physical body that interacts with the world (Wilson, 2002). She explains that perhaps the roots of modern-day cognition are situated cognitions taking place in the context of task-relevant inputs and outputs and under task demands and time limitations.

In Sheila Reindl's (2001) account of women's recovery from bulimia nervosa (i.e., an eating disorder marked by dysregulated eating, binge/purge behaviors, and intense body dissatisfaction), the central feature of recovery was development of a sense of self. The emphasis matters—"here the word *sense* is as important as the word *self*" (Reindl, 2001, p. 9). There is an important distinction to make between conceptually understanding the self and the embodiment of self. In a series of case studies, Reindl (2001) aptly demonstrated the critical importance of having a felt sense of one's being in this world and the risks that arise when one does not have this sense.

Emotional Self

The emotional self is the seat of an individual's feeling self. A substantial amount of research and practice demonstrates the importance of cognitive processing in emotional and self-regulation. The realm of emotions is often considered the seat of the challenge. In fact, people need to effectively regulate their emotions to function in society (Heatherton, 2011). The failure of emotional regulation can result in aggression, violence, and other behaviors detrimental to social ties and connections. Further, emotional regulation is tied to healthy psychological functions and lack of emotional regulation is associated with several mental disorders (Heatherton, 2011).

Emotions are a very physical experience. Citing a long history of research, Herbert and Pollatos (2012) suggest that the foundation of our feelings is comprised of neural representations of the body or somatic markers that serve to evoke feeling states that influence both cognition and behavior. Similar to the sensory-motor activation that occurs during conceptualization, or use of concepts, the representation of body signals and the meta-representation of the state of the body create a sense of emotion in the self, or emotional awareness (Herbert & Pollatos, 2012). These are higher cognitive processes that function through perceptual symbols rooted in lived experience (Herbert & Pollatos, 2012). In a reciprocal dynamic, cognitive conceptualization reactivates sensory-motor states that occur when an individual is within an experience in the world (Herbert & Pollatos, 2012). The body is central to the experience of the self and is the seat, or container, for both the emotional and cognitive aspects of self.

Cognitive Self

The cognitive self is the thinking and understanding aspect of the self. This is the aspect of self that is most easily identifiable to individuals in Western culture. In 1637, René Descartes coined the phrase "Cogito, ergo sum," or "I think, therefore I am" (Descartes & Cress, 1998). In practice, therapists often experience this to be true for their clients. That is, clients identify their running, inner narrative, or ongoing thought processes, as the entire self. This is a circumscribed view of the self, far from the ARMS model we are presenting here (Cook-Cottone et al., 2013b). This aspect of self, the individual narrator, is an important component of the thinking, cognitive self. Here we conceptualize this as the seat of our inner narrator and consciousness processor. This is the aspect of the cognitive self that knows and creates our life story and the part of self at work when we are trying to purposefully understand or process information. It is one component of the cognitive self. The cognitive aspects of self also include the perceptual and the conceptual facets of self well delineated by Daniel Siegel in his text *The Mindful Therapist: A Clinician's Guide to Mindsight and Neural Integration* (2010).

First, it is important to highlight the narrative, thinking self. Consistent with the layperson's current overidentification with the thinking self, throughout the history of modern psychology various schools of thinking have also overly identified with cognitions. In essence, the mind, our narrative thinking self, is viewed as a tool to control emotions and physiological urges and desires. There may be something to this. It rings true for all of us in our day-to-day experience as well as in ongoing research. Regulation of thought or thought suppression has long been studied by cognitive neuroscientists (Heatherton, 2011). In fact, inhibition is a core feature of self-regulation, a process by which individuals "initiate, adjust, interrupt, stop, or otherwise change thoughts, feelings, or actions in order to effect realization of personal goals or plans or to maintain current standards" (Heatherton, 2011, p. 364). In this way, thoughts matter, a lot.

Our narrative experience is also the holder of our personal story, our memories. Our personal story, well integrated or not, can be a very powerful influence in our functioning (Cook-Cottone & Beck, 2007). As we develop, our personal narrative evolves. This is the story we hold of our lives. Most people do this unconsciously, that is, without intention. The brain simply integrates events as they have occurred into our current life narrative. This narrative is like a river in that it integrates life experiences as well as the stories we are told about ourselves by parents, friends, and loved ones (Cook-Cottone & Beck, 2007). Most of us take it for truth. There are many aspects of our narratives that are authentically, organically true in terms of a connection to what has actually happened to us. However, there are other aspects that are shaped by perceptions, stories, and biases (Siegel, 2010). These narratives are often who we think we are and we may or may not be correct. This can be an important component to address in working toward self-regulation.

For example, years ago I worked with a young woman who was a precocious child, a challenge to her overwhelmed and somewhat unskilled mother. She was told for decades about how difficult she was.

Stories were told to exemplify this bias and photos were served up as examples. Under careful examination, this portrayal was both true and untrue. In contrast to what she explained to me, I saw before me a very pleasant, bright, and passionate young woman determined to make a difference and help others. In our lived experience as client and therapist, things were not as she described. As we worked, my client was able to discover how her view of herself as difficult, the one storied to her by her mother, created an obstacle for her for many years. Once reframed and reintegrated as part of a bigger picture, a more comprehensive story of a bright, precocious, gifted child who could be challenging to adults (especially adults not equipped to handle her gifts), she was able to more effectively set goals for her future and more clearly perceive her current circumstances.

The cognitive self includes our perceptual and our conceptual understanding as well. Neuropsychologists have come to understand that our experiences change what we see and how we see things. Experience neurologically shapes us. This is often conceptualized via Hebb's rule summarized as "Neurons that fire together wire together" (Hebb, 1949). The mindful approach to psychology interfaces well with the neuropsychological approach in that both acknowledge that there are internal triggers, based on experience, that can shape our current awareness (Grabovac, Lau, & Willett, 2011; Siegel, 2010). Siegel (2010) describes our perceptual bias as moving us away from an open plane of perceptual possibility in which all things have the equal probability of being seen and perceived as is. Experiences, memories, and expectations move us toward a more constricted perceptual field marked by plateaus of probability, metaphors for the increased likelihood that we will see and perceive the world in ways consistent with our life experience and expectations.

Finally, there are the conceptual aspects of the cognitive self. Our conceptual understanding is built from both lived experience and learned knowledge. Within the context of this model, this is the aspect of the self that we think about when we consider what we know. It is our understanding of facts and can be biased from both our own perceptual limitations as well as by the nature of the content knowledge to which we have been exposed (Siegel, 2010). A friend of ours is a music teacher. He sees the world differently than I do. As a song is played on the radio, he hears similarities to traditional composers and influences of various genres of music. He knows these things given his training and his experiences. I hear the song. I make connection with the lyrics, perhaps enjoy the beat, and I can usually tell if it is a 1980s remix. However, my hearing is wholly different from his hearing. Interestingly, for our music teacher friend to be in pure presence and mindfulness with a particular song, he may struggle more than I to let go of what he knows. Conceptual knowing, like other aspects of self, can both contribute to and create obstacles for our growth.

External Aspects of Self

The external aspects of the representational self reflect the external demands placed on and supports provided to the internal self. Between the two, internal and external experiences of self, is the embodied experience of self. The embodiment that occurs in our lived experience may be reflective of core internal needs and intentions, or it may reflect the demands of the external system (Cook-Cottone, 2006; Heatherton, 2011; Schultz & Ryan, 2013). For example, Sheila Reindl (2001) theorizes that individuals with bulimia nervosa have split off the neediest parts of themselves. As conceptualized by the ARMS model, the physiological and emotional needs of a patient go unmet as they are split off or neglected by a patient (Cook-Cottone, 2006). Instead of creating an awareness and validation of these needs and consequently addressing them, the patient ignores or suppresses them as she is busy engaging in the needs, wants, and expectations of those in her family or community. She may even be ashamed or completely unaware of her own physiological and emotional needs, and may have no cognitive tools to access or regulate them.

Danny, our case study, lives this dynamic. She is externally focused on her boyfriend and his behaviors and desires to the neglect of her own experiences. She is focused on looking right and managing his and others' perceptions of her as she ignores her own needs for food, water, and even rest. She shows no hint of a cognitive awareness of her struggle, and her personal narrative is very externally focused, with Danny as an object in her own story. That is, she is his girlfriend, her boss's disappointment, and her mother's burden. She has no sense of her internal self and overvalues the role of her context in lived experience. Although Danny needs balance, she may come by the predisposition for external focus quite honestly.

In Kopp's early paper on self-regulation, she defines it as an ability to change ongoing behavior in response to events and stimuli in the environment, and flexibility of control processes that meet changing situational demands (Kopp, 1982, p. 202). Essentially, the evolution of humankind has depended on individuals being able to adapt to and accommodate the threats and demands of the external environment (Heatherton, 2011). Our ancestors who were able to solve external problems and adapt to their social environment were most likely to survive, reproduce, and pass on their genetic material (Heatherton, 2011).

Belonging and attunement with our social environment are fundamental to survival and well-being (Heatherton, 2011).

Schultz and Ryan (2013) refer to external regulation as the most controlled form of regulation as individuals contend with external contingencies through which they are both punished and rewarded. Heatherton (2011) described self-regulation as necessary for functioning within the social world. One example is introjected acts. Introjected regulation is a concept closely related to extrinsic motivation (Schultz & Ryan, 2013). Introjected acts are those acts performed in service of real or anticipated contingent approval or disapproval (Schultz & Ryan, 2013). An individual may control behavior in order to avoid guilt and/or projected disapproval or to gain esteem or ego enhancement (Schultz & Ryan, 2013). For example, Danny makes herself throw up in an attempt to regulate her weight and appearance in order to gain approval and continued acceptance by her boyfriend.

Our external systems extend beyond family and close friends to include our community and cultures. These influences can be neutral, validating, or risk enhancing. They can counteract one another or they can aggregate (Cook-Cottone, 2006; Cook-Cottone et al., 2013b). For example, Danny is quite vulnerable to media influences extolling an overly thin, idealized image of women (Cook-Cottone et al., 2013b). She is especially vulnerable to the influence of media due to having grown up with her mother, a retired fashion model, and her father, a local television news anchor. In her family, appearance is considered to be social capital. Her community was an influence as well. She was raised in an upper-middle-class neighborhood in a school culture that also emphasized appearance. Girls competed to wear the most recent fashion, some even taking on jobs after school just to keep up. For Danny, the layers of influence and risk run deep and have aggregated over time. She has internalized these conceptualizations of beauty, feels that they are very important to life success, and now primarily experiences herself as an object of the gaze and evaluation of others (see objectification theory, e.g., Fredrickson & Roberts, 1997).

When the external system is validating, supportive, and attuned to the emotional, cognitive, and physiological well-being of an individual, the representation of self is experienced in such a way that the self functions to serve the internal aspects of self and to engage in healthy, functional, and productive ways with the external environment (Cook-Cottone, 2006; Heatherton, 2011). In this way, the representation of self is an open, malleable system. Conceptualizing the self this way allows both clients and therapists to be present with the ability of new experiences to sculpt the self (Siegel, 2010).

SUMMARY

The attuned and embodied experience of self reflects an awareness and validation of the internal aspects of self (i.e., physiological, emotional, and cognitive) as well as managing and functioning within the external experiences of the self (i.e., family, community, and culture). Yogic and mindful approaches are presented as effective tools for facilitating this integration. As seen in the case studies of Mathilde and Zuri, mindful and yogic practices provide an embodied experience that enhances and develops the internal aspects of self, and help individuals live more effectively within their external context. These approaches allow for and can enhance the sense of attunement one experiences within the outer and inner aspects of self. The cognitive structure and tools provided by yogic and mindful approaches provide both a framework and active practice for patients to move toward mental health and away from risk and disorder.

Importantly, these practices are embodied. They are lived experiences. As patients practice, they create new neurological realities, new ways of being. Finally, both yogic and mindful approaches are increasingly valued in popular as well as medical cultures, as patients can access these supports without stigma and with the support of a physician and/or psychiatrist.

REFERENCES

Brown, K. W., & Ryan, R. M. (2003). The benefits of being present: Mindfulness and its role in psychological well-being. *Journal of Personality and Social Psychology, 84,* 822–848.

Bryant, E. F. (2009). *The yoga sutras of Patanjali: A new edition, translation, and commentary.* New York, NY: North Point Press.

Chernin, K. (1985). *The hungry self: Women, eating, and identity.* New York, NY: Random House.

Cook-Cottone, C. P. (2006). The attuned representation model for the primary prevention of eating disorders: An overview for school psychologists. *Psychology in the Schools, 43,* 223–230.

Cook-Cottone, C. P., & Beck, M. (2007). A model for life-story work: Facilitating the construction of personal narrative for foster children. *Child and Adolescent Mental Health, 12,* 193–195.

Cook-Cottone, C. P., Kane, L., Keddie, E., & Haugli, S. (2013a). *Girls growing in wellness and balance: Yoga and life skills to empower.* Stoddard, WI: Schoolhouse Educational Services.

Cook-Cottone, C. P., Tribole, E., & Tylka, T. (2013b). *Healthy eating in schools: Evidence-based interventions to help kids thrive.* Washington, DC: American Psychological Association.

Descartes, R., & Cress, D. A. (1998). *Discourse on method*. Cambridge, MA: Hackett Publishing.

Fredrickson, B. L., & Roberts, T. A. (1997). Objectification theory. *Psychology of Women Quarterly, 21,* 173–206.

Gandhi, M. (2009). *The Bhagavad Gita according to Gandhi*. Berkeley, CA: North Atlantic Books.

Grabovac, A. D., Lau, M. A., & Willett, B. R. (2011). Mechanisms of mindfulness: A Buddhist psychological model. *Mindfulness*. doi: 10.1007/s12671-011-0054-5

Greenwood, T. C., & Delgado, T. (2013). A journal toward wholeness, a journey to God: Physical fitness as embodied spirituality. *Journal of Religion and Health, 52,* 941–954.

Heatherton, T. F. (2011). Neuroscience in self-regulation. *Annual Review of Psychology, 62,* 363–390.

Hebb, D. (1949). *The organization of behavior*. New York, NY: Wiley & Sons.

Herbert, B. M., & Pollatos, O. (2012). The body in the mind: On the relationship between interoception and embodiment. *Topics in Cognitive Science, 4,* 692–704.

James, W. (1884). On some omissions of introspective psychology. *Mind, 9,* 1–26.

Karoly, P. (1993). Mechanism of self-regulation: A systems view. *Annual Review of Psychology, 44,* 23–52.

Kopp, C. B. (1982). Antecedents of self-regulation: A developmental perspective. *Developmental Psychology, 18,* 199–214.

Linehan, M. M. (1993). *Cognitive-behavioral treatment of borderline personality disorder*. New York, NY: The Guilford Press.

Molden, D. C., & Dweck, C. S. (2006). Finding "meaning" in psychology: A lay theories approach to self-regulation and social development. *American Psychologist, 61,* 192–203.

Osho. (2003). *Body mind balancing: Using your mind to heal your body*. New York, NY: St. Martin's Press.

Piaget, J., & Inhelder, B. (1969). *The psychology of the children*. New York, NY: Basic Books.

Piran, N. (2001). Re-inhabiting the body from the inside out: Girls transform their school environment. In D. L. Tolman & M. Brydon-Miller (Eds.), *From subjects to subjective: A handbook of interpretive participatory methods* (pp. 218–238). New York, NY: New York University Press.

Piran, N., & Cormier, H. C. (2005). The social construction of women and disordered eating patterns. *Journal of Counseling Psychology, 52,* 549–558.

Piran, N., Levine, M. P., & Steiner-Adair, C. (1999). *Preventing eating disorders: A handbook of interventions and special challenges*. Philadelphia, PA: Brunner/Mazel.

Reindl, S. M. (2001). *Sensing the self: Women's recovery from bulimia*. Cambridge, MA: Harvard University Press.

Ryan, R. M., & Deci, E. L. (2000). Self-Determination Theory and facilitation of intrinsic motivation, social development, and well-being. *American Psychologist, 55,* 68–78.

Schultz, P. P., & Ryan, R. M. (2013). The "why,"' "what," and "how" of healthy self-regulation: Mindfulness and well-being from a Self-Determination Theory perspective. In B. D. Ostafin, M. D. Robinson, & B. P. Meier (Eds.), *Handbook of mindfulness and self-regulation*. New York, NY: Springer.

Siadat, Z. D., Hasandokht, T., Farajzadegan, Z., & Paknahad, Z. (2013). Effects of multicomponent lifestyle modification on blood pressure control in health centers: Design of the study. *Journal of Research in Medical Sciences, 18,* 308–321.

Siegel, D. J. (1999). *The developing mind: Toward a neurobiological understanding of intrapersonal experience.* New York, NY: The Guilford Press.

Siegel, D. J. (2010). *The mindful therapist: A clinician's guide to mindsight and neural integration.* New York, NY: W. W. Norton.

Thompson, J. K., Heinberg, L. J., Altabe, M., & Tantleff-Dunn, S. (1999). *Exacting beauty: Theory, assessment, and treatment of body image disturbance.* Washington, DC: American Psychological Association.

Wilson, M. (2002). Six views of embodied cognition. *Psychonomic Bulletin & Review, 9,* 625–636.

❧ 2 ☙

The Dysregulated Self
From Craving, to Consumption, to Disorder

The urgency I felt, the pressure of the unknown force made my hands shake . . .
I felt the longing and it was not for food . . .
It was larger even than food, a hunger bigger than appetite . . .
Something about it terrified me.—KIM CHERNIN (1985, p. 151)

*E*mbodied self-regulation is a biologically rooted and socioculturally influenced practice. Foremost, our biological and genetic predispositions matter. No matter the context, there are great biological variations from person to person that affect various systems of our bodies and how these systems work, or do not work, together. For some, the mind and body are well integrated and self-regulation is spontaneous and automatic, requiring little or no effort or attention. For others, integration and self-regulation do not spontaneously manifest, or there has been a disruption of the process. For those who struggle, development of self-regulation requires awareness, intention, skill development, and practice. When there is no intentional, consistent cultivation of a more regulated way of being, the default is dysregulation. The challenge goes beyond our internal predispositions, defenses, and reactions. As explained in Chapter 1, there is a co-construction, a mutual influence among the internal and external aspects of self. Self-regulation and the mind–body connection exist within interpersonal, social, and cultural contexts (Fredrickson & Roberts, 1997; Porges, 2011; Siegel, 2007). Behaviors that move us toward understanding of and connection to the body are constructed through sociocultural practices and discourses (Fredrickson & Roberts, 1997; Porges, 2011; Siegel, 2007). Our relationships with our bodies, mind and body integration, and self-regulation all convey, to some degree, social meaning. They involve the here and now as well as our own personal history. Mind and body integration reflects the context within which we have developed and now function. At this point in Western history, there are substantial and powerful influences that discourage mind and body integration and individual self-regulation. For example, mass media abounds with marketing of pain medications, alcohol, and material goods. Ads pair happiness and life satisfaction with airbrushed, unrealistic beauty standards, excessive leanness, unbridled consumption, and substance use. It is no wonder we are challenged. We construct our selves within this context. That is, an individual's self-regulation manifests as the interaction between biological makeup and these types of social cultural practices and discourses. It is nature *and* nurture, as we are undeniably influenced by the environment within which we have been raised and now function.

This chapter describes that pathway from dysregulation to disorder as illustrated through the lens of struggles such as eating disorders, shopping addiction, self-harm, and gambling (e.g., Hartston, 2012). As captured by *The New York Times* piece titled "Dysregulation Nation" by Judith Warner (2010), "Today we might be called a nation of dysregulation. The signs that something is amiss in our inner mechanisms of control and restraint are everywhere." Warner lists increasing rates of eating disorders, obesity, drug addiction, and adolescents unable to sustain attention, regulate anger, or moderate their pain. Warner describes human struggle as an insatiable hunger. Warner's hunger echoes deep into and throughout history. We hear it in the words of Buddha: "Suffering [is] a ravenous appetite to find peace and security in places it can't be found" (Kabatznick, 1998, p. 2) and in Chernin's (1998) *The Hungry Self*. It is a dysregulation that has only seemed to grow deeper with the passage of time (Warner, 2010). As our culture becomes more expert at marketing to our inner hungry selves, risk for struggle and disorder increases. Our inner selves, our sense of embodied self-regulation, are challenged and for some, lost. To explicate this process and how it can present clinically, this chapter provides an overall model of the pathway to risk and disorder. Factors that may be important to review with your clients are covered and defined. Following a review of the risk factors and theories of risk, particular disorders are reviewed to highlight and detail points.

LOSS OF THE EMBODIED SELF: WHAT PUTS SOMEONE AT RISK?

Dysregulation of the self can present in many forms. When individuals are not self-regulated there are several ways that this shows up in their lives. We see this in Danny, the 24-year-old law clerk who struggles with her eating, drinking, and shopping (Hartston, 2012; see Chapter 1). For various reasons, Danny is at high risk. Research tells us that depending on genetic vulnerability, personal experiences, and environmental factors, some individuals struggle (Hartston, 2012). Dysregulation presents quite differently due to the complexity of the causal and influencing variables. For some people it shows up in mood regulation and they become depressed or overly anxious. There are other individuals who feel stuck in a behavioral battle with their eating (like Danny), with some developing eating disorders or weight concerns. Another set of individuals struggles to control consumption in other ways such as in compulsive shopping or gambling (Hartston, 2012). There are many ways that deficits in self-regulation can interfere with our clients' lives. Accordingly, addressing, teaching, and supporting self-regulation skills and practices within the therapy session can enhance therapeutic outcomes substantially (Linehan, 1993) and deter the reduction in one disorder (e.g., substance use) migrating to an increase in another disorder (e.g., eating disorder).

The scope is wide and reaches as far as those disorders that have a substantial genetic and biological etiology (e.g., bipolar disorders) to struggles of typical individuals working to get through the day (e.g., trouble overeating at dinner, having an extra glass of wine, struggling to integrate daily exercise). This text addresses behavioral dysregulation that ranges from the typical to the clinical, including the subclinical. The scope of the text incorporates trouble with self-regulation with roots in difficulty managing emotions, moods, and anxiety; ineffective cognitive schemata and habits; and a social or contextual component (Heatherton & Wagner, 2011). Specifically, this text addresses self-regulation problems that can trigger or maintain eating struggles and disorders, substance use and abuse, self-harm, compulsive gaming, and compulsive shopping and gambling (Hartston, 2012). Although some of the information in this text may be helpful for those struggling with disorders that are more biological than sociological in nature (e.g., bipolar disorder, severe mood disorders), these disorders are not the focus of the book. To be clear, specific disorders are not the heart of this text. Rather, the cultivation of embodied self-regulation and the path to wellness and integration is the emphasis.

The Model of Embodied Self-Regulation: Vulnerability to Disorder

In the case of risk and disorder, there is a mis-attunement that occurs between an individual's internal systems (i.e., physiological, emotional, and cognitive systems) and the external context (i.e., micro- [family], exo- [community], and macrosystems [culture]; Cook-Cottone, 2006). When considering this therapeutic approach to understanding self-regulation struggles, we accept the internal experience as valid. In this way, it is a phenomenological approach. The manifestation of an embodied sense of self begins with an individual's lived experience: body, emotions, and thoughts. As explained in Chapter 1, when the internal self exists within an attuned and validating external context, mental health is supported. In mindful and yogic terms, this would be seen as individuals living in their truth, their satya (Anderson & Sovik, 2000).

In the case of risk and disorder, the internal experiences of self, the phenomenological real self, is not seen, validated, or supported. In the case of risk and disorder, the internal self is rejected, denied, ignored, or neglected. For those at risk, the experience of the internal self is not embodied or represented even to those closest to them. These individuals are not living in their truth (i.e., satya, an authentic expression of self), and they may or may not be aware of this. When this occurs, the internal self is left without representation or embodiment (Cook-Cottone, 2006). Without representation or embodiment, there can be no real attunement with the external context. For example, if the people around you do not know or see how you are feeling or struggling, or what you need, it is very difficult if not impossible for them to acknowledge, validate, respond, or support.

We see this in Alexandra (Alex), age 28. She is what many call a *people pleaser*. She is always working to do the right thing, wear the right clothes, and be the person that a young woman should be. Alex is very externally focused and works hard to look good. Her family circumstances have influenced her. Her dad is an alcoholic and her mom enables him. She has learned from behaviors modeled by her parents to ignore her inner world and adapt to the needs and demands of those around her. She has watched her mom work at a job she hates and stay married to a man who breaks his promises on a weekly basis. Growing up, there were times when Alex doubted her own sanity. She knew full well her dad had done serious things while drinking (e.g., crashed the car, left the gas stove on in the kitchen). To cover, her mom made up story after story as if it were the truth. If Alex questioned things, her mom would become very angry with her. Alex learned not to question. She learned to silence the feelings and thoughts that were telling her otherwise (i.e., her truth, her satya) and to listen to her mom (Piran & Cormier, 2005). Now, at 28, she is married to Brandon, who drinks too much and is a constant critic of Alex. On the outside, they appear to be a beautiful young family. Alex works hard to be better, prettier, and funnier, and take perfect care of their two children. Truth is, she shops all of the time. Maintaining her *effortlessly perfect* facade takes a lot of work and a lot of money (Hinshaw & Kranz, 2009).

It seems that no matter how much she shops, she still feels empty inside. Things are at a breaking point. Her credit cards are up to $60,000 and she can't keep up payments anymore. Not one person knows about any of it. Well, no one but Alex.

Alex is stuck in this self-perpetuating, self-reinforcing cycle of feeling empty and alone and reaching to something outside of herself to meet a need that simply cannot be met in this way (Cook-Cottone, 2006; Figure 2.1). For some, the attempts at self-regulation are externalized. In these lived, embodied experiences, Alex feels like her body, emotions, and thoughts are aligned with what she is doing. When she is shopping or donning her new attire, it feels like her needs are being met. However, Alex has many clothes, some with tags still on them, collecting dust as they hang, untouched, in her closet. Her immediate sense of happiness when she buys and first wears an item is merely a distraction from her lack of connection with her real, internal self and absence of attunement in her life. Shopping won't ever fix it, and things are likely to get much worse.

Distinct from traditional views of self-regulation, embodied self-regulation posits that self-regulation must be embodied and manifested within lived experience (see Table 1.1). Accordingly, for those who

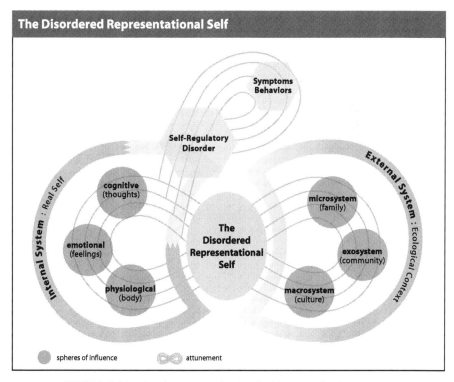

FIGURE 2.1 Disordered representational self with externalized symptoms.

struggle with self-regulation, risk includes a disconnection with the body and/or a disconnection from lived experience. For example, Danny, whom we met in Chapter 1, may decide to go into therapy to address her struggles. She may spend months working with her therapist to understand her past and its role in her current struggles. She may spend session after session reframing her cognitive perceptions of her experience. She may work on her cognitions and set goals for herself in areas like career, relationship, and negotiating emotions. However, until she embodies a new way of being in her lived experience, change will likely prove elusive. To be clear, it is important, even critical for some patients to understand their historical context and current situation, be aware of their cognitive and emotional responses to their experience, and set goals reflecting great clarity in what they are working toward. Still, none of it matters in terms of change until it is embodied, until it is practiced.

It is the loss of an embodied experience of a nurtured, healthy, and attuned self that places people at risk for self-regulation problems. Svenaeus (2013) refers to this as the experience of an "inauthentic" life (p. 84). There are intrapersonal (within the self), interpersonal (within relationships), and environmental (within a larger social context) factors that increase risk for disconnection with the self. Many known risks are associated with one or more internal and external factors. Several of the factors are described here. This is not intended to be an all-inclusive list. Rather, it is a list to illustrate the challenges associated with loss of embodied self-regulation. The following sections are included as possible points of didactic education for your patients. Understanding the challenges to self-regulation can be very helpful as the work to integrate and practice mindful and yoga interventions.

Alterations in Reward Areas of the Brain
(Internal—Physiological, Emotional, and Cognitive)

Patients who have genetic predispositions to reward sensitivities can benefit from awareness of this risk and its implications. Difficulties with disorders associated with problems in self-regulation are theorized to be associated with disturbed neurotransmission involving serotonergic, dopaminergic, and/or opioid systems (e.g., Black, 2007; Davis & Carter, 2009). For example, drugs of abuse typically hyperstimulate the dopamine (DA) and other reward areas, essentially hijacking the brain (Hartston, 2012). Researchers have made a case for behavioral addictions in which no external substance is ingested functioning similarly (e.g., compulsive buying; Black, 2007; Davis & Carter, 2009). In the case of both substance and behavioral addiction, the individual becomes dependent on the physiological brain responses associated with engagement in the substance (e.g., alcohol or cocaine) or the behaviors (e.g., shopping or gambling, compulsive overeating; Davis & Carter, 2009). Hartston (2012) explains how the brain does not distinguish between DA released due to drugs or experiences (real or imagined). Pleasurable experiences are associated with increased release of DA in two areas of the brain: the nucleus accumbens (NAcc) and the ventral tegmental area (VTA; Davis & Carter, 2009; Hartston, 2012). For some people, behaviors can act like hyperstimulating drugs. Researchers continue to explore the exact mechanism of action. Of note, some behavioral and substance addictions are known to work in a less direct way, causing hyperstimulation of the DA in the VTA and NAcc through a reduction in activity of the DA-inhibiting gamma-aminobutyric acid (GABA) neurons (Hartston, 2012). Others argue that the DA activity may be more involved in the wanting of the reward, whereas the GABA, opioid, and serotonin pathways are associated with the actual reward (Davis & Carter, 2009).

For most people, the process happens over time. When addictive substances are ingested or hyperstimulating behaviors are repeated over time, neuroadaptation occurs. Specifically, there is a down-regulation of the DA receptors that serves to maintain a homeostatic level of neurotransmission in the presence of the excessive DA release. Hartston (2012) describes this neuroadaptation as a hallmark of addiction. In some individuals, the repetition of the behavior triggers lasting changes in the DA reward pathway. At this point, craving can increase to levels above the individual's ability to intervene in the addiction-driven behavior. We see this in Alex's attempts to stop shopping in the face of the financial hardship it places on her family. She tries to stop and feels as if she cannot.

Once neuroadaptation has occurred, there are fewer receptor-binding opportunities (Hartston, 2012). Despite increases in DA, the net DA transmission rate is decreased. This manifests behaviorally as increased craving for the behavior, desire for more frequent exposure to the behavior to both feel good and to avoid feeling bad. Reward deficiency syndrome can occur, in which the individual experiences a constant state of withdrawal, feels depressed, and no longer finds everyday activities rewarding. Like those with substance addictions, a person who is behaviorally addicted struggles to feel rewards inherent in normal life experiences. When he or she is not able to engage in desired behaviors (e.g., shopping, gambling, playing a video game), feelings of depression, craving, and obsessive thinking are experienced. Like other addictions, those with behavioral addictions can go to extremes to experience exposure to their behaviors. Behavioral addictions are associated with self-deception, self-neglect, legal problems, role failure, and relationship loss (Hartston, 2012). Hartston (2012) notes that factors that increase the likelihood of changes in the DA pathways include easy accessibility, or a high likelihood of frequent engagement, and vulnerability to addiction (i.e., genetic predisposition, previous neuroadaptation, or reward deficiency syndrome).

Emotional Sensitivity and Control (Internal—Emotional, Cognitive, and Physiological)

Many of my patients present as emotionally sensitive. Additionally, nearly all of them have come to believe that this is a bad thing, that there is something wrong with them. It may be messages that they received from their parents, "You are too sensitive. Calm down!" It may be cultural standards and expectations. It may be due to history of a negative experiences associated with the expression of emotionality. It may be for all of these reasons. As such, I often spend a good part of the initial sessions explaining emotional sensitivity and commence ongoing work to address emotional control and regulation within the context of acceptance of the patient's emotional experience. That is, I introduce emotional sensitivity as a gift that provides a great range of internal experience and comes with added responsibility to self-regulate and manage.

Emotional control or regulation has been conceptualized in terms of both emotional sensitivity and as a regulatory process. The emotional sensitivity model involves two phases. First is the person's immediate, raw response to an event relevant to emotions (Koole, Van Dillen, & Sheppes, 2011). Second is the person's ability to cope with his or her initial emotional response (Koole et al., 2011). The primary response is related to his or her levels of sensitivity, which can be both genetically and experientially driven. The secondary response can be influenced by the development of skills or the utilization of supports. The secondary response can serve to either up-regulate or down-regulate the emotional experience. Here, emotional regulation skill development can be an important factor for individual outcomes. The process model of emotional regulation involves four stages (Koole et al., 2011). Table 2.1 details the process at each stage (Koole at al., 2011).

For example, at stage 1, an individual can carefully select situations that are less triggering or limit the exposure to triggering situations. This can occur in a down-regulating or up-regulating manner and can work to serve the problematic behavior or serve as a pathway to well-being and mental health. Alex, in our previous case study, makes errors at each stage that serve her spending problems. First, at stage 1, Alex is careless about the situational context. She regularly goes to the mall, peruses shopping catalogs, and views online shopping web pages. She has applications on her phone and computer that link her to specific shops and social networks designed to push products at consumers (e.g., Pinterest, Etsy). At

TABLE 2.1   The Process Model of Emotional Regulation

Stage of Emotion Generation	Process (Regulation of Emotion Generation)
Stage 1	Situational triggers encountered (e.g., situational selection, situational modification)
Stage 2	Attention/inattention to emotionally relevant features (e.g., attention deployment)
Stage 3	Cognitive appraisal of the situation (e.g., cognitive change)
Stage 4	Emotions expressed in behavior (e.g., response modulation)

stage 2, an individual can carefully select to what he or she attends. For Alex, when she is shopping she tends to ignore the price of objects, as the cost gives her anxiety and interferes with the immediate benefits of her shopping. Stage 3 involves shifting the cognitive process. Alex uses her cognition to rationalize and support her buying habits and to enhance the excitement of the shopping. She has quotes on her daily planner about the fun of shopping (e.g., "Shopping is cheaper than a psychiatrist," and "Whoever said money does not buy happiness did not know where to shop"). She engages in shopping in order to increase her feelings of excitement and fun, simultaneously avoiding feelings of anxiety and sadness. Finally, Alex is fully engaged in her feelings of excitement and thrill as she actively purchases an object. Each step has served to up-regulate her positive feelings of excitement and fun and to down-regulate anxiety and sadness.

Dysregulation of affect has been implicated in nearly all of the psychological disorders (Haedt-Matt & Keel, 2011). Psychopathology can result from the inability to control, or down-regulate, negative emotions (Nolen-Hoeksema, 2012). Problems with emotional control have been associated with specific brain functions. Heatherton (2011) cites extensive neuropsychological research concluding that dysfunctional amygdala (associated with the limbic or emotional activation system) and prefrontal (associated with cognitive mediation of behavior) circuitry in mood disorders highlights the importance of emotional regulation for psychological well-being.

Individuals who have difficulty with self-regulation often have deficits in emotional regulation and/or control. Regularly, they feel incapable of handling the negative thoughts and feelings associated with experiencing distressing emotions such as anger, loneliness, anxiety, rejection, and grief. When triggered by an internal cognitive event (e.g., a troubling memory) or an external experience (e.g., perceived peer rejection) the individual feels overwhelmed by the emotions associated with the event.

This is seen in self-injury, spending too much money, engaging in risky behavior, and using alcohol or food for comfort (Heatherton & Wagner, 2011). Specifically, the presence of negative feelings is often reported as a trigger for the behavior (Heatherton & Wagner, 2011; Nock, 2010). For some, this is partially due to what researchers call a genetic predisposition for high emotional/cognitive reactivity (Adrian, Zeman, Erdley, Lisa, & Sim, 2011; Nock, 2010). For others, this struggle is associated with a history of abuse or family hostility or criticism (Nock, 2010). In these cases, it is believed that the emotional experience is overwhelming and is accompanied by substantial physiological arousal. Further, for some there may have been inadequate environmental learning to manage these intense emotions (Adrian et al., 2011). That is, rather than teaching positive coping and self-regulation techniques, parents or caregivers punish, minimize, deny, or engage in conflict (Adrian et al., 2011). Note that you will read about the mindful and yogic approaches to emotional regulation in later chapters.

Negative affect has been explored in terms of its relationship with problem behaviors. For example, the affect regulation model of binge eating posits that maladaptive behavior (e.g., binge eating) functions to decrease negative emotions (Haedt-Matt & Keel, 2011). Similar theories have been posited for self-injury, substance use, pathological gaming, eating disorders, gambling, and excessive shopping. In theory, an individual experiences an increase in negative emotions. Distressed, the individual is triggered to binge eat (or use, buy, game, etc.). The symptoms, in this case binge eating, alleviate the individual's negative affect, as he or she is comforted and distracted. Through a negative reinforcement process (i.e., the aversive stimuli is removed via engagement in the behavior, thereby reinforcing the behavior), the behavior is maintained and the likelihood that it will recur is increased (Haedt-Matt & Keel, 2011). In an extensive meta-analysis, Haedt-Matt and Keel (2011) found that despite what individuals who binge eat may believe, following the binge eating there is (a) no reduction in negative affect and (b) no change or a possible increase in negative affect. Notably, this does not indicate that during the binge there may or may not be a relief from negative affect as theoretically posited. More research is needed to explore the pathway from emotional trigger, within and through engagement in the problematic behaviors, to behavioral outcomes both proximal and distal.

An associated construct, cognitive control, plays a role in self-regulation via action selection, response inhibition, performance monitoring, and reward-based learning (Ridderinkhof, van den Wildenberg, Segalowitz, & Carter, 2004). Action selection is deciding what action to take. A closely related process, response inhibition, refers to the suppression of actions that are inappropriate in a given context and that interfere with goal-driven behavior (Mostofsky & Simmonds, 2008). Specific brain mechanisms have been implicated in these processes (Mostofsky & Simmonds, 2008; Ridderinkhof et al., 2004). The frontal cortex and the presupplementary motor area are associated with both action selection and response inhibition (Mostofsky & Simmonds, 2008). The medial frontal cortex has been found to be involved in performance monitoring and reward-based learning (Ridderinkhof et al., 2004). The lateral and orbital frontal divisions of the prefrontal cortex are involved in the implementation of the appropriate adjustments during the process (Ridderinkhof et al., 2004).

Cognitive control and emotional control meet in restraint theory. Specifically, restraint theory posits that for those who are restricting or suppressing their behavior (e.g., chronic dieting), negative emotions can serve as the affective disinhibitor. We see this in the case of Danny (see Chapter 1), a 24-year-old woman who struggles with bulimia nervosa (BN) much of the time. When she is not actually symptomatic with BN, she is chronically dieting. That is, she manages her eating through rigid cognitive control of each calorie she puts in her body and each calorie she burns at the gym. When engaged in cognitive overcontrol she is not symptomatic for BN. Danny's slips, or relapses, manifest when she can no longer manage the rigid overcontrol. Difficulty negotiating negative affect is the psychological last straw. It is often after a fight with her boyfriend or trouble at work that she becomes overwhelmed and disinhibited, and subsequently binges (Haedt-Matt & Keel, 2011).

Expectancy and Escape Theories (Internal—Cognitive)

It is important to explore your clients' expectancies associated with their struggles with self-regulation and problematic behaviors. Expectancy and escape theories argue that dysregulated behaviors are cognitively facilitated by either an individual's expectancy regarding engagement in the behavior or by helping a person avoid thinking about his or her current life pressures. Specifically, expectancy theory posits that problematic behaviors associated with dysregulation are maintained through an individual's belief that engaging in the behavior will feel good (Haedt-Matt & Keel, 2011). Expectancies are developed through an individual's learning history. For example, as a little girl, Alex saw her father come home from his challenging job as the owner of a sandwich shop. He was consistently stressed and discouraged by lack of profits. After taking off his coat, he'd head right for a glass and some scotch, exhaling as he poured. She learned by watching that people are relieved when they look outside of themselves (e.g., alcohol, binge eating, gambling, or shopping) for release. As she vowed to never drink, Alex exhales as she shops. Expectancy theory holds that the behaviors are maintained not through the actual reduction of negative affect following the behavior. Rather, the reinforcing power is in the expectancies (Haedt-Matt & Keel, 2011).

Many of my clients are not necessarily pursuing problematic behaviors as much as they are working to escape from some component of their current reality. The escape theory first proposed by Heatherton and Baumeister (1991) suggests that individuals use maladaptive behaviors like binge eating or shopping to escape from current awareness. We can refer back to Alex. She is deeply in debt. Her husband is a financial advisor. The tension she experiences as she hides her debt from her husband is unbearable. When she is shopping, her attention narrows, moving away from the tension with her husband, away from her perfectionistic tendencies and the ideal image she is working to present, and toward the moment, this current moment, as she shops. The constriction in attention and the ability to be present in the immediate moment allows for escape from aversive self-awareness. Lowered self-awareness is experienced as an escape, a relief, and is therefore reinforcing her shopping behavior (Haedt-Matt & Keel, 2011).

Impulsivity and Decision Making (Internal—Physiological and Cognitive)

Much like differences in reward and emotional sensitivities, you will work with clients with substantial variations in impulsivity. Many clients with higher levels of impulsivity present with an associated lack of awareness of both their impulsivity and how this shows up in their day-to-day decision making and overall self-regulation. This is a critical aspect of self to explore, explain, and address in treatment goals. As you will read in the chapters on techniques, both mindfulness and yogic methodologies can be helpful in increasing self-awareness of impulsivity and the role it plays in your clients' functioning.

Self-regulatory difficulties have been associated with impulsivity and deficits in awareness of internal body states (Davis & Carter, 2009; Heatherton & Wagner, 2011). Specifically, impulsivity is defined as the diminished ability to inhibit behavior when an alternative behavior or no behavior would have more positive outcomes. The International Society for Research on Impulsivity defines impulsivity as "behavior without adequate thought, the tendency to act with less forethought than do most individuals of equal ability and knowledge, or a predisposition toward rapid, unplanned reactions to internal or external stimuli without regard to the negative consequences of these reactions" (International Society for Research on Impulsivity, 2014). Impulsivity is a key element in faulty decision making (Davis & Carter, 2009). Herbert and Pollatos (2012) recently reviewed research exploring risk and decision making. Their findings suggest that deficits in the generation, representation, and processing of physiological arousal are strongly associated with more risk and disadvantageous decision-making behavior. We see this in Joe. Joe is 20 years old, a sophomore in college. He plays offense on his college hockey team. His hockey coach is consistently mad at him for not thinking, seeming to forget plays, and taking shots at the goal without passing. He is seen on the team as a wild card, an unpredictable risk taker. He is struggling with his alcohol use and has been in several fights both on the ice and off. He has been mandated to see a college counselor. Joe tries to explain that he has no idea why he makes these mistakes. He explains that it feels like it "comes out of nowhere." Behaviorally, deficits in decision making are clear, as problematic behaviors are automatically selected above neutral or health-enhancing behaviors. These deficits can be involved in other forms of problematic behavior such as eating difficulties and problematic shopping. Researchers in the area of impulsivity and poor decision making have identified several neurological correlates (Davis & Carter, 2009). Specifically, recent evidence suggests that impulsivity and faulty decision making may play an important role within reward-based contexts relative to mundane, monotonous contexts (Davis & Carter, 2009).

Deficits in and Rejection of the Body, Bodily States, and Body Image (Internal—Physiological, Emotional, and Cognitive)

As I work in my private practice primarily with patients who have eating disorders or struggles with eating, I frequently see clients present for initial sessions with a substantial disconnection from the body. Further, if they do have a sense or an experience of the body, it is more often than not characterized by dissatisfaction and critical judgment. The problems range from complete disconnection and a lack of awareness to rejection and substantial distortions in body image. Across all disorders and struggles associated with self-regulation, a patient's relationship with, feelings toward, and thoughts about his or her body are important to address. It is here that the physiological foundation of emotional and physical experience and mental health occurs. Early sessions should begin here and goals toward embodied self-regulation should continuously bring awareness back to the body.

Phenomenologically, we are our bodies (Svenaeus, 2013). When development and experience are normal, individuals do not necessarily notice or think about their bodies when they are busy functioning in the world (Svenaeus, 2013). This includes a relative sense of proprioceptive and kinesthetic awareness as well as the natural allowing of life-supporting functions such as respiration, digestion, and elimination (Svenaeus, 2013). According to Svenaeus (2013), for some, the body is experienced as "uncanny" (p. 84). A term not often utilized in the United States, *uncanny* refers to the sense of being controlled by something foreign. The body is seen as an unruly, irrational, shameful aspect of the self that is separate from the soul and therefore alien to the true self (Bordo, 1993). When the body is experienced in this way, embodiment is elusive. The body is experienced as a source of labor and distress. For some time, theorists have linked rejection of the body and body states to disorder. For example, over 20 years ago Bordo wrote of the roots of anorexia nervosa (AN) lying in a long-standing, historical disdain for the body (Bordo, 1993; Svenaeus, 2013).

Behavioral difficulties associated with a disrupted connection with the body include smoking to curb appetite and weight gain, plastic surgery, self-harm, and even sexual activity without negotiation for self-protection and the experience of desire (Black, 2007; Piran & Cormier, 2005). Researchers have identified key brain structures and processes implicated in monitoring internal body states associated with emotional processing and reactivity as well as self-regulation of feelings and behavior (Herbert & Pollatos, 2012). Further, there may be an interaction with gender. Fredrickson and Roberts (1997) argue that women may be more at risk for alienation and distancing from their own bodies. They cite research suggesting that women may be less accurate than men in detecting internal physiological sensations (e.g., heartbeat, stomach contractions, blood glucose levels; Fredrickson & Roberts, 1997). Further, a lack of awareness of bodily signals can manifest in deficits in emotional awareness, or alexithymia. Alexithymia is a syndrome in which an individual presents with a marked inability to identify, describe, regulate, and express emotions (Herbert & Pollatos, 2012). Moreover, deficits in emotional awareness are seen as core to alexithymia. Disordered eating has been associated with difficulty in this area. For example, Herbert and Pollatos (2012) describe studies in which individuals with eating disorders have reduced capacity to accurately perceive body signals such as cardiac signals. In general, reduced internal awareness is associated with increased risk for dysregulation.

For over 35 years, Thomas Cash has devoted his life to the psychology of physical appearance (2008). Through both research and practice he has garnered a wealth of applicable knowledge regarding body acceptance and body image. Body image refers to how an individual personally experiences embodiment. Body image involves more than a mental picture of what an individual looks like. It also involves an individual's personal relationship with his or her body (Cash, 2008). Body image involves self-perceptions, beliefs, thoughts, feelings, and actions related to an individual's physical appearance (Cash, 2008). Poor body image has been associated with low self-esteem and self-worth, challenges with gender identity, interpersonal difficulties, sexual dysfunction, depression, eating disorders, plastic surgery, excessive shopping, and chronic dieting (Cash, 2008). I have found *The Body Image Workbook* (Cash, 2008) to be extremely helpful in the evaluation of body image issues as well as in the step-by-step treatment of these issues. The workbook includes self-assessments that help clients evaluate their own body image, thoughts about body image, body image distress and importance, body image coping, and body image quality of life.

Abstinence Violation, Cue Exposure, Poor Distress Tolerance, and Self-Regulatory Resource Depletion (Internal— Physiological; External—Familial, Community, and Cultural)

Helping your clients understand why they slip despite their goal setting and intentions is critical in work toward embodied self-regulation. Exploration of abstinence violation, cue exposure, distress tolerance, and self-regulatory resource depletion can help clients develop strategies for success as well as a sense of self-compassion for their struggles.

Abstinence violation (i.e., falling off the wagon or lapse-activated consumption) is another interesting behavioral process to consider. In a groundbreaking and replicated study, Herman and Mack (1975) created an experience in which the dieters were experimentally required to consume a milkshake (i.e., a rich, high-calorie food) as part of a supposed taste test. After the taste test, the nondieters ate comparably less than the dieters. Paradoxically, the dieters ate more, as the small indulgence resulted in disinhibition of dietary restraint. Similarly, cue exposure has been shown in both animal and human studies to trigger behavioral inhibition (Heatherton & Wagner, 2011). For example, someone who is making an effort to quit drinking may struggle more at dusk , a time when he or she usually has a glass of wine before dinner. The bottle opener, wine glasses, a partner having a glass of wine, and even the ritual of preparing dinner can all serve as cues stimulating increased craving, changes in heart rate, and activity-implicit cognitions that make abstinence more challenging (Heatherton & Wagner, 2011).

Poor distress tolerance and self-regulatory resource depletion are related to self-regulatory failure. Distress tolerance is the ability to experience uncomfortable feelings and physiological arousal without reacting in a maladaptive manner. Self-regulation requires that an individual be able to tolerate distress and remain engaged with his or her goal (e.g., sobriety, healthy eating, relationship maintenance). Distress tolerance is one of four major components of dialectical behavioral therapy (DBT; Linehan, 1993) and is covered in Chapter 11 reviewing mindfulness-based techniques.

Self-regulatory resource depletion refers to the process in which the cognitive faculties associated with self-regulation become fatigued (Heatherton & Wagner, 2011). In this way, an individual working hard to be disciplined and study for an exam for several hours may subsequently struggle to resist the temptation to eat a second cupcake. This fatigue may also be involved in fatigue in managing distress, consequently reducing one's capacity for distress tolerance. It is important to note that those who have strong emotional sensitivity, a tendency toward prolonged experiences of negative affect, or a predisposition to intense affective experiences can experience fatigue as they work to manage their emotional experience. Accordingly, more frequent self-regulatory failure may occur as they struggle to maintain effort and tolerate distress as they fatigue. Research is needed to explore these relationships. (For more on self-regulatory failure, see Wagner and Heatherton [2011].)

Problems Associated With Patterns of Goal-Directed Behaviors (Internal—Cognitive; External—Familial and Community)

Traditional self-regulatory techniques are centered on achievement of goals and goal-directed behaviors. In embodied self-regulation, the focus is on cultivating and creating a healthy and embodied experience as one works toward goals (see Chapter 1). In order to enhance self-acceptance and increase client success, it can be helpful to review typical problems associated with goal-directed behavior. This can help you identify, with your client, areas the client has struggled with in the past and identify potential future challenges. Further, knowledge of these common pitfalls and challenges assists in cultivating a sense of self-compassion within your clients.

Karoly (1993), in his seminal paper on the mechanisms of self-regulation, explicated failures in self-regulation. Specifically, patterns of goal-directed activity aimed at either behavioral maintenance or change were not successful when there was: (a) failure to initiate (b) premature termination and (c) persistence of patterns of behavior beyond the life span of utility. Karoly posits several mechanisms that can account for the failure in self-regulation. For example, he describes defensive evaluation and avoidance (DEA), in which an individual is facing a "difficult, high-stakes, self-relevant and socially discernable outcome" (Karoly, 1993, p. 43). In this case, an individual discards the goal in the face of poor progress, externalizing the cause of failure in order to preserve self-esteem. For Alex, described earlier, her efforts to finish graduate school while married to an alcoholic husband resulted in her quitting two semesters before finishing. Rather than acknowledging the faults and challenges in her own family and facing her childhood of growing up the child of an alcoholic, she begins to talk negatively about her graduate program, criticizing her progress and eventually dropping out, telling her friends the program was not worth her efforts. In this way, her self-esteem is protected and she no longer pursues the goal.

Karoly (1993) cites other mechanisms of DEA, including rationalization, downward social comparison, self-sabotage, self-deception, and compensatory self-inflation. Downward social comparison allows an individual to justify foregoing self-regulation toward a goal as he or she elevates self in comparison to others who do, or have done, less. In self-sabotage and self-deception, individuals get in their own way, creating obstacles to success. For example, working toward recovery in substance abuse requires scheduling in enough time to go to therapy or support groups, engaging in healthy behaviors such as moderate exercise, and resting. Overscheduling daily activities or taking on additional tasks can make working toward sobriety nearly impossible.

Compensatory self-inflation, another obstacle to self-regulation, manifests as the individual uses rationalizations such as "I am too good for this" or "I don't need this kind of menial work." The inflation of self accompanies the devaluation and abandonment of goals. Other obstacles include lack of accountability (Karoly, 1993). Accountability is believed to enhance the likelihood of success and is thought to be part of the mechanism of change involved in group interventions such as Alcoholics Anonymous. Many coaching techniques require the participants to socially announce goals in order to increase accountability. Finally, Karoly (1993) cites lack of self-awareness and self-monitoring as additional goal-disengagement mechanisms. In this case, an individual simply consciously or unconsciously withdraws from an aware state. For example, suppose Alex (described earlier) decides to set a goal to reduce her shopping budget to $200 per month. She begins her month very aware, writing her goal down in her journal and referring to it daily. After a week, her journal "ends up" underneath the novel she is reading for book club. She does not review her goal or think about it often. The week after that her friend asks her to do a little shopping with her. At this point, Alex is no longer actively thinking of her goal, her journal is now three books deep on her dresser, and she agrees to go shopping. It is the middle of the third week in which Alex spends $330 at an expensive dress shop and $270 at her favorite shoe store to buy the matching heels. The process was a gradual disengagement of awareness.

Poor Communication and Self-Silencing (Internal—Cognitive and Emotional; External—Familial and Community)

Difficulties with self-regulation, particularly emotional regulation, are associated with poor communication (e.g., self-injury; Nock, 2010). Those who share or voice their experience and elicit support fare better. Self-silencing is a behavior that occurs within the context of relationships. In literature, self-silencing was beautifully portrayed in Maya Angelou's *I Know Why the Caged Bird Sings* (1970). Maya silences herself after sexual abuse and its traumatic consequences. We see this also in the case of Alex's mom as she struggles to live with an alcoholic husband. In research, self-silencing has been predominantly explored among girls and women (Piran & Cormier, 2005). Essentially, self-silencing is viewed as part of larger relationship problems within which one individual puts the needs of others before his or her own. It is believed that in most cultures females are raised to silence their thoughts, feelings, and needs in order to maintain close relationships (Gilligan, Rogers, & Tolman, 1991; Piran & Cormier, 2005). Research suggests that self-silencing does in fact place individuals at risk. For example, in a study of nearly 400 young women, Piran and Cormier (2005) found that self-silencing was able to predict scores on eating disorder measures.

Gender and Sex (Internal—Physiological; External—Cultural)

Sex and gender play important roles in the internal and external challenges experienced by clients. Often, patients do not discern between the two constructs. At birth, sex is assigned as either male or female based on physiological markers. Gender is viewed as a socially constructed experience of the self as male or female. In private practice, I have noticed that patients tend to have little awareness of the influence of sex or gender on the experience of self. It can be empowering and validating for patients to learn about the unique experience of males and females as well as the cultural influences known to affect both men and women. Following are a few aspects of sex and gender that can be helpful to consider. For patients to whom this is more relevant, you may consider integrating research on sex and gender issues or bibliotherapy into the treatment plan.

Researchers are exploring sex differences in areas like impulsivity and behavioral control. For example, in an extensive meta-analysis on sex differences in impulsivity, Cross, Copping, and Campbell (2011) found that there seem to be differences in how the body regulates impulses across sexes. For example, although both sexes may experience impulses, women may have a greater sensitivity to anxiety about the punishing consequences of risky action that acts as a deterrent. Further, Cross et al. (2011) found that impulsivity appears to be less unitary than once believed and that sex differences emerge depending on the task that is employed to measure it. For example, men had greater difficulty concentrating, focusing attention, and carefully problem solving solutions to interpersonal problems, and showed a lesser tendency to consider the future. Conversely, women were more likely to report that impulse control was disrupted by negative affect or that they felt regret for impulsive actions. Finally, Cross and colleagues (2011) noted that impulsivity is distinct from sensation seeking, in which men show marked, relative elevations.

Emotional regulation also appears to vary by sex. In Western cultures, women are widely viewed as the more emotional sex, with increased tendency to experience, ruminate upon, and express emotions (Nolen-Hoeksema, 2012). Men are seen as having a tendency to suppress or avoid experiencing and expressing emotions (Nolen-Hoeksema, 2012). Women have also been found to engage in more emotional regulation strategies (Nolen-Hoeksema, 2012). For example, men have been found to use more autonomic, conscious emotional regulation and to be more likely to drink alcohol to cope. Women have been found to engage in more reappraisal, problem solving, acceptance, distraction, and the seeking of social support (Nolen-Hoeksema, 2012). Overall, research implicates biological and physiological sex differences that likely play a role in self-regulation.

Gender also plays a role. Relative to physiological sex, our experience of gender is more socioculturally constructed. Fredrickson and Roberts (1997) were among the first to address the disconnect between gender differences and the experience of the biological body (see their work on self-objectification). Similarly, Piran and Cormier (2005) argue that discussions about the mind and body disruption need to be contextualized in the experience of gender. Throughout history, gender differences have been socioculturally based, having had much more to do with differential socialization of boys and girls, social status, and power held by men and women in society (Daniel & Bridges, 2010; Fredrickson & Roberts, 1997). To be specific, gender, in contrast to sex (i.e., a genetically identifiable trait), is a socially constructed concept influenced by shared societal beliefs and dominate norms evident in the social discourses (Fox, 1997; Piran & Cormier, 2005). Powerful cultural and political institutions have great influence in the construction of gender. Throughout history and across cultures, there has been a shifting social construction of what it means to be men and women. That is, as cultures evolve and change, so does conceptualization of gender. This is true for gender roles, behavioral expectations, and in terms of the experience of the body.

For example, many theorists have examined the shift to the functionality of women and their bodies during World War II and the return to an emphasis on submissive and objectified bodies during times of peace (Piran & Cormier, 2005). Further, recent studies exploring risk have found that men and women may experience various risks differently, with some factors affecting one gender and not the other (e.g., self-objectification; Daniel & Bridges, 2010). In 2009, Stephen Hinshaw described the experience of the developing female in Westernized culture as the *triple bind* (Hinshaw & Kranz, 2009). Girls are expected to: (a) be good at all of the traditional "girl stuff," (b) be good at most of the traditional "guy stuff," and (c) conform to a narrow, unrealistic set of standards that allows no alternative. We can add an additional aspect to create the *quadruple bind*. That is, it should all be done in a manner that appears effortless.

Invalidating Environment and Loneliness (External—Familial, Community, and Cultural)

Marsha Linehan (1993) was among the first to explicate the importance of validation of experience for mental health. Research suggests that familial responses to a child's emotional displays play a critical role in an individual's subsequent emotional awareness, expression, regulation, and coping (Adrian et al., 2011). In an invalidating environment there is a failure to treat others with attention, understanding, and respect (Linehan, 1993). Invalidating environments are not necessarily abusive environments. For example, a child inclined to draw and paint may be born into a family in which both parents and the other siblings are highly athletic and enjoy outdoor sporting events and large crowds. The mismatch between the child's preferences and tendencies and those of the other family members can create a potentially invalidating environment if the parents and siblings are not careful to attend to, work to understand, and respect the artistic and quiet nature of the family member. When a child's experience is discounted, ignored, seen as bothersome, or otherwise invalidated, there can be a negative impact on his or her interpersonal development. It is believed that familial invalidation is associated with difficulties with down-regulation of emotional arousal. That is, those who are not validated within the family context experience greater emotional arousal of longer duration. Accordingly, invalidation can also play a role in psychosocial functioning as individuals struggle to regulate emotions within the context of interpersonal interactions (Adrian et al., 2011).

Loneliness is an unpleasant experience derived from deficiencies or problems in a person's network of social relationships (Lemmens, Valkenburg, & Peter, 2011). An individual may experience loneliness when there is an unfulfilled desire to have friends, a difference between actual social status and desires of social status, and/or insufficient affective bonding (Lemmens et al., 2011). In a longitudinal study exploring the onset of pathological gaming (defined and discussed further in the "Pathological Gaming and Internet Addiction" section later in this chapter), Lemmens and colleagues (2011) found that loneliness was both a cause and a consequence of pathological involvement with video games. That is, a person who is already feeling socially isolated and alone, has low social competence, and has low self-esteem will be at higher risk for pathological gaming and involvement will increase feelings of loneliness.

Media Influences (External—Cultural)

Media influences have been most thoroughly investigated in the area of eating disorders, although media plays a role in presenting environmental cues or triggers for problem behaviors such as substance use, excessive shopping, pathological gaming, and gambling. Specifically, in regard to eating disorders, Svenaeus (2013) stated, "Most narratives of anorexia seem to start with a scenario in which a young girl suddenly understands by way of comments or behaviors of others that she is too fat" (p. 85). The development of a healthy attuned self is a challenge within today's media culture. Hinshaw and Kranz (2009) write, "Different ways of becoming a woman [or a man], relating to society, or constructing an authentic self—have been virtually erased by the culture" (p. 8). Cultural ideals disseminated through media outlets (e.g., television, movies, commercials, magazines, web pages, media ads) continue to project overly thin, lean, or hypersexualized ideals as synonymous with success and happiness (Svenaeus, 2013).

Neuromarketing has evolved with advances in brain research (Hartston, 2012; Morin, 2011). Neuromarketing involves the use of scientific brain research to potentiate the effectiveness of product marketing using physiological and brain measurement techniques, including functional magnetic resonance imaging (fMRI), electroencephalograms (EEG), skin moisture levels, heart rate, breathing patterns, eye movement, and pupil dilation (Hartston, 2012; Morin, 2011). Each year, firms spend over $400 billion in advertising campaigns, with an increasing focus on neuromarketing (Morin, 2011). Firms have spent tens of billions of dollars on research leading to over $100 billion in advertising using such findings. Critics state that the goal is to bypass the conscious, rational decision-making brain functions and to maximize excitement, emotional attachment, brand identification, reward pathway activation, medial prefrontal identification, and oxytocin stimulation. In this way, impulsive purchasing behaviors may be influenced in ways that individuals are not fully aware of or informed about (Hartston, 2012). Marketers argue that people cannot fully articulate their preferences when asked explicitly (Ariely & Berns, 2010). They suggest that the consumer brain holds "hidden information about their true preferences" (Ariely & Berns, 2010, p. 284). Hartston (2012) provides a few examples of scientifically informed marketing, such as incorporating the color red and playing music designed to slow a shopper's pace in stores and increase impulsive purchases. The ethical issues associated with neuromarketing are many. For example, companies may not be primarily concerned with the best interests of the consumer, and neurological information can be used to exploit specific neurological traits of subgroups of individuals (e.g., those prone to impulsivity, addictions, or compulsive behavior) and utilize peripheral routes of influence (e.g., sex appeal for selling beer; see Ariely and Berns [2010] for a review).

For example, Santos, Seixas, Brandao, and Moutinho (2012) studied a theory of perception of brand using fMRI as participants view brand logos. They conclude that the particular areas of the brain activated when participants viewed logos (i.e., medial frontal pole, paracingulate gyrus, frontal orbital cortex, frontal medial cortex, and hippocampus) were self-reflexive, suggesting that participants were thinking about what others might be thinking. That is, brands function like social currency in which individuals assess one another (Santos et al., 2012).

Self-Objectification Theory (Internal—Cognitive; External—Cultural)

Self-objectification has been implicated in the onset of eating disorders because it contributes to the risk factors—body dissatisfaction and drive for thinness. In a sense, self-objectification is a shift in the "I" in "I need." To explain, self-objectification begins with objectification. Objectification of an individual involves being treated as a body, or a collection of body parts, that is valued predominantly for its utilization by others (Fredrickson & Roberts, 1997). In this way, the body is seen as it exists for the benefit of another's consumption or gaze (Svenaeus, 2013). That is, the body exists for the utility and pleasure of another. Rather than focusing on authentic internal needs that satisfy the body, emotional and cognitive aspects of self, the individual regulates the body in order to manifest an external appearance that others will want. The individual believes that this is what he or she wants, when in reality the individual is regulating the physiological self in terms of what he or she believes others want to see.

There are three aspects to the objectifying gaze: (a) occurrence within interpersonal and social encounters (e.g., a woman checking out a man's abdominal muscles) (b) visual media depictions of social encounters (e.g., an ad for a car that sexualizes a man watching a woman walk by) and (c) media spotlights of bodies and body parts aligned with an implicitly sexualizing gaze (Fredrickson & Roberts, 1997). The process of internalization is critical to risk. The sociocultural influences and practices result in a shift in the way the self is perceived. At the psychological level, individuals adopt a view of self in which the observer's perspective is internalized. They see themselves as they would be seen, or objectified, by others. Over time, individuals not only internalize this way of seeing themselves, it becomes how they experience themselves in lived actions. It is expected that the process of human identity development involves identification of gender-related and body-related discourses (Figure 2.2; Piran & Cormier, 2005).

Generally speaking, self-objectification as explicated by Fredrickson and Roberts (1997) illustrates the internalization of and later identification with social discourses. Ultimately, when an individual self-objectifies, he or she has internalized the media and cultural objectification of bodies. That is, the individual has integrated the cultural attitudes, values, standards, and opinions regarding the body. At the level of identification, an individual embodies, in lived experience, these constructs.

Self-objectification changes the way we experience ourselves. The experience of self, the flow of consciousness, is disrupted as the individual works to maintain both an inner self and a socially mediated self.

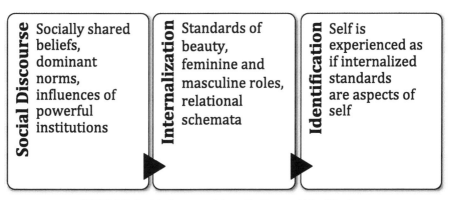

FIGURE 2.2 Social discourse, internalization, and identification.

A dual consciousness is manifest (Fredrickson & Roberts, 1997). In cases of complete identification there is a risk of wholly losing the sense of the authentic self and living only as the objectified self. As delineated by the Attuned Representational Model of Self (ARMS; Cook-Cottone, 2006; see Chapter 1), the self is constructed and organized in attunement of the external systems. The experience of the internal self (physiology, emotions, and cognitions) is aligned to the external demands, needs, and ideals of an individual's environmental context. The true needs of the physiological, emotional, and cognitive self are ignored, neglected. Fredrickson and Roberts (1997) argue that the vigilance and focus delegated to self-conscious body monitoring may relegate fewer perceptual resources for attending to the inner body experience. In more extreme cases of identification, an individual may lose access to his or her own inner physical experiences (Fredrickson & Roberts, 1997).

Not surprisingly, self-objectification has been shown to predict eating-disordered behavior among young women (Piran & Cormier, 2005). As individuals self-objectify, they often begin to restrict food, diet, and engage in other behaviors such as excessive exercise or plastic surgery, all intended to change the size and shape of the body. Dieting and restrained eating may be associated with a disconnection from the body, as both require suppression of hunger signals. It is believed that this can lead to a generalized insensitivity to internal body signals (Fredrickson & Roberts, 1997; Heatherton, Polivy, & Herman, 1989). Recent research suggests that self-objectification, as currently measured, may not be as relevant for men (Daniel & Bridges, 2010). For example, Daniel and Bridges (2010) explored self-objectification among college-age males and found that internalization of media ideals was the strongest predictor of a drive toward muscularity, with self-objectification having no impact. More research is needed to better understand how this construct is experienced across genders.

DYSREGULATION EMBODIED

Self-regulatory failure is believed to be a core feature of many social and mental health problems (Heatherton & Wagner, 2011). As you can see in Figure 2.1, both external and internal factors, alone or working together, can create a mis-attunement, lack of attunement, or failure of attunement between the external presentation of self and the internal regulation of self. When this occurs, the internal self (i.e., emotional, cognitive, and physiological) is at risk for functioning in service of symptoms or disorder. For example, as we saw with Alex in the earlier case study, she is driven primarily by her dysregulated behaviors manifesting a self that is not able to authentically and effectively interact with her family or community. There is a failure of effective, embodied, self-regulation. We can achieve some sense of the scope of the problem by looking at the rates of subclinical and clinical levels of disorders that have dysregulation as part of their etiology.

Dysregulated Eating

We need to eat at least three to five times a day. Food is increasingly designed to be exactly what we desire, with researchers working hard to develop even more foods that we will actually crave (Kessler, 2013). Food consumption is one of the key areas in which difficulties with dysregulation show up for many people. The *Diagnostic and Statistical Manual of Mental Disorders,* Fifth Edition (*DSM-5*; American Psychiatric Association [APA], 2013) describes feeding and eating disorders as a persistent disturbance in eating or eating-related behavior that changes the way an individual consumes food. The eating disorders that are most relevant to this discussion are AN, BN, and binge-eating disorder (BED).

Anorexia Nervosa

In Westernized countries, 12-month prevalence rates of AN among young females are at approximately 0.4%; rates for males are much lower, with the clinical population exhibiting a 10:1 female-to-male ratio (APA, 2013). The pursuit of excessive thinness is believed to be a part of the search for identity, which has been collapsed onto control of the body—its weight, size, and shape (Svenaeus, 2013). Individuals with AN restrict food or energy intake below levels needed to perform daily requirements and maintain a healthy body weight. As a result, those who struggle with AN have a significantly low body weight. They also exhibit an intense fear of gaining weight and becoming fat, despite their low weight. Further, patients often show a disturbance in the way in which their body weight and/or shape is experienced (e.g., feeling big or huge when in fact they are underweight for their height). They also place an undue influence of their body weight on their own self-evaluation, thinking it is one of the most important aspects of self. Last, there is a failure to acknowledge the seriousness of their behavior and low weight (APA, 2013).

Bulimia Nervosa

In Westernized countries, the 12-month prevalence rates of BN among women are at 1% to 1.5% (APA, 2013). Like AN, BN appears to have a

10:1 female-to-male prevalence ratio, with rates peaking from later adolescence to young adulthood. The disorder is characterized by recurrent episodes of binge eating (i.e., eating abnormally large amounts of food in a short amount of time) that occur with a subjective sense of a lack of control over eating (APA, 2013). Those who struggle with BN engage in recurrent compensatory behaviors to prevent weight gain that are risky to health and considered self-destructive (e.g., self-induced vomiting, diuretic and/or laxative misuse, fasting, and excessive exercise; APA, 2013). At the clinical level, the binge-and-purge behavior occurs one or more times per week. At lower levels the behavior occurs one to three times per week, and within the extreme level there can be an average of 14 or more episodes per week (APA, 2013). As in AN, the process of self-evaluation in BN involves an overemphasis on body weight and shape.

Binge-Eating Disorder

BED has a 12-month prevalence rate among adults of 1.6% for women and about half that rate for men (APA, 2013). Those with this disorder binge eat as described for BN, with the same sense of lack of control over their eating (APA, 2013). The *DSM-5* carefully describes what qualifies as a binge-eating episode to make a distinction between binge eating and the overeating associated with typical weight gain (i.e., ingested energy exceeds expended energy). To be considered a binge-eating episode, most of the following criteria must be met: (a) rapid eating (b) uncomfortable fullness (c) substantial ingestion of food without hunger (d) high frequency over time (i.e., at least once per week for at least 3 months) and (e) it is not associated with BN or AN (APA, 2013).

Researchers have identified that the compulsive overeating (excessive consumption or food addiction) component of BED has compelling similarities to conventional drug addiction (Davis & Carter, 2009). Davis and Carter (2009) proposed that compulsive overeating be included as an addictive disorder in the *DSM*. It is argued that behavioral addictions include those behaviors associated with natural rewards. Further, with the recent changes in the chemical makeup of food—the relative increases and chemical alterations in potency in ingredients such as sugar and fats—it is believed that there has been a potency-related increase in the addictive potential of food (Davis & Carter, 2009). Behavioral markers associated with other addictive behaviors also manifest in compulsive eating, such as loss of control, tolerance and withdrawal, craving, and relapse (Davis & Carter, 2009).

Other Specified Eating Disorders and Subclinical Eating Disorders

The *DSM-5* category of unspecified feeding or eating disorder is utilized when an individual's symptoms are generally characteristic of a feeding or eating disorder and cause clinically significant distress and impairment in functioning. Despite distress and/or impairment, the individual does not meet the full criteria for one of the specific disorders of feeding or eating (APA, 2013). The *DSM-5* provides five examples of presentations for the other-specified designation: (a) atypical AN; (b) BN of low frequency and/or limited duration; (c) BED of low frequency and/or limited duration; (d) purging disorder that involves purging to lose weight in the absence of binge eating; and (e) night-eating syndrome, which is marked by recurrent episodes of eating at night following the onset of sleep or after the evening meal. As this is a new category for the *DSM-5*, prevalence rates are not available. However, older estimates suggest that 8% to 15% of adolescent women manifest subclinical levels of eating-disordered behavior (e.g., Austin, 2000). For more on self-regulatory failure and eating disorders, see Herman and Polivy (2011).

Self-Injury

Self-injury is the direct and deliberate harm of the body in the absence of conscious suicidal intent (Adrian et al., 2011; Nock, 2010). It is often referred to as nonsuicidal self-injury (NSSI). Review of the literature suggests that prevalence rates vary, with community samples finding rates from 13% to 45% among adolescents and lower rates among adults (i.e., less than 5%; Nock, 2010). Self-injury is distinct from the engagement in behaviors that indirectly cause self-harm to some degree (e.g., drinking alcohol, smoking tobacco, eating unhealthy foods). Note, in these other cases (e.g., smoking), the indirectly self-injurious or self-defeating behavior is done in the pursuit of enjoyment, and the self-harm is an unfortunate side effect (Nock, 2010). The most commonly reported methods of NSSI are cutting or carving one's skin with a sharp instrument (e.g., knife or razor), scratching or scraping the skin to the point of bleeding, burning of the skin, inserting objects under the skin, hitting or biting oneself, picking at wounds, and pulling one's own hair (Nock, 2010). The frequency of the behavior ranges substantially, with respondents in school-based samples reporting that they have engaged in self-injury 10 or less times in their lives and individuals from inpatient samples reporting more than 50 episodes in the past year (Nock, 2010).

Like other disorders described in this chapter, individuals who struggle with self-injury think about self-injury when distressed and feel compelled to engage in the behaviors (Nock, 2010). Researchers believe that the self-injurious behavior is self-soothing in nature or an attempt to regulate an affective experience (Nock, 2010). Researchers believe that social modeling and a desire for self-punishment may be unique risk factors for self-injury (Nock, 2010). Finally, researchers have posited the pain analgesia hypothesis, in which the self-injuring episode is associated with minimal, or the absence of, pain. It is not clear if this is due to lower pain sensitivity, habituation to pain, or an associated release of opiates. Of note, self-injury is associated with risk for other maladaptive behaviors, such as drug and alcohol use and eating disorders (Nock. 2010).

Shopping Addiction/Compulsive Buying Disorder

Uncontrolled, problematic buying behavior has been referred to by several different names: uncontrolled buying, compulsive shopping, addictive buying, excessive buying, and compulsive buying disorder (CBD; Black, 2007; Koran, Faber, Aboujaoude, Large, & Serpe, 2006). Compulsive buying involves frequent preoccupation with buying, seemingly irresistible or intrusive impulses to buy, buying items that are not needed, buying items that are not affordable, shopping for longer periods than intended, and spending more money than intended (Black, 2007; Koran et al., 2006). Further, the individual experiences adverse consequences associated with the buying behavior. Finally, the buying behavior is associated with marked distress, impaired social occupational functioning, and/or financial problems (Koran et al., 2006). These symptoms are often associated with feelings of guilt and remorse, excessive debt, bankruptcy, familial conflict, separation and divorce, and engagement in illegal activities (e.g., embezzlement, fraud; Koran et al., 2006). Individuals with CBD tend to shop by themselves (Black, 2007). Prevalence rate estimates in the United States vary substantially, with rates reported as low as between 1% and 2% to estimates around 15% among smaller samples (Black, 2007; Koran et al., 2006). In a large national sample, prevalence was estimated at 5.8% (Koran et al., 2006). For more on self-regulatory failure and spending, see Faber and Vohs (2011).

Pathological Gaming and Internet Addiction

Pathological gaming and *Internet addiction* are relatively new terms. These terms reflect pathological involvement with video games, on or off the Internet, and the broader conceptual category of pathological engagement with Internet-based activities (Ferguson, Coulson, & Barnett, 2011). There is substantial disagreement regarding the prevalence rates and diagnostic criteria. An extensive meta-analysis of studies suggests that the overall prevalence rate of pathological gaming is 3.1% (Ferguson et al., 2011). Diagnostic approaches vary, with some researchers suggesting a pathological gambling analogy and others encouraging an interfering model. In the latter, gaming is seen as pathological when it interferes with life needs and responsibilities (e.g., issues in role fulfillment, school or work problems, relationship issues, and/or feelings of personal distress; Ferguson et al., 2011). Notably, Lemmens et al.'s (2011) longitudinal study of 851 adolescents found that adolescents' time spent playing video games was not related to their psychosocial well-being, presenting the argument that it is important not to overstate the dangers of playing computer and video games.

Gambling Addiction

Gambling disorder is included in the *DSM-5* as a non–substance-related addictive disorder. According to the *DSM-5*, gambling disorder involves persistent and recurrent patterns of gambling behavior that lead to clinically significant impairment or stress. The terms *problem gambling* and *pathological gambling* are sometimes used to describe subclinical levels of behavior (Lorains, Cowlishaw, & Thomas, 2011). Individuals with gambling disorder show a need to gamble with increasing amounts of money in order to achieve the desired level of excitement. The individual might become restless or irritable when trying to cut down or stop the gambling behavior. Often, the person has made repeated unsuccessful efforts to control, cut back, or even stop the gambling behavior. When not gambling, individuals with gambling disorder are preoccupied with gambling. As in other disorders associated with dysregulation, the individual may gamble to help negotiate uncomfortable or stressful feelings. The behaviors are frequently associated with lying to cover up the gambling or the problems that are associated with gambling. Frequently, those who struggle with this disorder experience financial, relational, and occupational problems (APA, 2013). Gambling problems are associated with other mental health disorders, including mood disorder, anxiety, bipolar disorders, and substance use disorders (Lorains et al., 2011). The *DSM-5* lists prevalence rates at 0.2% to 0.3% for the general population, and some researchers list rates a bit higher at 1.1% to 3.5% (APA, 2013; Lorains et al., 2011).

Substance Use Disorders

According to the *DSM-5*, the essential feature of substance use disorders is a variety of symptoms (i.e., cognitive, behavioral, and physiological) that reflect the individual's continued use of a substance despite significant substance-related problems. The manual cites 10 classes of substances associated with the disorder, including alcohol, cannabis, hallucinogens, inhalants, opioids, sedatives, stimulants, caffeine, tobacco, and other (or unknown). Critical to diagnosis, the disorder is associated with underlying alterations in brain functioning that may persist beyond intoxication, leading to repeated relapse, craving, and a sense of feeling triggered when exposed to drug-related stimuli (APA, 2013). Those who struggle with substance use disorder show impaired control regarding use of the substance. That is, once they start using they are unable to moderate the amount, frequency, and/or duration of the use. There is a sense of loss of control. Also, those who struggle often show frequent and persistent attempts to control or stop use. As noted in the *DSM-5*, those who use a substance spend a substantial part of their time seeking and using the substance, to the detriment of other life activities (APA, 2013). Social impairment typically arises as use of the substance interferes with the individual's ability to fulfill major life roles and he or she withdraws in order to use the substance.

Risky use of a substance is also seen at clinical levels. In this case the individual uses the substance in situations or at levels that are considered physically dangerous (APA, 2013). It is not the existence of a problem that matters in this case; rather, it is the failure to abstain from using despite the difficulty it causes in the person's life. Further, those who use, depending on the substance, may begin to experience tolerance, in which case they must use increasing amounts of the substance in order to secure the desired effects (APA, 2013). Withdrawal can also occur, in which blood or tissue concentrations of the substance decline and the individual begins to experience uncomfortable and sometimes dangerous symptoms of the withdrawal. The individual can become extremely motivated to secure and ingest the substance in order to relieve the withdrawal symptoms (APA, 2013). Prevalence rates vary across the substance categories. For example, prevalence rates are reported at 8.5% for alcohol use disorder, 1.5% for cannabis use disorder, 0.1% for hallucinogen use disorder, and 0.47% for opioid use disorder (APA, 2013). For more on self-regulatory failure and addiction, see Sayette and Griffen (2011).

CONCLUSIONS

As revealed through this chapter's discussion of the model of dysregulation, the risks and theories of risk, and the associated disorders, the challenge for clinicians may seem nearly insurmountable. Answers come both from recent advances in research and ancient texts. This book invites you to integrate the scientific progress in the field of yoga and mindfulness with practical techniques that will move your clients forward. These are on-the-mat and on-the-cushion as well as off-the-mat and off-the-cushion techniques.

In Buddhist mythology there is an image depicting the futility of pursuing one object of desire after another; it is called the *Hungry Ghost* (Kabatznick, 1998). The Hungry Ghost pursues desires blindly, taking the form of a believable inner voice that says, "This will make you feel better. Buy this fancy thing. Drink this drink. Eat of these foods and all will be well." Kabatznick (1998) describes how feeding the ghost only increases its demands, and its powers. The more you feed it, the more it wants. It doesn't care what you consume—it just wants. Once one thing is consumed, the desire moves to the next. Once one desire is controlled, the compulsion moves to the next. The Hungry Ghost, like the ignored and unvoiced internal self, cannot be satisfied.

In my work with clients in private practice, I call this *symptom shapeshifting*. Patients move from eating-disordered behavior, to cutting, to drinking and use of other substances if the underlying mechanisms of self-regulation have not been addressed in a healthy way. The external objects, desires, or attempts at regulation do not satisfy. As one is addressed, the individual simply shifts to the next. It is our work to help clients learn healthy and effective techniques and practices that engage, regulate, and respond to the internal self. The following chapters explain and explicate conceptual, narrative tools as well as practical embodied practices that will calm the Hungry Ghost. It is believed that perhaps the ghost does not want to be fed, but wants to be seen. Once seen, the ghost rests.

Use the worksheet on the next page to help your clients review their current internal and external challenges and assets (see Figure 2.3, Disordered Representation of Self Worksheet). You may want to review the risk factors and symptoms discussed in this chapter with clients as relevant to their struggles. Have your clients begin by listing their internal challenges and assets, including any physiological predispositions or current difficulties (e.g., genetic predisposition to addiction), emotional aspects of self (e.g., emotional sensitivity), and cognitive aspects of self (e.g., adoption of media ideals, perfectionism, or body image difficulties). Next, ask them to complete the external challenges and assets, beginning with family and close friends, moving to community, and ending with cultural challenges and assets. Finally, ask them to fill out the middle column. This column should detail what they do that affects their self-regulation. For example, a client might note that she drinks a few glasses

This worksheet is designed to bring mindfulness to (a) your challenges and assets both internally and externally, and (b) how your behavioral choices, challenges, and assets align. Complete the internal and external columns of the worksheet first. Next, fill in the center column. What do you do on a regular basis that affects your self-regulation? Be sure to include the behaviors that enhance self-regulation as well as those that increase dysregulation. Make connections (draw arrows) where you see influences. For example, you may notice that your drinking affects your relationship with your children, your physical well-being, and your mood (i.e., emotional self). You may also notice that when you go to yoga, you feel better (i.e., physical and emotional self) and you feel more connected to your family and community. Discuss the connections you have made with your therapist.

Internal	Your Embodied Journey Starting Point	External
(Physiological, Emotional, and Cognitive)	*List the things you do.*	(Family, Community, and Culture)
List your challenges and assets.	*List the things that enhance your self-regulation and the things that cause dysregulation.*	*List your challenges and assets.*
My Physical Self		My Family and Close Friends
My Emotional Self		My Community and Work
My Thinking Self		My Culture

FIGURE 2.3 Disordered representation of self worksheet.

of wine each night or binge drinks on the weekends. Another might note compulsive shopping or feeling out of control when she plays video games. When listing behaviors that seem to contribute to self-regulation, a client might add that she runs, does yoga, or has a weekly tea date with a dear friend. Next, have your clients make connections. They can do this by drawing single-direction or bidirectional arrows. For example, a client might notice that her shopping and associated lying about the shopping are having a negative impact on her relationship with her husband as well as causing her substantial emotional stress. Another client might note how her weekly tea date helps her feel more connected, physically relaxed, and clear-minded. The objective of the activity is to bring awareness to challenges, assets, and the behaviors that affect self-regulation. The forthcoming chapters detail mindful and yogic approaches that can be embodied and integrated into your clients' behavioral repertoires in order to further enhance self-regulation. Of note, as you will read in Chapter 3, these practices are beneficial for therapists too. Consider completing this worksheet to inform your own practice.

REFERENCES

Adrian, M., Zeman, J., Erdley, C., Lisa, L., & Sim, L. (2011). Emotional dysregulation and interpersonal difficulties as risk factors for nonsuicidal self-injury in adolescent girls. *Journal of Abnormal Child Psychology, 39,* 389–400.

American Psychiatric Association. (2013). *Diagnostic and statistical manual of mental disorders* (5th ed.). Arlington, VA: American Psychiatric Publishing.

Anderson, A., & Sovik, R. (2000). *Yoga: Mastering the basics.* Honesdale, PA: The Himalayan Institute Press.

Angelou, M. (1970). *I know why the caged bird sings.* New York, NY: Bantam Books.

Ariely, D., & Berns, G. S. (2010). Neuromarketing: The hope and hype of neuroimaging business. *Nature Reviews Neuroscience, 11,* 284–292.

Austin, S. B. (2000). Prevention research in eating disorders: Theory and new directions. *Psychological Medicine, 30,* 1249–1262.

Black, D. W. (2007). A review of compulsive buying disorder. *World Psychiatry, 6,* 14–18.

Bordo, S. (1993). *Unbearable weight: Feminism, Western culture, and the body.* Berkeley, CA: University of California Press.

Cash, T. (2008). *The body image workbook: An eight-step program for learning to like your looks* (2nd ed.). Oakland, CA: New Harbinger Publications.

Chernin, K. (1985). *The hungry self: Women, eating, and identity.* New York, NY: Random House.

Chernin, K. (1998). *The woman who gave birth to her mother: Tales of transformation in women's lives.* New York, NY: Penguin Books.

Cook-Cottone, C. P. (2006). The attuned representation model for the primary prevention of eating disorders: An overview for school psychologists. *Psychology in the Schools, 43,* 223–230.

Cross, C. P., Copping, L. T., & Campbell, A. (2011). Sex differences in impulsivity: A meta-analysis. *Psychological Bulletin, 137,* 97–130.

Daniel, S., & Bridges, S. K. (2010). The drive for muscularity in men: Media influences and objectification theory. *Body Image, 7,* 32–38.

Davis, C., & Carter, J. C. (2009). Compulsive overeating as an addiction disorder: A review of theory and evidence. *Appetite, 53,* 1–8.

Faber, R. J., & Vohs, K. D. (2011). Self-regulation and spending: Evidence from impulsive and compulsive buying. In K. D. Vohs & R. F. Baumeister (Eds.), *Handbook of self-regulation: Research, theory and applications* (2nd ed.). (pp. 537–550). New York, NY: Guilford Press.

Ferguson, C. J., Coulson, M., & Barnett, J. (2011). A meta-analysis of pathological gaming prevalence and comorbidity with mental health, academic, and social problems. *Journal of Psychiatric Research, 45,* 1573–1578.

Fox, C. (1997). The authenticity of intercultural relations. *International Journal of Intercultural Relations, 21,* 85–103.

Fredrickson, B. L., & Roberts, T. (1997). Objectification theory: Toward understanding women's lived experiences and mental health risks. *Psychology of Women Quarterly, 21,* 173–206.

Gilligan, C., Rogers, A. G., & Tolman, D. (1991). *Women, girls, and psychotherapy.* New York, NY: Hawthorn Press.

Haedt-Matt, A. A., & Keel, P. K. (2011). Revisiting the affect regulation model of binge eating: A meta-analysis of studies using ecological momentary assessment. *Psychological Bulletin, 137,* 660—681.

Hartston, H. (2012). The case for compulsive shopping as an addiction. *Journal of Psychoactive Drugs, 44,* 64–67.

Heatherton, T. F. (2011). Neuroscience in self-regulation. *Annual Review of Psychology 62,* 363–390.

Heatherton, T. F., & Baumeister, R. F. (1991). Binge eating as escape from self-awareness. *Psychological Bulletin, 110,* 86–108.

Heatherton, T. F., Polivy, J., & Herman, C. P. (1989). Restraint and internal responsiveness: Effects of placebo manipulations of hunger on eating. *Journal of Abnormal Psychology, 98,* 89–92.

Heatherton, T. F., & Wagner, D. D. (2011). Cognitive neuroscience of self-regulation failure. *Trends in Cognitive Sciences, 15,* 132–139.

Herbert, B. M., & Pollatos, O. (2012). The body in the mind: On the relationship between interoception and embodiment. *Topics in Cognitive Science, 4,* 692–704.

Herman, C. P., & Mack, D. (1975). Restrained and unrestrained eating. *Journal of Personality, 43,* 647–660.

Herman, C. P., & Polivy, J. (2011). The self-regulation of eating: Theoretical and practical problems. In K. D. Vohs & R. F. Baumeister (Eds.), *Handbook of self-regulation: Research, theory and applications* (2nd ed.). (pp. 522–536). New York, NY: Guilford Press.

Hinshaw, S., & Kranz, R. (2009). *The triple bind: Saving our teenage girls from today's pressures.* New York, NY: Random House.

International Society for Research on Impulsivity. (2014). *What is impulsivity?* Retrieved from http://www.impulsivity.org/index.htm

Kabatznick, R. (1998). *The zen of eating: Ancient answers to modern weight problems.* New York, NY: The Berkley Publishing Group.

Karoly, P. (1993). Mechanisms of self-regulation: A systems view. *Annual Review of Psychology, 44,* 23–52.

Kessler, D. A. (2013). *Hijacked: How your brain is fooled by food.* New York, NY: Random House.

Koole, S. L., van Dillen, L. F., & Sheppes, G. (2011). The self-regulation of emotion. In K. D. Vohs & R. F. Baumeister (Eds.), *Handbook of self-regulation: Research, theory and applications* (2nd ed.). (pp. 22–40). New York, NY: Guilford Press.

Koran, L. M., Faber, R. J., Aboujaoude, E., Large, M. D., & Serpe, R. T. (2006). Estimated prevalence of compulsive buying behavior in the United States. *American Journal of Psychiatry, 163,* 1806–1812.

Lemmens, J. S., Valkenburg, P. M., & Peter, J. (2011). Psychosocial causes and consequences of pathological gaming. *Computers and Human Behaviors, 27,* 144–152.

Linehan, M. (1993). *Skill training manual for treating borderline personality disorder.* New York, NY: Guilford Press.

Lorains, F. K., Cowlishaw, S., & Thomas, S. A. (2011). Prevalence of comorbid disorders in problem and pathological gambling: Systematic review and meta-analysis of population reviews. *Addiction, 106,* 490–498.

Morin, C. (2011). Neuromarketing: The new science of consumer behavior. *Society, 48,* 131–135.

Mostofsky, S. H., & Simmonds, D. J. (2008). Response inhibition and response selection: Two sides of the same coin. *Journal of Cognitive Neuroscience, 20,* 751–761.

Nock, M. K. (2010). Self-injury. *Annual Reviews in Clinical Psychology, 6,* 339–363.

Nolen-Hoeksema, S. (2012). Emotion regulation and psychopathology: The role of gender. *Annual Review of Clinical Psychology, 8,* 161–187.

Piran, N., & Cormier, H. C. (2005). The social construction of women and disordered eating patterns. *Journal of Counseling Psychology, 4,* 549–558.

Porges, S. W. (2011). *The polyvagal theory: Neurophysiological foundations of emotions, attachment, communication, and self-regulation.* Norton Series on Interpersonal Neurobiology. New York, NY: W. W. Norton.

Ridderinkhof, K. R., van den Wildenberg, W. P. M., Segalowitz, S. J., & Carter, C. S. (2004). Neurocognitive mechanisms of cognitive control: The role of the prefrontal cortex in action selection, response inhibition, performance monitoring, and reward-based learning. *Brain and Cognition, 56,* 129–140.

Santos, J. P., Seixas, D., Brandao, S., & Moutinho, L. (2012). Neuroscience in branding: A functional magnetic resonance imaging study on brands' implicitly and expressed expressions. *Journal of Brand Management, 19,* 735–757.

Sayette, M. A., & Griffen, K. M. (2011). Self-regulatory failure and addiction. In K. D. Vohs & R. F. Baumeister (Eds.), *Handbook of self-regulation: Research, theory and applications* (2nd ed.). (pp. 505–521). New York, NY: Guilford Press.

Siegel, D. J. (2007). *The mindful brain: Reflection and attunement in the cultivation of well-being.* Norton Series on Interpersonal Neurobiology. New York, NY: W. W. Norton.

Svenaeus, F. (2013). Anorexia nervosa and the body uncanny: A phenomenological approach. *Philosophy, Psychiatry, and Psychology, 20,* 81–91.

Wagner, D. D., & Heatherton, T. F. (2011). Giving in to temptation: The emerging cognitive neuroscience of self-regulatory failure. In K. D. Vohs & R. F. Baumeister (Eds.), *Handbook of self-regulation: Research, theory and applications* (2nd ed.). (pp. 41–63). New York, NY: Guilford Press.

Warner, J. (2010, June 18). Dysregulation nation. *The New York Times,* pp. A11–A12.

The Mindful and Yogic Self
Embodied Practices

Man is not fully conditioned and determined but rather determines himself
whether he gives into conditions or stands up to them.
In other words, man is ultimately self determining.
Man does not simply exist but always decides what his existence will be,
what he will become in the next moment.—VIKTOR FRANKL (1959, p. 131)

BETWEEN STIMULUS AND RESPONSE

As well stated in the quote at the beginning of this chapter, humans are self-determining. Frankl (1959) describes the power of mindful awareness and embodied action as he refers to the moment-by-moment choices we all make. It is to the moment-by-moment experience that this text now shifts focus. This chapter serves to transition you to the following chapters addressing mindful and yogic approaches to the care and treatment of your clients and to your own life. In Chapters 1 and 2 you were introduced to the Attuned Representational Model of Self (ARMS): embodied self-regulation (Chapter 1) and the disordered self (Chapter 2). These chapters explicated how the integrated model of self (ARMS) reflects an ongoing process of attunement, integration, and construction of the self. Further, we saw in Chapter 2 that when there are challenges, obstacles, or dysfunction in either an internal or external domain, the regulation of the self can be disrupted or complicated. We now explore how the process of embodied self-regulation is preventive and prescriptive. In both mindful and yogic approaches, the experience of self is considered self-determined and embodied through practice (Ajaya, 1983; Prabhavananda & Isherwood, 2007). The practices help create the space required to cultivate an experience of self that will serve you. As you and your clients engage in mindful and yogic practices, you will become increasingly aware, cultivate inquiry and understanding, and create an intentional experience of self through choice. Based on the writings of Viktor Frankl and the ideas presented within the context of the Buddhist Psychological Model (BPM; Branson & Gross, 2014; Frankl, 1959; Grabovac, Lau, & Willett, 2011), the following selection speaks directly to embodied self-regulation:

> *Between stimulus and response there is a space.*
> *In that space, you have the power to choose a response.*
> *In your response, lies your growth, freedom, and possibility.*

This chapter reviews the unique aspects of the role of mindfulness and yoga in therapy, explores the definition of self in both mindful and yogic traditions, and defines the 12 embodied practices of mindful and yogic self-regulation.

UNIQUE ASPECTS OF MINDFUL AND YOGIC APPROACHES TO PRACTICE

Both yogic and mindful conceptualizations of the self view the self as existing in the space between stimulus and response. It is between both the internal and external triggers that individuals experience the self. That is, despite of, or without regard for, internal or external contingencies, consequences, or rewards, we can construct the self. The active process of constructing, experiencing, and regulating the self involves practice. Both mindfulness and yogic traditions provide systems, conceptualizations, and sets of practices that give individuals access to who they really are. In yoga this is referred to as your true nature (Prabhavananda & Isherwood, 2007). Yogic and mindfulness approaches differ from traditional, Western psychotherapy in three key ways (see Chapter 1 for a comparison of embodied self-regulation and traditional self-regulation models):

1. The therapist is a practitioner of mindful and yogic practices.
2. The client is not viewed as broken and acceptance is essential.
3. Mindful and yogic approaches involve the cultivation of healthy self-regulation practices.

The Therapist Is a Practitioner

As you read through the following chapters, I ask you to contemplate your own experience and your own practice. In previous chapters, I have used case studies and examples to illustrate points and struggles. As we move toward Part II of this text, we also shift to seeing the therapist as an additional source of wisdom and insight. That is, you and your experience with mindfulness and yoga are integrated into your learning and practicing of these methodologies. Perhaps distinct from what are considered traditional approaches to Western psychotherapy, yogic and mindful approaches *require* the practitioner to be on the path. As a therapist using these techniques, you are expected to speak from an authentic experience of practice and struggle (a part of practice). As a result of your practice, when you speak, you speak from a knowing of this journey and the challenges it holds. McCown, Reibel, and Micozzi (2010) call this authority. This authority comes from a living it, loving it, and knowing it that can only come from dutiful practice. What does this look like in day-to-day life? This means that you have commitment to consistent, formal practice that mirrors the frequency, intensity, and duration expected of your clients (McCown et al., 2010). To glean therapeutic benefits of yoga practice, one should practice three times a week for a duration of at least an hour for a period of more than 6 weeks (Cook-Cottone, 2013). To teach yoga, certification is recommended, along with a foundation of steady practice of 2 years. See Yoga Alliance (www.yogaalliance.org) for questions about yoga certification and registration as a yoga instructor. Yoga Alliance sets standards and provides information for yoga teachers and teacher-training programs. Regarding meditation, one should engage in some form of meditation daily for at least 90 days prior to teaching meditation or speaking about it from any sense of authority (McCown et al., 2010).

The Client Is Not Viewed as Broken and Acceptance Is Essential

The most important role of the therapist does not lie in fixing or solving problems but in helping clients tolerate the difficulties, uncertainty, and pain in their lives (Germer & Siegel, 2012). Bien (2006) explains that the goal of mindful therapy is to help the patient successfully relate to his or her emotional life and all of his or her experience in a new way. Typically, in Western culture, we are taught to judge as bad any wanting, needing, sadness, worry, anxiety, and so forth. Accordingly, we work to eliminate any wanting, needing, sadness, worry, anxiety, and so forth. Mindful and yogic approaches are different. As you and your clients illuminate each circumstance, solution, or struggle with awareness, with acceptance, and without resistance of what is, you will begin to experience an increase in positive and healthy emotions and a decrease in suffering (Bien, 2006). To illustrate, two key practices of mindful awareness and nonattachment can help ease your response to difficult experiences. First, you simply notice the experience, allowing it to simply be. You notice if it increases in intensity and recedes. Second, you do not try to gain control or power over it. You allow it. That is, you notice it (mindful awareness) and simply let it be (nonattachment).

The Cultivation of Healthy, Self-Regulation Practices

Advances in neuroscience have helped illuminate exactly what our way of being is doing to our brains. In *Buddha's Brain: The Practical Neuroscience of Happiness, Love, and Wisdom,* Hanson and Mendius (2009) report that what flows through your mind sculpts your brain. Such conceptualizations go back to Aristotle, who described action, or doing, as a pathway to becoming (e.g., Aristotle is often quoted as saying, "We become what we repeatedly do"). Bien (2006) notes that in Buddhist teaching, it is held that the mind takes on the quality upon which it dwells. In this way of seeing struggle, the work against something difficult, negative, or painful only gives the difficulty more energy (Bien, 2006). With more energy and practice, the negative aspects of experience gain strength and begin to shift how your brain habitually responds to experience (Bien, 2006). Conversely, you can use your mind and your thought processes to change your brain for the better (Hanson & Mendius, 2009). Much more on mindfulness, as well as a set of practices, is presented in Chapters 4, 5, and 6. Further, for an easy-to-understand review of the neuroscience underlying the changes seen in mindfulness practices, see Hanson and Mendius (2009).

THE MINDFUL AND YOGIC SELF

With a clear understanding of how embodied self-regulation differs from traditional approaches to self-regulation (Chapter 1), a model of the embodied, regulated self (Chapter 1), and risk factors associated with dysregulation and the associated disorders (Chapter 2), we are ready to conceptualize the mindful and yogic *self*. The dominant conceptualization of the self in Western psychology is the view of the self as an object (Ryan & Brown, 2003). From the roots of object-relations theory in the early part of the 20th century, the term *self-concept* arose to describe the appraisals one has of him- or herself and the associated attributes (Ryan & Brown, 2003). The associated concept, self-esteem, is comprised of the evaluative schemata associated with self-concept (Ryan & Brown, 2003). In this way of thinking, your client is an object, a thing, with various attributes, which can be good or bad. Distinctly, mindful and yogic approaches see this act of seeing self as object and the accompanying self-evaluation as a key source of suffering. In fundamental ways, mindful and yogic traditions view the self differently.

The roots of mindfulness and yogic conceptualizations reach back thousands of years and intermingle, informing each other (Ajaya, 1983; Simpkins & Simpkins, 2011). Mindful and yogic approaches share conceptualizations of self and the methods for reaching self-realization and enlightenment. In both traditions, there are multiple schools of thought and practice, many key texts, and thousands of texts interpreting and applying original texts (Ajaya, 1983). Specifically, this text serves to honor mindful and yogic traditions with a focus on the practical methodologies, or practices, that can help cultivate embodied self-regulation. Suitably, the definition of self is viewed within this practical context.

Mindfulness and Self

In mindfulness-based approaches the self is viewed as the witness or observer of experiences. For example, Hanson and Mendius (2009) describe the "apparent self" as "perhaps the single greatest source of suffering" (p. 204). In Buddhist and mindfulness teaching, the self is not viewed as an unchanging entity that moves through life aggregating experiences while remaining constant (Bien, 2006; Hanson & Mendius, 2009). Nevertheless, Buddhist teaching asks the individual to reflect on the apparent self (Bien, 2006; Hanson & Mendius, 2009). So, who or what is the mindful self? Is it the observer? If your answer is "yes," then Bien (2006), author of *Mindful Therapy: A Guide for Therapists and Helping Professionals*, asks, "Does this observer-self then cease to exist [when one stops observing]?" (p. 151). Bien (2006) questions, if the self can move in and out of existence, is it more like a process than an entity? Answering from a mindfulness-based perspective, the answer is "yes." You (the self) are the process (Ryan & Brown, 2003). Hanson and Mendius (2009) suggest that these processes, the self, exist in patterns that are anchored in the brain and experienced by the mind.

You will read about the Buddhist Psychological Model in Chapter 4 (Grabovac et al., 2011). Within this model, there are three aspects of experience that, when not accepted and allowed, cause suffering: (a) the notion of not-self (b) impermanence and (c) nonattachment (Grabovac et al., 2011; Hanson & Mendius, 2009). These three concepts can be utilized as a perspective from which to consider the idea of self. First, mindful approaches view identification with the self as one of the main causes of suffering (Hanson &

Mendius, 2009). The sense of "I" is associated with many approaches to everyday existence that lead to negative affect and decreased feelings of well-being, such as taking things personally, a need to differentiate from others, overemphasis on achievement and competition, acquisition of material items and wealth, and an overemphasis on appearance and ability. This does not mean that you and your patients are no-thing(s), or nothing (Bien, 2006). Within this context, you are not an object of some kind; rather, you are a process (Bien, 2006).

Holding on to an apparent self creates a struggle against impermanence. Impermanence is the acknowledgment of the truth that everything changes, always. That is, things you have now, you will not have later (e.g., youth, material items, ability, beauty). Your relationships are of the nature to change and will always be changing. Who you are within those relationships will also change and will always change. There are many more ways to consider the concept of impermanence. Mindful approaches see the acknowledgment and acceptance of impermanence, especially as it relates to your sense of self, as critical to growth and well-being (Hanson & Mendius, 2009).

Last, nonattachment is the notion that letting go of the need to pursue or avoid something will be beneficial to your growth and well-being (Hanson & Mendius, 2009). Marsha Linehan (1993) was one of the first Western therapists to embrace these concepts and integrate them into treatment. Distress tolerance and emotional regulation, two components of her program, hold nonattachment as a foundation of skill development. For example, if your client is feeling a strong, deeply uncomfortable feeling, an effective strategy is to let it be, observe it, and neither work hard to accept or avoid it (i.e., nonattachment). In terms of self, your client will benefit from nonattachment—the experience of self, the apparent self, moves in and out of emotional and material experiences; the lesser one attaches to these experiences, the greater one's sense of well-being will be. Conversely, if your client attaches to a moment of joy, happiness, or a material item, the fear of its loss is on the other side of the coin. Chapter 4 will cover these concepts in more detail. For now, it is important to understand that the apparent self is happier when nonattachment is a practice.

Some of you who are reading this section may feel that the concept of not identifying as "I," lacking a sense of permanence, and not attaching to anything (i.e., a person, feeling, or item) seems dissociated, disconnected, even pathological. As described, independent of the whole, it can seem that way. Notably, there are practices such as mindful awareness, compassion, and loving-kindness that are part of the mindfulness approach that work with these three practices (i.e., not-self, impermanence, and nonattachment) to create an engagement in, and awareness of, each living moment of your and your clients' lives. As you read through and practice mindful techniques, you will come to realize that when one is free from overidentification with self, fear of impermanence, and a need to attach or avoid each feeling, person, and thing, a much richer, happier, and satisfying experience of life is possible.

To illustrate, Zuri, the 13-year-old girl you met in Chapter 1, struggles to be present sometimes. Her mom is an alcoholic, and Zuri worries about her all of the time. Her counselor at school, Mrs. Markham, has helped her to understand alcoholism and has encouraged her to go to meetings to learn more about alcoholism. Mrs. Markham also helped Zuri sign up for the after-school yoga program with Miss Amanda. Zuri often tells Mrs. Markham that she thinks that her mom's drinking is her fault. She comes to this thought as a result of her lived experience. She explains that her mom often tells her that if she and her brothers were better behaved she wouldn't need to drink so much. In fact, Zuri explains, when her mom leaves to go to the bar she often does it right after she gets mad at Zuri and her brothers. Zuri explains that she becomes so anxious when her mom leaves that she can barely breathe. She says, "I am scared." She thinks, "Mom left because I am bad." She thinks she will not be okay if her mother is not there to make things okay. She becomes completely overwhelmed.

Mrs. Markham utilizes the aspects of mindfulness to help Zuri self-regulate. First, as Zuri tells Mrs. Markham, "I am scared," Mrs. Markham reflects, "You are feeling a lot of anxiety," immediately shifting identification as the feeling (e.g., "I am _____") to a process of observing the experience of feeling a strong feeling (e.g., "I am feeling _____"). Next, she asks Zuri to tell her about the anxiety, when it happens, how it happens, and how the anxiety feels in her body (e.g., "Does your heart rate increase? Are there sensations in your body? Does your breath change?"). Focus on the body and on experience increases connection for Zuri between body and mind (McCown et al., 2010) while allowing an experience of interpersonal attunement as Mrs. Markham shares a focus on Zuri's experience and validates Zuri's anxiety. Embracing impermanence and the notion that everything comes and goes, Mrs. Markham then asks Zuri to slow her breath and count to four as she inhales and five as she exhales. They practice this together. She asks Zuri to notice how her body may feel different as she breathes (e.g., heart rate, breath, sensations in her belly). Mrs. Markham helps Zuri understand that feelings come and go (i.e., impermanence), that anxious feelings seem to be triggered when Zuri's mom leaves, and that this makes total sense. It is scary when your mom leaves, angry, to go out drinking. Her work with Zuri is designed around giving Zuri tools to manage her emotional experience. In this way, Zuri is able to experience the self as a malleable, evolving process. (Note that as any good school counselor would do, Mrs. Markham explores any child neglect and related issues. These techniques are embedded within standard good practice.)

Yoga and Self

Similar to mindfulness-based techniques, yoga was developed as a means for cultivating a higher consciousness and transcending self through mental and physical discipline and practice (Simpkins & Simpkins, 2011). The practices of yoga are ancient, passed down through generations as teachers taught their students verbally and through practice. This is called the guru tradition (Simpkins & Simpkins, 2011). Five major texts can be considered the philosophical foundations of yoga: the Vedas, Upanishads, Bhagavad Gita, Vedanta, and Yoga Sutras. Within the past 25 years, as with mindfulness-based techniques, applications of yoga practice have evolved to meet the needs of current-day practitioners. Many schools of yoga have risen from Eastern traditions and now thrive in Western culture (Ajaya, 1983). Further, yoga has increasingly become viewed as a tool for developing health and wellness (e.g., McCall, 2007). As a sign of the changing role of yoga in Western culture, the *International Journal of Yoga Therapy* was added to the Medline database within the past 5 years.

According to the Yoga Sutras, egoism or attachment to ego (e.g., "I") is one of the causes of suffering (Yoga Sutra 2.3, Prabhavananda & Isherwood, 2007). More specifically, egoism, or a focus on I, is considered an obstacle to self-realization (Prabhavananda & Isherwood, 2007). In yoga, obstacles are considered to be those things that obscure our access to what is within us, our inner light, or our inner access to connection, attunement, and contentment (Prabhavananda & Isherwood, 2007). In this way, ego (i.e., I), referred to as the lowercase "s" *self* or *ego self*, is an obstacle to your true nature, your connected uppercase "S" *Self* or soul Self. The soul Self, or yogic Self, is conceptualized as our connection to all things (note that the word *yoga* means "to unite, or yoke") and it is deep within us, sometimes obscured by obstacles. The ego self is akin to the "apparent self" described in mindfulness. The soul Self is akin to seeing the self as a process, as described previously. In yoga, one works to reveal the true Self. The practice of yoga, all eight limbs, is designed to gradually remove these obstacles to reveal the Self, one's true nature (Prabhavananda & Isherwood, 2007).

In private practice, I have found the yogic conceptualization of the Self very helpful. Many patients enter therapy convinced that they are empty inside or missing something (Weintraub, 2004). Self-regulation difficulties seem to anchor on this belief as patients attempt to fill this space or meet this emptiness. In their efforts to fill and satisfy a perceived emptiness, they binge, shop, crave, gamble, drink, and use. Because there is no empty space to fill, their efforts fail to satisfy, serving only to further dysregulate. When a patient presents in this way, I introduce the yogic conceptualization of self, saying, "You may find this interesting. In yoga philosophy, there is no emptiness inside of you. In yogic thinking, you have an inner light that connects you to the universe, or your conceptualization of God. In yoga, the difficulty is that our access to our inner light has been obscured with obstacles. These obstacles are things such as ways of thinking, lack of connection with our bodies, or behaviors such as drinking or using. In yogic thinking, the focus is on slowly removing these obstacles so that you can have access to what is already light inside of you, your true nature." This approach can be empowering for patients, giving them hope.

Both the mindful and yogic approaches to self shift attention away from perfecting, refining, or fixing the "I" or enhancing the ego, toward practicing the process of being. The identification with the self, or "I," is viewed as a source of challenge and suffering. Both traditions see the self as complete and whole as it exists in the here and now, moment by moment. As you work with your clients, you too can help them shift their focus from I, or ego, toward the process of being.

THE 12 EMBODIED PRACTICES OF THE MINDFUL AND YOGIC SELF

As a practitioner wanting to integrate mindful and yogic approaches into your mental health practice, you may feel overwhelmed by the thought of having to select and review the most fitting traditional texts (e.g., Yoga Sutras) or the most appropriate recent interpretation of the traditional texts (e.g., *The Four Immeasurables: Practices to Open the Heart* [Wallace, 2010]; *Yoga for Emotional Balance: Simple Practices to Help Relieve Anxiety and Depression* [Forbes, 2011]). The 12 embodied practices were organized to distill these readings, traditional through recent, into a practical set of 12 essential practices to facilitate embodied self-regulation. The 12 embodied practices, listed in Table 3.1, are briefly reviewed here. These practices detail the pathway to developing the skills inherent in the mindful and yogic self as a way of negotiating both internal and external challenges of daily life (Figure 3.1).

TABLE 3.1   The 12 Embodied Practices

Practice 1: Be mindfully aware.

Practice 2: Honor your breath and physical experience.

Practice 3: Live in inquiry.

Practice 4: Accept impermanence.

Practice 5: Cultivate nonattachment.

Practice 6: Discern what is not-self.

Practice 7: Allow what is with nonjudgment.

Practice 8: Prioritize self-care.

Practice 9: Be of your values.

Practice 10: Observe compassion for self and others.

Practice 11: Maintain equanimity.

Practice 12: Cultivate loving-kindness and joy.

The following chapters break down mindful and yogic conceptualizations and detail specific practices referring back to these 12 practices as central organizing themes. Consider this your starting place. Continued study of traditional and current texts is encouraged as you progress on your path of self-development and refine your work with your clients.

Practice 1: Be Mindfully Aware

Mindful awareness is a way of being—"a way of inhabiting one's body, one's mind, one's moment-by-moment experience" (Shapiro & Carlson, 2009, p. 5). More obviously central to mindfulness-based practice, mindful awareness is also fundamental to yoga. In fact, one of the Yoga Sutras' first teachings is as follows: "Yoga is the control of the thought-waves in

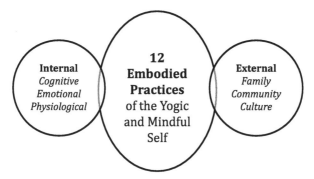

FIGURE 3.1 The self as 12 embodied practices.

the mind" (Yoga Sutra 1.2; Prabhavananda & Isherwood, 2007, p. 14). Mindful awareness is the state of being attentive to and aware of what is taking place in the present (Brown & Ryan, 2003). Siegel (2010) describes mindful awareness as a conscientious and intentional approach to what we do that allows us to be creative with possibilities. It involves an awareness of the present moment without judgment. It is a flexible, receptive, and open presence (Brown & Ryan, 2003; Siegel, 2010). Mindful awareness necessitates single-mindedness (Grabovac et al., 2011). According to the BPM, an individual can truly be aware of only one object at a time. Consciousness is viewed as a stream of awareness, a rapid series of sense impressions and mental events that arise and pass away (Grabovac et al., 2011). Recent research has found mindful awareness to be associated with a variety of positive outcomes, including sense of well-being and increased self-knowledge (Brown & Ryan, 2003). Before anything, you must be mindfully aware. With awareness, possibility abounds.

Practice 2: Honor Your Breath and Physical Experience

Breath and physical experience are the key components of embodied self-regulation. The breath is the bridge between the body and the mind. Breath is central to yogic teachings. For example, Yoga Sutra 1.34 reads, "The mind may also be calmed by expulsion and retention of the breath" (Prabhavananda & Isherwood, 2007, p. 70). Further, over 30 years of research tells us that the breath is the antidote for the stress response. It is the access point to the relaxation response first describe by Herbert Benson in 1976. Your breath aligns with your internal activation, your feeling state, and your state of arousal. You have both control of your breath and involuntary, automatic breath (Simpkins & Simpkins, 2011). This fundamental truth of voluntary and involuntary roots to breath control is the source of the power of intentional breath (Simpkins & Simpkins, 2011). Breath control can assist the shift out of psychological activation, down-regulate the chronic stress response, and move an individual into the relaxation response (Simpkins & Simpkins, 2011; Weintraub, 2012). In these ways and more, the breath is very powerful.

Like breath, the physical experience must also be honored as critical to healing and preventing struggle (McCown et al., 2010). The experience of physiological self is as relevant to mental health as the cognitive and emotional aspects of self (Cook-Cottone, 2006). Embodied approaches to self-regulation view the role of physical practice as key to well-being and emotional growth. Experiencing body sensations as they arise and pass away, without judgment, helps us disembed our immediate experience from our stories about the experience (McCown et al., 2010). Over time, a practice of bringing awareness to the body and away from the "privileged cognitive domain" helps lead us to new possibilities unencumbered by limited beliefs and past impressions (McCown et al., 2010, p. 145). Emphasis on embodiment brings awareness to internal sensation (i.e., interoception) and can deepen a sense of resonance with others (McCown et al., 2010). Without embodied practice, there can be no change.

Finally, emotions are a composite of cognitive and physiological experiences. They live in the mind and body. Emotional memories are both seated in the brain and remembered in the body. To access and process emotions, the body must be part of the methodology. Anchoring feelings where they reside, within the physical self, self-awareness, leading to greater likelihood of effective self-regulation. That is, the body is key to effectively processing and regulating emotional experience (Bennett, 2002; Siegel, 2010). Overall, steady physical practice, physical self-care, and awareness and active processing of the physiological aspects of emotional experience create a physical foundation for self-regulation.

Practice 3: Live in Inquiry

Yogic and mindful practices view life as the journey of the seeker of knowledge (Wallace, 2011). That is, you and your clients are on a path of self-inquiry (Bennett, 2002). Wallace (2011) reminds us that "the search for insight and wisdom is not done for the sake of knowledge itself; it is a search to deepen our experiential understanding" (p. 5). To be in inquiry means to come from a place of not knowing (McCown et al., 2010). That is, you are curious about the presemantic experience, before words and concepts, of the present moment (McCown et al., 2010). Each present-moment experience is an opportunity to learn and grow. The Sanskrit word *Svadhyaya* refers to self-study as a path to deeper self-knowledge (Weintraub, 2012). Inquiry and curiosity cultivate an attitude of openness and nonjudgment. Curiosity moves you away from a withdrawal and defense mode of processing and toward engagement and approach (McCown et al., 2010). Presemantic inquiry questions would sound like this: "What am I noticing in my body?" or "What am I noticing in the current moment?" Inquiry questions can help guide behavior as well. For example, Shapiro and Carlson (2009) ask us to inquire, "What is most conducive to my own and others' well-being?" (p. 6) or "What would best serve my intentions right now?" In this way, the process of growth is fluid, responsive, nonjudgmental, ongoing, and open.

Practice 4: Accept Impermanence

Impermanence is a central tenet of mindful practices (Grabovac et al., 2011; Shapiro & Carlson, 2009). Our experiential worlds are made up of both sense impressions and mental events triggered by both internal and external stimuli (Grabovac et al., 2011). Sense impressions and mental events are transient. That is, they arise and pass away. Nothing is permanent—no thing, person, sensation, feeling, thought, or circumstance. Yet we live as if everything in our world is permanent, static, and unchanging (Shapiro & Carlson, 2009). Even the self is impermanent (Hanson & Mendius, 2009). Due to the neurological construction of experience in the brain, the self seems to be permanent and continuous (Hanson & Mendius, 2009). In fact, the self is a series of thousands of overlaying sense impressions and mental events (Grabovac et al., 2011; Hanson & Mendius, 2009). Suffering is believed to come from the lack of acceptance of and resistance to impermanence (Bien, 2006).

Practice 5: Cultivate Nonattachment

Grabovac et al. (2011) identify the habitual reactions of attachment and aversion as central to suffering. Specifically, Yoga Sutra 2.7 defines attachment as that which dwells upon pleasure or the pursuit of that which gives you pleasure (Prabhavananda & Isherwood, 2007). Further, Yoga Sutra 2.8 defines aversion as that which dwells upon pain, or avoids pain (Prabhavananda & Isherwood, 2007). We can manifest attachment and aversion toward things, feelings, thoughts, people, and circumstances. Yoga Sutras 1.12 and 1.15 address nonattachment, describing it as a means of stilling the thought waves of the mind (Yoga Sutra 1.12) and as a pathway to the "freed one." Specifically, Yoga Sutra 1.15 reads, "Nonattachment is self-mastery; it is freedom from desire for what is seen or heard" (Prabhavananda & Isherwood, 2007, p. 26).

The BPM and the Yoga Sutras describe nonattachment in terms of the thought process. As you meditate or practice, you can become attached to the thoughts, feelings, or sensations that arise. In your mindfulness work (i.e., yoga and meditation), you can cultivate nonattachment. That is, you simply notice the thoughts, feelings, or sensations as they arise in and pass out of your awareness without engagement or proliferation (Grabovac et al., 2011; Prabhavananda & Isherwood, 2007). This practice then serves you when external objects or desires enter your consciousness (e.g., a new car, a lover). With practice, you can be present with, and not attached to, your experience. Other Yoga Sutras refer to nonattachment and attachment (e.g., 1.16, 1.19, 2.3), suggesting that as nonattachment is achieved, all craving ceases.

Practice 6: Discern What Is Not-Self

Shapiro and Carlson (2009) and Bien (2006) explain that the concept of impermanence can be extended to the understanding of self. That is, all things change—including the self. In essence, there is no stable entity called the self. Bien (2006) describes the self as a river with nothing to hold on to, nothing permanent or unchanging. In this manner, there is nothing to defend (Bien, 2006). That is, we are not the car we drive, the salary we make, or even the nose on our face. These all change. This can be freeing in that at any given moment we can cultivate the self we would like to be, our intentional self. Bien (2006) explains it this way: Imagine that there are two people sitting on the bank of a flowing river. They watch the river flow by; the water ripples and swirls around rocks. One of the people watches, fascinated by the energy of the water, the peaks and valleys in the waves, the mist as it rises off of the clashes between water and rocks. She is happy and content as she watches. The other is agitated and angry. He wishes that the water would stop; it is going too fast. He desires to see rocks over the waves and that the mist would stop landing on his face. Interestingly, neither of the two observers change the river.

You are the process, and this need not include the reaction to it. You are no *thing*—no object—you are a process, an ever-changing, ever-evolving process (Bien, 2006). The discerning or not discerning of this distinction makes the difference. Yoga Sutra 2.3 describes egoism as an obstacle that causes suffering (Prabhavananda & Isherwood, 2007). Specifically, a focus on I or the lowercase "s" or apparent self is a contributor to suffering (see Yoga Sutra 2.6). With egoism you have something to defend and something to lose (e.g., status). You have a need to differentiate from others and a need to compare seeing the ego relative to others. In many ways, seeing the ego, I, or apparent self as self creates suffering.

Practice 7: Allow What Is With Nonjudgment

Embrace all that arises (Shapiro & Carlson, 2009). Another cause of suffering is resisting what is actually happening (Bien, 2006; Shapiro & Carlson, 2009). In Buddhism, it is believed that we suffer not from what is happening but due to our relationship with what is happening (Shapiro & Carlson, 2009). Buddhist teacher Shinzen Young (1997) created a mathematical equation to explain the relationship between suffering and resistance (Bien, 2006; Shapiro & Carlson, 2009):

$$Suffering = Pain \times Resistance$$

Pain is that which we cannot control. It can be many things—a physical sensation, a relational loss, or a material loss. Pain can be small (a delay at the grocery store) or overwhelming (the loss of a loved one). Resistance is ours to manage, and therefore so is the suffering. For example, if you are delayed at the grocery store (low level of pain), yet manifest large amounts of resistance, you can experience a great amount of suffering while waiting in line. Conversely, you may experience great pain (e.g., a cancer diagnosis) and yet allow what has happened to be and acknowledge it for what it is—you will experience manageable pain (Shapiro & Carlson, 2009).

Allowing what is requires nonjudgment. As well described in Grabovac et al.'s (2011) article on the BPM, suffering stems from the labeling of mental events of sense impressions as pleasant or unpleasant. These feeling tones (i.e., pleasant, unpleasant, or neutral) are concomitant to the awareness of any object (i.e., sense impression or mental event). There is an automatic pulling toward the pleasant and a pushing away from the unpleasant. These feeling tones often pass by quickly beneath our consciousness. However, at times, they can serve as a trigger to a chain reaction of thoughts, emotions, and actions that can lead to suffering. It is the judgment of the object as good or bad that can begin this chain to suffering. Shapiro and Carlson (2009) define nonjudgment as a process of impartial witnessing and observing of the present moment without evaluating or categorizing. In essence, allowing what is requires an open presence, the absence of judgment.

Practice 8: Prioritize Self-Care

Self-care is a multifaceted process that includes the care of the physical, emotional, and cognitive self within the context of our families, friends, and community. To engage in self-care you must cultivate self-awareness and a set of daily practices that are firmly integrated into your routine. There is an entire chapter in this book dedicated to the practice of self-care (Chapter 12), which speaks to its importance in well-being and mental health. The components of self-care include nutrition, hydration, rest, self-soothing, exercise, environmental accommodations, anticipation of challenges, and preparation, as well as good medical and dental care. Of critical importance is physical health. Without physiological health, it is difficult to maintain psychological health or emotional regulation (Cook-Cottone, Tribole, & Tylka, 2013). More recently, self-care has become a focus in mindful and yogic practice—perhaps because the treatment provider and the provider's own journey are considered an important part of the treatment process (Shapiro & Carlson, 2009). Through the process of cultivating self-care, providers and patients learn to tend to themselves in a kind and healing way. For both the patients and the practitioners, this results in a greater ability to provide attention, loving-kindness, and care to those lives we touch (Shapiro & Carlson, 2009).

Practice 9: Be of Your Values

Both mindful and yogic traditions include a code of ethics for practitioners to follow. In mindfulness approaches, adherence to the ethical practices is thought to reduce mental proliferation and increase concentration and mindfulness (Grabovac et al., 2011). Leading a life of ethics allows practitioners to experience less guilt and fewer doubts, which can be the source of mental proliferation (Grabovac et al., 2011). Within the mindfulness tradition there is the noble Eight-Fold Path (Bien, 2006). This is a path of eight practices: right view, right thinking, right speech, right action, right livelihood, right mindfulness, right diligence, and right concentration (Bien, 2006). In yogic traditions, these are described within limbs 1 and 2 of the eight limbs of yoga (Simpkins & Simpkins, 2011). Limbs 1 and 2 are called the Yamas and the Niyamas, respectively. The Yamas are the restraints, or the things not to do, and the Niyamas are the observances, or the things to do. The Yamas include ahimsa (nonharming), satya (not lying), asteya (not stealing), brahmacharya (restraint), and aparigraha (nonattachment). The Niyamas include shaucha (purity), santosha (contentment), tapas (austerity), pranitara (attentiveness to self-study and reflection on matters of meaningful spirituality), and ishvara pranidhana (devotion to a higher value; Simpkins & Simpkins, 2011).

Practice 10: Observe Compassion for Self and Others

The Yoga Sutras and mindfulness traditions refer to compassion as one of the four immeasurables or aspirations (i.e., compassion, equanimity, loving-kindness, and joy; Prabhavananda & Isherwood, 2007; Wallace, 2010, 2011). Compassion is defined as the integration of the ability to feel empathy for the suffering of oneself and others as well as an accompanying desire to act to alleviate the suffering (Shapiro & Carlson, 2009; Wallace, 2010). An important distinction between compassion and loving-kindness is that in compassion one is a witness to the suffering of others, feels empathy, perhaps even loving-kindness, *and* yearns to alleviate the suffering (McCown et al., 2010; Wallace, 2010). Self-compassion involves the ability to see one's own suffering, feel loving-kindness toward the self, and work to address the suffering with warmth and kindness (Shapiro & Carlson, 2009). It has three components: (a) offering understanding and kindness to oneself (b) viewing your own experiences as part of the larger human experience and (c) remaining present with your painful thoughts and feelings without overidentifying with them (McCown et al., 2010; Neff, 2003). Compassion and self-compassion are the antidotes to cruelty (Wallace, 2010).

Practice 11: Maintain Equanimity

Another of the four immeasureables, equanimity can be defined as impartiality or even-mindedness (Hanson & Mendius, 2009; Wallace, 2010). As things pass through our experiences, we stay even-keeled, steady; we aren't easily thrown off balance (Hanson & Mendius, 2009). It is important to make a distinction between equanimity and indifference or a lack of caring (Wallace, 2010). Equanimity can be attained through mindful awareness of, inquiry regarding, and an allowing of our sense impressions, mental events, and feelings. Equanimity is an even, steady presence with what is, without the flight into rumination, emotional overwhelm, or attachment. Hanson and Mendius (2009) describe equanimity as the mental mudroom, the entry room of the house where people place their muddy boots, rain coats, and lacrosse sticks. It is with equanimity that your initial reactions to things (e.g., I like that, I don't like that) are left in the mud room so that the inside of your home, your mind, remains clean and of peaceful clarity (Hanson & Mendius, 2009).

I work on equanimity when I achieve an asana, or yoga posture, upon which I have been working. I have noticed that this is an experience in which I tend to lose a sense of equanimity. When I was first able to hold flying pigeon, I became very excited and happy, as I had worked hard and practiced many hours to master the asana. My practice then becomes a cultivation of the aspiration of equanimity. I feel my feelings of happiness, joy, and pride, yet I breathe and work to not attach to them. This is not an easy task for me. I notice that the next time I practice I worry that I might not be able to replicate flying pigeon. I become aware of my attachment to the achievement of this pose. To cultivate equanimity, I leave the pose out of my practice; I bring my awareness to my breath and my physical experience, over and over, letting go of my *need* to attach to flying pigeon. Notably, throughout this whole process, flying pigeon is the current object of my experience, my growth. It is valuable not as an asana that I achieved at some point, but as an experience that shined a light on my equanimity practice. Flying pigeon, it is a good day. No flying pigeon, it is a good day.

Practice 12: Cultivate Loving-Kindness and Joy

Loving-kindness and joy are the final two of the four immeasurables or aspirations (Wallace, 2011). Loving-kindness helps develop the capacity for empathy and connection. Loving-kindness involves attending to others with a quiet and open heart (Wallace, 2011). Loving-kindness is a healing form of love (Siegel, 2010). Loving-kindness is the feeling of compassionate concern for, genuine interest in, and engagement with another (Siegel, 2010). Hanson and Mendius (2009) make a distinction between compassion and loving-kindness: "If compassion is the wish that beings not suffer, kindness is the wish that they be happy" (p. 157). Loving-kindness is present all of the time and ranges from acts such as helping a stranger to the deep love you feel for a partner or child (Hanson & Mendius, 2009).

Empathetic joy is the act of rejoicing in the well-being of others (Wallace, 2010). Joy comes easily when we are with those we love and our friends. To cultivate joy, you simply bring the person into your mind and reflect on the virtuous qualities of his or her life, considering the good and lightness that he or she has brought to the people in his or her life and the environment. You allow yourself to enter into that same joy, share it, and rejoice in it (Wallace, 2010). In private practice, I cultivate empathic joy when a patient has accomplished a treatment goal. I work with individuals who struggle with eating disorders, primarily. My patients frequently have goals to be symptom-free for a period of time. They work hard to cultivate healthy practices and to let the symptoms go as they cultivate a new way of being. When they share with me that they have accomplished 30, 60, or more days of symptom-free living, I ask them, "How do you feel?" I encourage them to describe the feeling, the experience in the body, in the present moment, and to review the journey. What manifests is a wonderful feeling of empathetic joy.

EXPLORING THE 12 EMBODIED PRACTICES OF THE YOGIC AND MINDFUL SELF

It can be helpful to make this exploration concrete for your patients and to provide them with a processing sheet that lists their challenges (see Chapter 2) and the potential strategies for growth (i.e., the 12 embodied practices). Using Figure 3.2, have your client list each of the challenges that manifest within the internal aspects of self (body, emotions, and thoughts) and the external aspects of self (family, community, and culture). Next, ask your client to draw arrows from the specific embodied practice that might be a possible support or alternative action for the challenge he or she has identified. Ask your patient to circle, star, or underline the practice he or she would like to know more about. Figure 3.3 provides a sample figure completed by someone who struggles with excessive substance use. In future chapters, specific activities and scripts

Internal Self Challenges	The 12 Embodied Practices	External Self Challenges
Cognitive (Thinking)	*Be mindfully aware* *Honor your breath and physical experience* *Live in inquiry* *Accept impermanence* *Cultivate nonattachment*	Family and Friends
Emotional (Feeling)	*Discern what is not-self* *Allow what is with nonjudgment* *Prioritize self-care* *Be of your values*	Community (e.g., School/Work)
Physiological (Body)	*Observe compassion for self and others* *Maintain equanimity* *Cultivate loving-kindness and joy*	Culture (e.g., Media, Social Pressures)

FIGURE 3.2 Exploring your challenges and the 12 embodied practices.

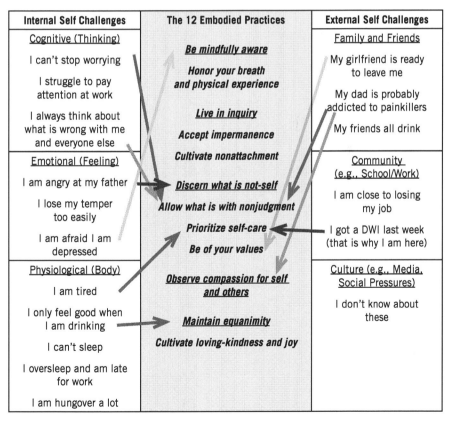

FIGURE 3.3 Exploring your challenges and the 12 embodied practices—client-completed example.
DWI, driving while impaired.

are provided for you to facilitate the active practice of a healthier, embodied experience of self.

Recall John, the 20-year-old young man who is struggling with his drinking and his father's addiction, described in an earlier chapter. He completed the sheet and placed arrows to the mindful practices that he think might help. As you can see in Figure 3.3, some of his challenges have no arrows. He is not sure what might help for these. Also, he does not have a sense of the cultural implications of drinking and drug use. He also underlined a few of the practices he thinks he would like to learn more about. This exploration sheet provides a nice starting place for the exploration of yogic and mindful practices.

SUMMARY

The mindful and yogic self is not a thing, or an object, but a process. The process of becoming a mindfulness and yoga-informed therapist involves (a) a commitment to the practices of yoga and mindfulness; (b) acceptance of your patients as on the path toward health and healing; and finally (c) building and practicing the knowledge and skills to support your clients on their journey in the development of a healthy and positive experience of self. The mindful and yogic self is distinct from the ego, or apparent self, and involves the cultivation of a set of skills or practices that help remove obstacles to one's true nature. These skills can be summarized in a set of 12 embodied practices: mindful awareness, honoring breath and physical experience, living in inquiry, accepting impermanence, cultivating nonattachment, discerning not-self, allowing what is with nonjudgment, prioritizing self-care, being of your values, observing compassion for self and others, maintaining equanimity, and cultivating loving-kindness and joy. These practices integrate a large body of knowledge passed down from both mindful and yogic traditions and reflect the core sutras of this text. Welcome to the journey.

REFERENCES

Ajaya, S. (1983). *Psychotherapy East and West: A unifying paradigm.* Honesdale, PA: The Himalayan International Institute.

Bennett, B. (2002). *Emotional yoga: How the body can heal the mind.* New York, NY: Fireside.

Benson, H. (1976). *The relaxation response.* New York, NY: Harper Torch.

Bien, T. (2006). *Mindful therapy: A guide for therapists and helping professionals.* Somerville, MA: Wisdom Publications.

Branson, C. M., & Gross, S. J. (Eds.). (2014). *Handbook of ethical educational leadership.* New York, NY: Routledge.

Brown, K. W., & Ryan, R. M. (2003). The benefits of being present: Mindfulness and its role in psychological well-being. *Journal of Personality and Social Psychology, 84,* 822–848.

Cook-Cottone, C. P. (2006). The attuned representational model for the primary prevention of eating disorders: An overview for school psychologists. *Psychology in the Schools, 43,* 223–230.

Cook-Cottone, C. P. (2013). Dosage as a critical variable in yoga research. *International Journal of Yoga Therapy, 2,* 11–12.

Cook-Cottone, C. P., Tribole, E., & Tylka, T. (2013). *Healthy eating in schools: Evidence-based interventions to help kids thrive.* Washington, DC: American Psychology Association.

Forbes, B. (2011). *Yoga for emotional balance: Simple practices to help relive anxiety and depression.* Boston, MA: Shambhala Publications.

Frankl, V. (1959). *Man's search for meaning.* Boston, MA: Beacon Press.

Germer, C. K., & Siegel, R. D. (2012). *Wisdom and compassion in psychotherapy: Deepening mindfulness in clinical practice.* New York, NY: Guilford Press.

Grabovac, A. D., Lau, M. A., & Willett, B. R. (2011). Mechanism of mindfulness: A Buddhist Psychological Model. *Mindfulness* [advance online publication]. doi: org/10.1007/s12671-011-0054-5

Hanson, R., & Mendius, R. (2009). *Buddha's brain: The practical neuroscience of happiness, love, and wisdom.* Oakland, CA: New Harbinger Press.

Linehan, M. (1993). *Cognitive-behavioral treatment for borderline personality disorder.* New York, NY: Guilford Press.

McCall, T. (2007) *Yoga as medicine: The prescription for health and healing.* New York, NY: Bantam Books.

McCown, D., Reibel, D., & Micozzi, M. S. (2010). *Teaching mindfulness: A practical guide for clinicians and educators.* New York, NY: Springer.

Neff, K. (2003). The development and validation of a scale to measure self-compassion. *Self and Identity, 2,* 223–250.

Prabhavananda, S., & Isherwood, C. (2007). *How to know God: The yoga aphorisms of Patanjali.* Hollywood, CA: Vedanta Press.

Ryan, R. M., & Brown, K. W. (2003). Why we don't need self-esteem: On fundamental needs, contingent love, and mindfulness. *Psychological Inquiry, 14,* 71–76.

Shapiro, S. L., & Carlson, L. E. (2009). *The art and science of mindfulness: Integrating mindfulness into psychology and the helping professions.* Washington, DC: American Psychological Association.

Siegel, D. J. (2010). *The mindful therapist: A clinician's guide to mindsight and neural integration.* New York, NY: W. W. Norton.

Simpkins, A. M., & Simpkins, C. A. (2011). *Meditation and yoga in psychotherapy.* New York, NY: John Wiley & Sons.

Wallace, B. A. (2010). *The four immeasurables: Practices to open the heart.* Ithaca, NY: Snow Lion Publications.

Wallace, B. A. (2011). *Minding closely: The four applications of mindfulness.* Ithaca, NY: Snow Lion Publications.

Weintraub, A. (2004). *Yoga for depression: A compassionate guide to relieve suffering through yoga.* New York, NY: Broadway Books.

Weintraub, A. (2012). *Yoga skills for therapists: Effective practices for mood management.* New York, NY: W. W. Norton.

Yoga Alliance. (n.d.). Retrieved from https://www.yogaalliance.org

Young, S. (1997). *The science of enlightenment* [Audio cassettes]. Boulder, CO: Sounds True.

The Mindful Self

CR 4 BO

Mindfulness
The Basic Principles

Zen comes as a reminder that
if we do not learn to perceive the mystery and beauty of
our present life, our present hour,
we shall not perceive the worth of any life,
of any hour.—HUSTON SMITH, IN KAPLEAU (1965, p. xiii)

AN ANTIDOTE

This chapter serves to introduce you to the basic principles of mindfulness as they can be applied to embodied self-regulation. In practice, I use the basic principles of mindfulness and yogic philosophy as a framework for helping patients understand their experiences. I do so because this framework allows for an attunement between cognition, emotions, body, family, and culture. That is, mindful principles allow for an authentic expression of self as well as an effective means for negotiating external circumstances and challenges. These principles are an antidote to our current cultural messages that promote and trigger dysregulation and, accordingly, increase risk for and maintain dysregulation-based disorders (e.g., disordered eating, self-injury, shopping addiction, pathological gambling, and substance use disorders). I have compiled a list of the messages that increase risk anchored on the risk factors identified in the research (see Chapter 2 on the dysregulated self). The dysregulating messages from our culture include:

• This is what an ideal body, emotional experience, life, romantic relationship, and community *look like*. Aspire to this.

- There is probably something wrong with you.
- You are not enough.
- A substance or chemical will help you feel better.
- The answer to your struggles is outside of you.
- You might feel better if you buy this, or this, or this . . .
- You should never feel uncomfortable.
- Feeling certain feelings is weak (e.g., sadness, grief, anger, jealousy).
- Everything should be easy.
- Don't ever fail. If you do, you are a failure.
- Don't tell people your fears, insecurities, needs, and so forth. Silence yourself. These things are secret and probably bad.
- You are a thing. See yourself as others might see you. You are an object to be admired, judged, and evaluated.
- Your life should be very exciting, all of the time.
- You should be effortlessly perfect.

There are more. These are some of the good ones. Many times, a client enters therapy with no explicit knowledge of these messages. Yet, the client has internalized them over the years. They run like automatic scripts governing thoughts, feelings, and actions. Unfortunately, without a conscious awareness of their presence, a power over them, and an alternative way of conceptualizing the world, these messages, or scripts, perpetuate dysregulated behaviors. Without tools (i.e., cognitive, emotional, and behavioral), it can be difficult to embody a healthy, authentic representation of self within the context of the external systems (i.e., family, community, and culture; see Chapter 1, Figure 1.1).

Mindfulness concerns clarity of awareness of one's inner and outer worlds (Brown, Ryan, & Creswell, 2007). This includes thoughts, emotions, and actions, as well as one's surroundings, as they exist moment by moment (Brown et al., 2007). Mindfulness traditions provide an alternative set of guidelines by which we can help our clients organize their understanding of their thoughts, emotions, and behavior, and the external context. For example, Mason is a 40-year-old lawyer and a partner at his firm. He has a bright and beautiful wife who is an English teacher at the local high school. He has been married for 13 years and has three children, all in elementary school. They own their house and have paid off their student loans. By all accounts he has made it. Yet, Mason is struggling. He drinks three, sometimes four, strong drinks a night. He sees all that they have not achieved and gets frustrated that he drives a Honda to work when the other partners have BMWs. He wonders if his wife is losing her looks and is actively considering calling a plastic surgeon for liposuction on his waistline. He doesn't understand why things are so hard. He wakes up feeling like "crap" every day, thanking the universe for the caffeine drinks he secretly drinks all day long. In a good life, with so much for which to be grateful, Mason ruminates on all that he does not have. He drinks his frustration away, failing to see the beauty in his present life, in his present hour. Mason is unaware of the degree to which internalized messages of success, emotional regulation, and beauty affect his emotions, decisions, and behaviors. It is time for a new way of understanding things.

Mindfulness practices are associated with many positive outcomes, including increased ability to self-regulate, as documented in empirical research and literature reviews (e.g., Brown & Ryan, 2003; Brown et al., 2007; Duckworth, Grant, Loew, Oettingen, & Gollwitzer, 2011; Shapiro & Carlson, 2009; Siegel, 2010). Specific processes that are enhanced include clarity of awareness; nonconceptual, nondiscriminatory awareness; flexibility in awareness and attention; an empirical stance toward reality; present-oriented consciousness; and stability and continuity of attention and awareness (Brown et al., 2007). These types of practices and ways of being are negatively associated with psychopathology, alexithymia, neuroticism, and overall psychological distress (Brown et al., 2007). With mindfulness practice, there is an increased sense of well-being, stronger affect regulation tendencies, greater awareness and understanding of emotions, and an increased ability to adjust unpleasant mood states (Brown & Ryan, 2003). Interestingly, the work of Brown and Ryan (2003) suggests that more mindful individuals show a stronger relationship between implicit and explicit affect than those less dispositionally mindful. Knowing oneself in this way is a key aspect to self-regulation and critical for the maintenance of a healthy, authentic representation of self.

MINDFULNESS

Mindfulness is a unique quality of consciousness, a receptive awareness of ongoing internal states, behavior, and external realities (Brown et al., 2007). It is accompanied by an open and distortion-free perception of what is (Brown & Kasser, 2005). It is distinct from the self-awareness (i.e., awareness of self-relevant thought) and self-focused attention (i.e., focus of attention on aspects of self; Brown et al., 2007) that we see to some degree in Mason's ruminations about his life and status. In a mindful mode of consciousness behaviors tend to autonomously regulate in accord with chosen interests and values rather than aligning with socially derived pressures (Brown et al., 2007). Mindfulness entails an unconditional presence and unconditional openness (Brown et al., 2007). Some suggest that mindfulness may be an anecdote to consumerism and messages from the media (e.g., Rosenberg, 2004). Reviews indicate that mindfulness has been associated with well-being and voluntary simplicity, a lifestyle shaped around intrinsically satisfying pursuits and expressions of self and away from material goals (Brown & Kasser, 2005). Awareness is defined as the conscious registration of stimuli associated with the five senses, the kinesthetic senses, and the functions of the mind (Brown et al., 2007). Mindful awareness is the first of the 12 embodied practices of yogic and mindful self-regulation (see Chapter 3).

According to Brown and colleagues (2007), mindfulness is primarily rooted in Buddhist psychology. These models of the mind are thought to have developed in northern India in the 5th through 3rd centuries BCE (Olendzki, 2012). Buddhist psychology in its essence is focused on the subjective perceptive experience (Olendzki, 2012). The focus on the attentional and awareness aspects of consciousness is conceptually similar to ideas advanced by several other philosophical and psychological traditions. These include ancient Greek philosophy, phenomenology, existentialism, transcendentalism and humanism in America, and naturalism as it was manifest in later Western European thought. McCown, Reibel, and Micozzi (2010) trace the European connection to Eastern spiritual thought and practice back to ancient Greece, around 327 to 325 BCE. In 1784, British scholars and magistrates of the Asiatic Society of Benga authored the first translations of Hindu scriptures from Sanskrit to English (McCown et al., 2010). What followed has been debated and criticized as *Orientalism*, or a Western perception and representation patronizing of the East (McCown et al., 2010; Said, 1978). The Romantics embraced Eastern culture as philosophically irrational and exotic (McCown et al., 2010). Poets and philosophers explored Eastern ideas as an alternative to existing predominant ideas of rationality and nationality, sometimes failing to represent the breadth, depth, and subtleties present in the full range of Eastern discourses (McCown et al., 2010). Arising from these roots, a movement toward the possibility of a transcendental reality developed. In the 1800s, Emerson and Thoreau, American writers, integrated Eastern concepts as they worked to understand the world and existence, powerfully shaping aspects of Western discourse (McCown et al., 2010).

The Zen boom of the 1950s and 1960s permeated both academic studies and popular culture, and the LSD Harvard studies marked the narrative of mindfulness interventions (McCown et al., 2010). The 1960s are considered a period of foundation and growth, with the 1980s and 1990s considered the "painful passage into maturity" (McCown et al., 2010, p. 54). What has transpired over these many years is considered the movement toward a universalizing and secularizing discourse (McCown et al., 2010). Tension continues as the practices and traditions are extruded through Western constructs such as the scientific method and practical applications. In my personal practice, I am working to understand and know the heritage of the practices that have brought great peace and happiness to me. In private practice with my clients, I share the knowledge I have accumulated over years of practice and study in a way that is effective for them. I work to make these life-changing practices accessible to those who need them. Sometimes, this involves a discussion of the heritage and history and sometimes it does not.

Linehan (1993) teaches her patients that a focus on right or wrong is not necessarily a useful line of inquiry. Rather, she teaches looking for what is effective, or as the Buddha might say, what relieves suffering. John Kabat-Zinn told a story about Ben Huan, a 98-year-old Chinese Chan master who had learned about mindfulness-based stress reduction (MSRB; Kabat-Zinn, 2013; see also Chapter 11). He commented, "There are an infinite number of ways in which people suffer; therefore there must be an infinite number of ways in which Dharma is made available to them" (McCown et al., 2010, p. xix). Current Western definitions of mindfulness and mindful practices, as they are described here, are derived from traditions, tensions, and an effort to create accessibility, or an opening to a whole new way of seeing and being in the world for patients as they show up in our offices. Purposefully, there is a Vygotskian scaffolding (Vygotsky, 1978) of Western language and culture integrated in order to provide a comprehensible methodology for use with those who are struggling with self-regulation issues.

Mindful practices are believed to strengthen the functioning of the prefrontal orbital cortex (PFC), which is known for executive control, inhibition, decision making, and purposeful intention (Hanson & Mendius, 2009). These practices strengthen access to the parasympathetic nervous system, which is recognized for calming the body and mind (Hanson & Mendius, 2009). They also help to cultivate positive emotional experience from the limbic system, the emotional center of the brain (Hanson & Mendius, 2009). Finally, these practices help create neurological integration within the brain, allowing for increased feelings of inner and outer harmony and attunement (Siegel, 2010).

In private practice, I often use Daniel Siegel's *River of Integration* to explain what living in a regulated manner might be like (Siegel, 2010). I grab a blank piece of paper and a pen and draw two lines from top to bottom and then make wavy lines running vertically between the two lines. This is the river. I write, along the center of the river, the word *INTEGRATION*. I explain that it is here that we feel our healthiest, make our best decisions, and connect most effectively with those in our lives. It is here that we can be truly present for ourselves and for others. I show the patient the two lines that demarcate the banks of the river of integration. I explain that there are ways to know that we are starting to fall out of integration or getting close to one of these banks. Our thoughts, emotions, and behaviors are our signs. If we become too close to the bank on the right, we are moving into *CHAOS*. I write the word *CHAOS* as I explain. Here, we see substance use, out-of-control eating, emotional extremes, increases in interpersonal struggles, gambling, and similar behaviors. Essentially, things begin to feel and be out of control. We have trouble with organization, details, and thoroughness. On the other bank lies *RIGIDITY*. We can tell when we are close to this bank because we become overcontrolled—there is possible food restriction, and/or withdrawal from others or a need to control others. Thinking becomes overly rulegoverned and we struggle to be flexible in problem solving. Many of my patients with eating disorders like to call these types of rigid behaviors "being perfect." I explain that calling these behaviors "perfect" is *romanticizing rigidity*.

On one occasion, after explaining the river of integration (Siegel, 2010) to a patient who was on the path toward recovery from a long history of anorexia nervosa (AN), I asked her what she thought of the model. How did it relate to her life? She was smiling as she explained to me that, yes, this fit. She said that for years she had careened from one bank to the other, never experiencing integration. She would go from chaos to overcontrol and back to chaos, with neither experience being tolerable for too long. She said, "I never touched a foot into the river of integration. I just zip-lined from one bank to the other." For several years now, I have shared this anecdote with the psychologists-in-training at the university with my client's blessing. This anecdote speaks to so many of us— practitioners and clients. That is, we take on rigid, unmanageable plans for self-regulation and then careen into chaos as we are unable to tolerate our own unreasonable dictates. Mindful, and yogic, practices can be approached in a gentle, manageable manner as a way to find the centerline of integration. These practices can help when you are on either bank, chaos or rigidity. I like to introduce these practices as being like a friend who is always there when you call, who never minds if it has been too long or is too much, who is just there to help manage the hard stuff and keep the good stuff in perspective. In fact, yogic and mindful practices were born out of a search for a more centered and integrated way of being.

THE THREE PILLARS OF BUDDHIST PRACTICE

It is said that more than 2,000 years ago, a young man named Siddhartha Gautama was born a prince and protected from many of the harsh realities of life (Bien, 2006; Gunaratana, 2001). During his early years, he lived in his father's lavish palace (Gunaratana, 2001). Later, as he traveled the world, he was exposed to sickness, death, poverty, and other earthly truths. Unable to comprehend the cruel nature of human existence, he succumbed to an existential crisis (Bien, 2006). It was when he met a holy man (Sadhu) that he saw a possible answer to his suffering. To become like the Sadhu, Siddhartha left his family, the palace, and all of his comforts and began a practice of training his mind (Bien, 2006; Hanson & Mendius, 2009). After extended contemplation, he came to realize that there were causes of suffering and a path to freedom from suffering (Hanson & Mendius, 2009). Later, known as the Buddha, he began the teaching of these principles and practices (Hanson & Mendius, 2009). Bien (2006) explains that the term *Buddhism* is essentially a Western construct. The teachings and practices that lead to the end of suffering are referred to as *dharma* in Sanskrit (Bien, 2006). The three pillars of Buddhist practice are part of these teachings: (a) virtue (b) mindfulness and (c) wisdom.

Virtue

Virtue involves "regulating your actions, words, and thoughts to create benefits rather than harm for yourself and others" (Hanson & Mendius, 2009, p. 13). To live in virtue means to live from your innate goodness as guided by your principles (Hanson & Mendius, 2009). The practice of virtue involves being virtuous no matter what others do (Hanson & Mendius, 2009). It is not an if–then proposal. It can be very helpful to have your clients identify their core virtues as guiding principles for their behavioral choices. Hanson and Mendius (2009) suggest that we all develop our own personal code of virtues. They suggest simple statements that can guide actions, such as "Listen more, talk less," "Be loving," "Do no harm," and "Be of truth" (p. 148).

To illustrate how this might look in practice with patients, in my work with individuals with eating disorders, I sometimes help patients explore the Golden Rule, or "Do unto others as you would have them do unto you." For the individuals with whom I typically work, this usually is a given—of course they would never hurt anyone else. As well explicated in Chapters 1 and 2, individuals with eating disorders are often so hyperattuned to those in their lives that they have lost a sense of themselves. They are more than happy to forego any connection with their thoughts and feelings to make someone else happy or comfortable, and to avoid conflict. For these patients, I reverse the Golden Rule: *Do unto yourself as you would do unto others.* I ask them if they would starve a friend and then yell at her for being lazy, fat, and disgusting. I ask them if they would stuff a friend with food, well after she was full, and then force her to purge or run 15 miles to undo what she had done. I ask them if they would have a friend forego her hopes and dreams to endlessly count calories and check her collar bones and hips to ensure that she was not too big. By looking at the virtue of *do no harm*, I help them cultivate a new way of conceptualizing the set of behaviors in which they are engaging as cruel, hurtful, and even abusive, as opposed to a disciplined pursuit of perfection (or romanticized rigidity). See also the discussion of embodied practice 9, be of your values, in Chapter 3.

Mindfulness

Mindfulness involves "the skillful attention to both your inner and outer worlds" (Hanson & Mendius, 2009, p. 13). In Buddhist tradition, the mind is viewed much like the other sense organs (e.g., ears, eyes, skin; Olendzki, 2012). Each of the senses has an object. For example, the nose is smelling scents and the eyes are seeing things. In this way, the mind is thinking, which is considered knowing with the mind (Olendzki, 2012). The objects of the mind include anything that can be cognized, such as thoughts, images, and memories (Olendzki, 2012). In mindfulness, we work toward bare attention (Brown et al., 2007). We acknowledge that we are of the tendency to quickly conceptualize what is happening. We construct, interpret, evaluate, assess, and connect what is happening with what we know (Brown et al., 2007). In mindfulness, we work to de-couple the nearly automatic tendency to intertwine attention and cognition (Brown et al., 2007). When the mind is in the mindful mode of processing, it does not compare, judge, categorize, evaluate, contemplate, reflect, introspect, or ruminate on experiences based on what is known (Brown et al., 2007). Rather, the mind is open and present with bare attention to input manifested by a simple noticing of what is happening (Brown et al., 2007).

Mindfulness is a big concept that is cultivated in many different specific practices as well as in our day-to-day activities. Shapiro and Carlson (2009) provided a helpful distinction between the uppercase "M" Mindfulness and the lowercase "m" mindfulness. The uppercase "M" Mindfulness is the fundamental way of being, of inhabiting your body and moment-by-moment experience (Shapiro & Carlson, 2009). The lowercase "m" mindfulness involves the formal practices (e.g., sitting meditation), or the ways in which one intentionally pursues the uppercase "M" Mindfulness (Shapiro & Carlson, 2009). The three pillars are referring to both the uppercase "M" and lowercase "m" as ways of being and the practices that will get you there.

McCown et al. (2010) describe four foundations of mindfulness. First, there is mindfulness of the body. This involves bare attention to the breath, then to the calming of the body, and finally to awareness of the body in sensation, postures, and movements in both formal practice and daily living (Kabat-Zinn, 2013; McCown et al., 2010). The second foundation is mindfulness of feelings in which bare attention is focused on the feeling tone that accompanies the experiences of each moment (Grabovac, Lau, & Willett, 2011; McCown et al., 2010). These are the feeling tones of unpleasant, neutral, or pleasant (McCown et al., 2010). In mindfulness practice, these feeling tones are simply noticed as they arise and pass away. The third foundation is the mindfulness of the mind (McCown et al., 2010; Siegel, 2010). Bare attention is focused on the activity, or processing of the mind, noticing shifts in states of awareness, concentration, and distraction (Kabat-Zinn, 2013). Finally, the fourth foundation of mindfulness is mindfulness of mind-objects. In this practice, bare attention is brought to the things the mind is thinking about. The mind-objects may come from within, such as sense-desires, anger, frustration, worry, doubt, memories, and so forth (McCown et al., 2010).

Brown et al. (2007) suggest that the disentanglement of consciousness from cognitive content may allow you and your patients to think with greater effectiveness and precision. When being mindful, the activity of conceptual thought can be purposefully engaged and disengaged by choice (Brown et al., 2007). Shapiro and Carlson (2009) refer to this as a shift to conscious responding versus automatic reactivity. In Buddhism, suffering is thought to arise from the habitual ways in which we react and the seemingly automatic grip of our mental habits (Shapiro & Carlson, 2009). With mindfulness, one can be aware of thoughts as just thoughts, aware of emotions as simply emotions (Brown et al., 2007; Kabat-Zinn, 2013). As stated in Chapter 3, it is in the nonreaction that we have choice, the ability to define who and what we are through our actions, and our freedom. See also the discussion of embodied practice 1, be mindfully aware, in Chapter 3.

Wisdom

Wisdom is applied common sense in which you come to understand what hurts and what helps, letting go of what hurts and strengthening what helps (Hanson & Mendius, 2009). Sternberg (2012) makes a distinction between abstract wisdom and personal wisdom. Abstract wisdom is knowing of the conceptual, theoretical, and even empirical spheres of knowledge. Personal wisdom is an attitude toward life. It is the openness to learning about yourself and how you react to and are in your world. Concentration and mindfulness turn into the practice of wisdom, or insight, when the focused mind is used to penetrate the illusions that create obstacles to insight (Olendzki, 2012). Olendzki (2012) suggests that there are four ways that we can turn our mindful practice into wisdom. First, by watching the arising and passing away of all phenomena, over and over, time and time again, we begin to notice that everything is impermanent (see following discussion of impermanence). Second, by considering experience from both the internal and external perspective, we notice the interaction and interdependency of the two. That is, experience is constructed from what is presented to us on the outside and our processing of it on the inside (Olendzki, 2012). Third, by reducing awareness to its barest form of attention (sans conceptualization, elaboration, or interpretation), we begin to see the world as it is, free of our constructed story of how it is (Olendzki, 2012). Fourth, growth in wisdom allows us to be present in each moment of experience without clinging or craving (Olendzki, 2012). Olendzki (2012) describes the heightened awareness that comes with wisdom as a pry bar that gets under the common assumptions and habitual responses that we bring to each moment. With this pry bar, we are able to loosen the attachment to them (Olendzki, 2012).

Sam is a 31-year-old lawyer, in the same field as Mason. However, at age 23 when he was nearing the end of law school he took a course called "The Mindful Lawyer." As part of the requirements of the course, Sam began the practice of meditation. At first he began for 5 minutes a day, later reaching his current, 8-year practice of 20 minutes a day. He also began to integrate the noticing that he did in meditation into his daily life. This was very useful, as he works in criminal law and there are many deeply concerning issues that arise each day in terms of the effectiveness of the system, fairness, truth, and, not surprisingly, justice. As a well-intentioned and good person, Sam finds his meditation and mindfulness practices to be one of the most powerful tools he has to combat suffering. His job is hard and the challenge is substantial. His practice lets him be in the moment, present for his clients, and effective. His practices also helped him to realize that he was not entirely happy in his work. He noticed that although he felt good about representing the accused in general, he needed more balance. His awareness led him to actively pursue virtue in his life. He contacted the law school and now volunteers at the free public law clinic, empowering victims of crime. Virtue, mindfulness, and wisdom continue to grow in his life as a direct result of his practice, and he is present to see this. See also the discussion of embodied practice 3, live in inquiry, in Chapter 3.

THE DHARMA SEALS: IMPERMANENCE, NONATTACHMENT, AND NOT-SELF

As one practices and gains wisdom, one begins to see the Three Dharma Seals—impermanence, nonattachment, and not-self—in each and every aspect of being. Grabovac et al. (2011) describe these as the three characteristics of Buddhist thought common to all sense impressions and mental events.

Impermanence

Everything changes (Kabat-Zinn, 2013; Shapiro & Carlson, 2009). Yes, all phenomena are impermanent (Bien, 2006; Kabat-Zinn, 2013). It is an essential aspect of the nature of reality and one of the first insights that surfaces with steady mindful practice (Kabat-Zinn, 2013; Shapiro & Carlson, 2009). Flowers sprout, blossom, and die. Humans are born, develop, grow old, and die. Businesses begin, grow, prosper, and eventually dissolve. Empires do the same. A difficult situation at work manifests, becomes uncomfortable, and resolves. It is the nature of things to arise and pass away. In terms of self-regulation, all sense impressions and mental events are transient in that they arise and pass away (Grabovac et al., 2011). We do not suffer because of all things being impermanent. We suffer because we resist or forget this fact (Bien, 2006; Kabat-Zinn, 2013).

When things are pleasurable, safe, and good, we cling. I remember when my oldest daughter grew out of her first set of clothes. She grew quickly and in a week or two of life, she moved from the 3- to 6-month-old clothes to the 6- to 12-month-old clothes. I became anxious and sad as I folded up her old clothes. I was utterly in love with her. I wanted to be able to hold her, cuddle her, and protect her forever. I was clinging, attached to the need for things to stay just the way they were—permanently wonderful. I knew exactly what I was doing. I recognized it for what it was. I honored the feeling and the memories of her in each of her little outfits. Then, I folded them up and stored them away. Truth be told, I was clinging to the off chance that she might have a little sister someday (which she did). She is now 16 years old and 2 years away from leaving for college. Sometimes when I look at her, I feel that same feeling that I felt when folding up the baby clothes. When I do, I focus on my breath and connect with the present moment. And so it goes, the practice of being completely present with impermanence (Kabat-Zinn, 2013).

Impermanence shows up differently when something is uncomfortable, challenging, or distressing. When something is uncomfortable, it is easy to react as if it is never going to end. Hence, being reminded of impermanence offers relief. When I am doing a difficult yoga pose or feeling resistance in meditation, I remind myself that the emotion or reaction I am feeling will arise and pass away. Similarly, Linehan (1993) asks patients to notice impermanence when they are working to tolerate distress. They are asked to watch an urge or an uncomfortable emotion arise and pass away, not reacting or allowing the sensation to trigger symptoms of dysregulating.

Katie is 17 years old. She has been diagnosed with AN and has subclinical obsessive-compulsive symptoms (e.g., ruminating, checking, counting, needing things to be even). She is quite anxious and tends to be perfectionistic. She demonstrates a lot of harm avoidance, withdrawing from conflict and avoiding interpersonal relationships. Her parents are medical doctors who met in medical school. Her younger sister was born at 23 weeks of gestation and is now 12 years old with cerebral palsy. Katie clings to everything. She is scheduled to go to college next year, yet she only feels safe with her mom, dad, and sister. She lives as if things will never change. Her sister will always be her baby sister. Her mom and dad will always be strong bright doctors who can fix everything. She doesn't want to go to college because she does not want anything to change. Change is bad. She learned that when her sister was born and almost died. She restricts her eating in an effort to manage things. If she can just stay small, little, it will all be okay.

Katie's treatment plan involves increasing her food intake from under 900 calories a day up to 3,000 calories a day in order to get her to a healthy weight, avoid inpatient treatment, and prepare for success at college. When she eats her meals she is overwhelmed by the full feelings. Her mother has taken a break from work to help Katie get through this rough patch. She prepares Katie's meals, sits with her while she eats, and practices impermanence with her as they digest their food together. Katie's mom reminds her that "this too shall pass" as Katie holds her belly, telling her mom she is so scared to be as full she as is. Katie's mom helps her breathe as she tolerates the feelings of overwhelm, letting her self be present in her own body. For Katie, accepting impermanence is a critical aspect of her recovery. See also the discussion of embodied practice 4, accept impermanence, in Chapter 3.

Nonattachment

Nonattachment is the process of not attaching to or attempting to avoid thoughts, feelings, emotions, people, things, and so forth. It begins at the most basic of levels. Each sense impression or mental event is reflexively paired with a feeling tone of positive, negative, or neutral. We naturally feel drawn to the positive or pleasurable feeling tones and are compelled to avoid the negative or aversive feeling tones. For example, Danielle, first introduced in Chapter 1, often shops when she is feeling distressed, bored, and unhappy. She has thousands of dollars of credit card debt on top of her student loans. She is in treatment for bulimia nervosa (BN) and hides her compulsive shopping from her therapist. When she sees a catalog for clothes, especially her favorite designers, she is drawn mindlessly toward it. She sees a pair of designer shoes and feels a positive, pleasurable feeling tone. She responds to that by reading the product description, picturing herself in the shoes. She is now drawn closer to the shoes. As she tries to tell herself that she can't afford the shoes, that $450 is too much and she is too far in debt as it is, she feels sadness and loss. That is, attached—she now feels a sense of loss for shoes that she has never owned, had not thought of until the 5 minutes previous, and now is struggling over not having them as her own.

Over time, habitual reactions such as attachment and aversion to the feelings of a sense impression or mental event, as well as a lack of awareness of this process, can lead to suffering (Grabovac et al., 2011). As you see with Danielle, her lack of awareness of the process and the failure to use any tools to reduce the attachment lead her to suffering, a self-perpetuating, mental proliferation that often leads her to make self-destructive shopping choices. See also the discussion of embodied practice 5, cultivate nonattachment, in Chapter 3.

Not-Self

Not-self is sometimes considered to be one of the most difficult mindful teachings for Westerners to understand (Shapiro & Carlson, 2009). In Western culture, we are very tied to who we are. We have a strong sense of identity. It is a part of our way of viewing human development. We have a "me" generation (i.e., the baby boomers) and entire decades in which people were "trying to find themselves" (i.e., 1970s). Contrary to these strongly held beliefs, mindfulness teachings tell us that there is no stable, unchanging entity that can be called *self* (Shapiro & Carlson, 2009). Specific to self-regulation, both sense impressions and mental events do not contain anything that could be called a *self* (Grabovac et al., 2011).

I often meet people in private practice who have identified wholeheartedly with a particular disorder. For example, they might say, "I am anorexic" or "I can't control myself." I watch their language for these statements to reveal a sense of a nonchanging, permanent self that is serving their disorder or struggle. When I hear a statement like this, I tell them what I noticed and ask them to reword the sentence in an empowering, malleable manner. For example, a patient can change "I am anorexic" to "I have struggled with food restriction when I feel overwhelmed." Another example is changing "I can't control myself" to "In the past, I didn't notice that I was triggered by clothing advertisements to shop." See also the discussion of embodied practice 6, discern what is not-self, in Chapter 3.

ALLOWING WHAT IS

Allowing is a term that I find easier to negotiate than *acceptance*. One of my doctoral students, who is also an effective life coach, Carla Giambrone, brought this interesting contrast to my attention during a discussion on acceptance. It is a subtle semantic difference. Yet I believe it is an important one. *Acceptance* is intended to mean an acknowledgment of or a cessation of resistance to something. However, in Western culture, *acceptance* has a connotation of agreement, whereas *allowing* suggests a clearer boundary between what you or I might consider acceptable and what is happening. Allowing suggests that although we are not going to resist this happening, thing, experience, or person, we are also not of acceptance with it. Allowing is the antidote to resistance. It is resistance that adds suffering to pain (Kabat-Zinn, 2013; Shapiro & Carlson, 2009). That which is already painful can become seemingly unbearable when resistance is added.

For example, John, a 20-year-old young man, is struggling with his own alcohol use. He grew up with a dad who was diagnosed with posttraumatic stress disorder (PTSD) after a harrowing car accident. His dad is now clinically depressed and takes way too many painkillers. His dad has real pain, both psychological and physical. However, John has a sense that his dad has become dependent on the painkillers, and he knows for sure that there are nights that his dad is essentially wasted on the drugs, head nodding, eyes half closed. He has tried to get his dad to admit, acknowledge, even talk about his painkiller use, to no avail. John even wrote his dad's doctor a letter telling the doctor about his worries and what he has observed at home. Still, nothing has changed. John is angry. He hates the feeling he gets when watching his dad nod off on the couch. He resents seeing other young men with their fathers fixing cars and running road races together. For some time now, John has used this stress as a reason to drink. He feels overwhelmed about his mom and dad's situation and sits down with a cold beer. Unfortunately, when John has one beer, he has six. He knows this. John is ready to talk about his drinking and deal with his father's drug use.

As my student, Carla, so eloquently described allowing, we can think of the thing that bothers us in a similar manner. Let's say you don't like dogs. You go to your friend's house and he has a dog. You see the dog. You have an associated feeling tone (i.e., aversion) when you see the dog (i.e., sense impression). It stops there. You are aware. You breathe. You center on your friend and the conversation. You allow the dog. He curls up on the floor a few feet away from you and you allow him to be there. You know he is there, yet you do not have a reaction to him. You allow what is. This will need to be John's practice. Distinct from enabling his dad's drug use, he will know it is there; he may continue to write notes to his dad's doctor and tell his dad he is worried. However, John will practice an allowing of what is that will give him the space to be present with his mom and dad as well as the freedom from reacting, a reacting that helps trigger his own drinking. See also the discussion of embodied practice 7, allow what is with nonjudgment, in Chapter 3.

THE FOUR NOBLE TRUTHS

The Four Noble Truths provide a road map for what is to be explored in mindfulness (Gunaratana, 2001; McCown et al., 2010). Gunaratana (2001) states that the Buddha himself saw the Four Noble Truths as key. The first two truths address identification of the problem and diagnosis of the problem. The second two truths provide the prescription or resolution to the problem (McCown et al., 2010). Bien (2006) says that if you understand the Four Noble Truths deeply, then you understand the essence of Buddhism.

The First Noble Truth: Understanding Suffering

The first Noble Truth is that *suffering is* (Bien, 2006; McCown, 2010). That is, dissatisfaction is unavoidable (Gunaratana, 2001). Suffering includes great loss and hardship as well as minor inconveniences. In suffering, we want something other than what we have. We might crave freedom from pain, ownership of material objects, a relationship, or acknowledgment. In general, this truth can be interpreted as unsatisfactoriness or suffering (in Sanskrit, *duhkha*; Wallace, 2011). That is, in life—my life, your life, our patients' lives—there is suffering, unsatisfactoriness, and anxiety. We come by it honestly. Human beings biologically function on a need-drive system in the continual regulation of homeostasis (e.g., hunger and the drive to eat, thirst and the drive to drink). Wallace (2011) suggests that in this way, for all biological beings, pain is essential. For example, if you did not get hungry, you might starve to death. If you did not feel the pain of heat, fire might burn you. He suggests that for living organisms, pain is a motivator, one stronger than the motivation for happiness. Although pain may be universal, suffering is not (Bien, 2006). It is our relationship to this pain that can create or enhance our suffering (Kabat-Zinn, 2013). Accordingly, the truth is that we are of the nature to suffer.

The Second Noble Truth: Suffering Has a Cause

The second Noble Truth is that suffering has a cause (Bien, 2006). In the careful noticing and bare attention, you see that there is a cause of the arising of suffering (in Sanskrit, *samudaya*; Wallace, 2011). The more that you notice, the more that you see that *everything* that there is, in the world, has the potential to create suffering due to craving and grasping (Wallace, 2011). It then makes sense that letting go of craving is a critical aspect of freedom or liberation from suffering (McCown et al., 2010).

The Third Noble Truth: Suffering Can Be Stopped

The third Noble Truth is that there is a possibility of cessation (in Sanskrit, *nirodha*) of craving and the freedom from suffering (Wallace, 2011). Affliction does not extend to the core and pure awareness can be revealed. Letting go of craving can result in cessation of suffering (McCown et al., 2010). This can be a very powerful concept, or cognitive reframing, for patients. It involves explaining the first three Noble Truths. This can ultimately be summarized as "pain is inevitable and suffering is optional."

In Chapter 1, you were introduced to Mathilde. She has many substantial challenges in her life. For example, she has a friend who is terminally ill. This is painful, very painful. Still, knowing that she is faced with this pain each and every day, Mathilde has decided to step up her yoga and meditation practice to help her cope. Also, she practices informal forms of mindfulness as she makes sure to carefully notice the flowers, the people, and the gorgeous architecture in Buffalo as she walks to and from yoga each day. She knows that she could easily make the experience of her friend's illness worse by trying to resist or avoid it. She knows that she could make this pain worse by adding substance abuse or another self-destructive behavior. This is why she stays present. As she holds her friend's hand and reads her chapters from a romance novel to support her during her treatment, Mathilde says to herself, "Pain is inevitable. Suffering is optional."

The Fourth Noble Truth: There Is a Way to Live That Prevents Suffering

The fourth Noble Truth is that there is an Eight-Fold Path (in Sanskrit, *marga*) to liberation. Bien (2006) refers to this as developing a lifestyle. There are ways of living that are not conducive to ending suffering. Mason is a good example of someone who has adopted a way of being that will not lead to freedom from suffering. These ways of living include his ruminations on what he does not have, concern for appearance and status, and substance use (Bien, 2006). The Eight-Fold Path is described next.

THE EIGHT-FOLD PATH

The Eight-Fold Path is a nonlinear process that helps you and your patients remove, or move beyond, the conditioned responses that obscure one's true nature (Allen, 2014; Bodhi, 1994). The search for this path is thought to be born out of suffering (Bodhi, 1994). Paradoxically, the path is primarily about unlearning our conditioned responses (Allen, 2014). Each area of the path provides a direction for the journey. Because it is a nonlinear path, one or more areas can be explored at once. The path is reflected in embodied practice 9, be of your values (see Chapter 3).

It is important to make a distinctions between and associations with the path and the ultimate goal: connection with your true nature. It is a finger pointing at the moon—don't confuse the finger for the moon (Allen, 2014). That is, some people get so caught up in the path that they forget that it is a methodology for accessing your true nature. Conversely, others becomes so focused on the goals that they forget the path. Recall, as noted in Chapter 1, Table 1.1, that the emphasis of embodied self-regulation is in honoring the process and the journey with an eye toward balanced and sustainable self-mastery. Both the journey and the goal are important, and the approach should be manageable and sustainable.

Each aspect of the Eight-Fold Path begins with the word *samma*. According to Allen (2014), the word *samma* means proper, whole, thorough, integral, complete, and perfect. Conceptually, it is related to the English word *summit* (Allen, 2014). In writings on the Eight-Fold Path you will frequently read the word *samma* translated to mean *right*. However, in this manner, *samma* does not necessarily mean right as opposed to wrong. Rather, it refers to a completeness of things. For example, if I were working on awareness, right awareness, and I was not quite there, I would not be wrong. I simply would not be complete with it (Allen, 2014). Gunaratana

(2001) interprets samma to mean a skillfulness or effectiveness. In this way, there is no moral judgment. Rather, one explores the effectiveness of what he or she is doing (Linehan, 1993). Bringing these ideas together, we can consider samma to refer to an effective, skillful path toward a completeness. Allen (2014) suggests that the eight aspects of the Eight-Fold Path be considered in terms of the following: What does this mean for your life right now? What is your direction, your guide, your path? See the discussion of embodied practice 3, live in inquiry, in Chapter 3.

Samma-Ditthi: Right Understanding or Complete Vision

Samma-ditthi is translated to mean complete or perfect vision, right view, or right understanding (Allen, 2014). It can also be translated as skillful understanding (Gunaratana, 2001). It is an ability to see clearly the nature of reality and the path of transformation (Allen, 2014). The right view is the beginning of the entire path, providing insight for all the other factors (Bodhi, 1994). This aspect of the pathway is intended to bring you and your patients to knowing the truth. Gunaratana (2001) explains that this aspect of the path has two components. First is the understanding of cause and effect (Bodhi, 1994). Second, the right view incorporates the Four Noble Truths: understanding suffering, understanding its origin, understanding its cessation, and understanding the way leading to its cessation (Bodhi, 1994).

Cause and effect, sometimes referred to as kamma (or karma), is the idea that acting in skillful, effective ways can lead to happiness and living in unskillful, ineffective ways can lead to unhappiness (Bodhi, 1994; Gunaratana, 2001). Everything that you or your clients say or do leads, inevitably, to an effect. If your client is searching for a good life with happiness, he or she must start choosing effective and skillful behavior. It requires cultivation over time. For embodied self-regulation this means seeing past the immediate rewards (e.g., a drink, drug use, shopping, self-harm, gambling). Rather, your client can engage in a skillful or effective practice that offers loving-kindness and compassion to someone who is suffering or struggling (Gunaratana, 2001). For example, David, age 54, is now an Alcoholics Anonymous sponsor. When his wife got sick with cancer 20 years ago, his drinking got out of control. A counselor at the cancer center recommended that he seek help. He did. Now, when he's triggered to drink again, he turns his intention toward helping others on the path to recovery. He goes to a meeting and shows loving-kindness and compassion to those who need it. He leaves each meeting stronger and sober. See also the discussion of embodied practice 12, cultivate loving-kindness and joy, in Chapter 3.

The second aspect of right view is understanding the Four Noble Truths (described earlier). As you can see, the embodied practices of the mindful path share many intersections and overlays. The practices are nonlinear and lead you, and your clients, always back to presence and mindfulness. Overall, the right view, or skillful understanding, requires that the seeker (i.e., me, you, and our clients) understands skillful behavior both in terms of the karma (i.e., cause and effect) and the Four Noble Truths in terms of how they fit into the overall scheme of the path (i.e., embodied self-regulation; Gunaratana, 2001)

Questions to Ask Your Clients

- Do you have a sense of cause and effect in your life? Explain it to me.
- How does your understanding of cause and effect inform your behavior?
- What does the phrase "Pain is inevitable, suffering is optional" mean to you?
- How might your understanding of suffering be related to your current struggle?

Samma-Sankappa: Right Intention or Perfected Aspiration

Samma-sankappa is translated to mean perfected aspiration or right intention, thought, or attitude (Allen, 2014; Bodhi, 1994). It can be thought of as skillful thinking (Gunaratana, 2001). As we know from years of cognitive behavioral therapy research, thinking can affect our well-being. The second aspect of the path offers a way of redirecting thoughts in positive and helpful directions (Gunaratana, 2001). Here, thinking includes your thoughts and any intentional mind state (Gunaratana, 2001). It involves the liberation of emotional intelligence in your life and acting from love and compassion (Allen, 2014). It includes monitoring thoughts for attachment (or desire), ill will, and harmfulness (Bodhi, 1994). When these types of thoughts are noticed, you simply replace them with wholesome thoughts such as letting go, allowing, acceptance, loving-kindness, and compassion (Gunaratana, 2001; see also the discussions in Chapter 3 of embodied practice 4, accept impermanence; embodied practice 5, cultivate nonattachment; embodied practice 7, allow what is with nonjudgment; embodied practice 10, observe compassion for self and others; and embodied practice 12, cultivate loving-kindness and joy).

Questions to Ask Your Clients

- Can you identify negative thinking patterns that may be influencing your current struggle?
- How often do you judge something as good or bad, right or wrong?

- Can you reframe your thinking to ask, "How effective is this behavior?"
- Can you reframe your self-evaluation with the level of compassion you might show a friend? What would that look like?
- How often do you use the phrases "I can't . . .," "I am . . .," and "It won't ever change"?
- Can you reword these phrases to say "I am working on . . ." and "My intention is . . ." ?

Samma-Vaca: Right Speech or Perfected Speech

Samma-vaca is translated to mean perfected or whole speech, right speech, or clear, truthful, uplifting, and nonharmful communication (Allen, 2014; Bodhi, 1994). Gunaratana (2001) refers to this aspect of the path as skillful speech. Unskillful speech would include speaking without thinking, lying, exaggerating, using harsh language, saying hurtful things or slander, speaking inconsiderably, engaging in idle chatter, and talking about others (i.e., gossip; Bodhi, 1994). Right speech includes speaking the truth, avoiding malicious talk, speaking kindly, ceasing gossip, and speaking mindfully (Gunaratana, 2001). See the discussions in Chapter 3 of embodied practice 1, be mindfully aware; embodied practice 9, be of your values; and embodied practice 10, observe compassion for self and others.

Questions to Ask Your Clients
- How often do you lie, gossip, exaggerate, use harsh language with yourself or others, or speak without consideration?
- When you do, what does that feel like in your body? What are the consequences? Does it bring you closer to others in your life or create barriers?
- How often do you speak kindly, offer compassion, support yourself or others, and speak the truth?
- When you do, what does that feel like in your body? What are the consequences? Does it bring you closer to others in your life or create barriers?

Samma-Kammanta: Right Action or Integral Action

Samma-kammanta is translated to mean integral action, right action, or an ethical foundation for life based on the principle of nonexploitation of oneself and others (Allen, 2014). Gunaratana (2001) refers to this aspect of the path as skillful action. In guidance similar to this aspect of the path, Buddha offered *Five Precepts* for skillful action: (a) abstain from killing

(b) abstain from stealing (c) abstain from speaking falsely (d) abstain from sexual misconduct and (e) abstain from misusing alcohol or other intoxicants (Bodhi, 1994; Gunaratana, 2001). On the Eight-Fold Path, the Buddha describes unwholesome action as any action that hurts another or the self (Gunaratana, 2001). Further, mindfulness is brought to action; the Buddha said, "All wholesome words, deeds, and thoughts, have mindfulness as their root" (Gunaratana, 2001, p. 127). See the discussions in Chapter 3 of embodied practice 1, be mindfully aware; embodied practice 8, prioritize self-care; and embodied practice 10, observe compassion for self and others.

Questions to Ask Your Clients
- What is your understanding of an ethical path? What are your rules to live by?
- How do these precepts line up with your understanding of God and religion?
- What role do these precepts play in your life and in your struggle?

Samma-Ajiva: Right Livelihood or Proper Livelihood

Samma-ajiva is translated to mean proper livelihood, right livelihood, or a livelihood based on correct action and the ethical principle of nonexploitation (Allen, 2014). "Our means of sustenance should not interfere with our spiritual development" (Gunaratana, 2001, p. 133). Recall David, age 54, the recovering alcoholic. When he quit drinking he became very aware of the deep conflict he was feeling in his professional life. He worked for a successful business that marketed toys for kids' meals at fast-food restaurants. When he was drinking, he laughed off the contribution that these plastic toys were making to the world's waste. Once he stopped drinking, he could no longer ignore the impact that these toys—which children either immediately threw away or played with for a few minutes before throwing them away—were having on the Earth. He addressed his conflict by attempting to influence the manufacturers into making recyclable toys, with no effect. Eventually, he began actively searching for another job. Within 7 months, he was able to find work with an eco-friendly supplier. This teaching holds that working a job that harms others is wrong because it (a) violates moral principles, and (b) harms you (Gunaratana, 2001). As counselors and therapists, we have found good work. This aspect of the path is an important consideration for our patients as they explore their work and how it affects themselves and others. See also the discussion of embodied practice 9, be of your values, in Chapter 3.

Questions to Ask Your Clients
- Are you satisfied in your work?
- Does the work you do each day align with your values?
- Does your work trigger or contribute to your struggle?
- What changes could you make in your work to bring it into closer alignment with your values?

Samma-Vayama: Right Effort or Full Effort

Samma-vayama is translated to mean complete or full effort, energy, or vitality (Allen, 2014). It is also referred to as right effort or diligence (Allen, 2014; Bodhi, 1994). Gunaratana (2001) refers to this aspect of the path as skillful effort. It involves consciously directing your life energy to the transformative path of creative and healing action that fosters wholeness (Allen, 2014). There are four parts. First, use determination and energy to prevent the arising of painful, unwholesome states of mind (e.g., greed, resentment, attachment; Bodhi, 1994; Gunaratana, 2001). Second, if an unwholesome state has arisen, work to overcome the state that has taken hold (Bodhi, 1994; Gunaratana, 2001). Third, replace unwholesome states with wholesome states (Bodhi, 1994; Gunaratana, 2001). For example, Mathilde, from Chapter 1, is very sad about her friend who is dying of cancer. There are times when she feels intense anger about the unfairness of her friend's situation. She feels this anger, yes. Yet, she does not let it take hold. She transforms the anger into energy that she uses to support her friend and to help with fundraisers, and if she is still feeling energy, she takes it to her yoga practice and processes it there. Fourth, manifest effort to continuously cultivate pleasing, wholesome mental states (Bodhi, 1994; Gunaratana, 2001). I often joke that yoga is my medicine and I must take it daily. In fact, I find this to be true. My daily practice brings forth a sense of well-being and happiness that begins each day. In this way, I am in right effort.

Questions to Ask Your Clients
- What intention do you bring to mind each morning to guide your efforts for the day?
- Do you notice when your mind has shifted to a negative state? Describe what you notice.
- What actions do you take to shift your mind to a more positive, effective way of processing? What have you tried? What have you found that works?
- What do you do daily, in a preventive way, that helps you cultivate a positive frame of mind?

Samma-Sati: Right Mindfulness or Complete Awareness

Samma-sati is translated to mean complete or thorough awareness. It is also called right mindfulness, which refers to the developing of awareness of things, oneself, feelings, thoughts, people, and reality (Allen, 2014; Bodhi, 1994). Gunaratana (2001) refers to this aspect of the path as skillful mindfulness. It is said that Buddha often told his disciples to "keep mindfulness in front" (Gunaratana, 2001, p. 193). That is, cultivate moment-by-moment awareness. We have covered mindfulness in this chapter as well as in embodied practice 1, be mindfully aware (Chapter 3).

Questions to Ask Your Clients

- At this present moment, describe to me your awareness of your body. Do you feel tension or relaxation throughout your muscles? Do you feel your feet grounded on the floor and your body in your chair? Do you feel your hands? Describe what you feel in your belly, your chest, your neck. Having a sense of your whole body, can you describe what you feel?
- At this present moment, what are you feeling emotionally? What words go with that feeling? What body sensations? Show me where you are feeling the emotions in your body right now.
- In this present moment, describe to me what is on your mind. Is your mind clear? Are you fully present?
- In this present moment, what are the objects of your mind? What are you thinking about? Is there a narrative, questions, distractions? Describe to me the current processes of your mind.
- During the day, how often do you have awareness of your body, your feelings, your mind, and the objects of your mind? Does one play a central role, leaving the others ignored? Are there triggers throughout your day to attend to one aspect of the self over another?
- What can you do to cultivate more presence of body, emotions, and mind?

Samma-Samadhi: Right Concentration or One-Pointedness of Mind

Samma-samadhi is translated to mean full, integral, or holistic samadhi. It is also referred to as concentration, meditation, absorption, or one-pointedness of mind (Allen, 2014). Gunaratana (2001) describes this aspect of the path as skillful concentration. Allen (2014) suggests that none of these translations is adequate. *Samadhi* literally means to be fixed, absorbed in, or established at one point; thus, the first level of meaning is concentration when the mind is fixed on a single object. Ultimately, this is samadhi in the sense of enlightenment or Buddhahood (Allen, 2014). It is the last essential step on the path to happiness (Gunaratana, 2001). The steps to skillful concentration follow (Gunaratana, 2001):

- Sit with the intention of cultivating skillful concentration.
- Give up all thoughts of attachment (e.g., ideas, people, work).
- Let go of awareness of past mistakes or errors.
- Cultivate thoughts of loving-kindness.
- Take several deep breaths.
- Focus your mind on an object of meditation (e.g., breath, candle, mantra).
- Concentrate on the present moment. Continuously bring your mind back to the present moment.
- If you think or feel unwholesome thoughts or feelings, cultivate loving-kindness and compassion for yourself and bring your awareness back to your object of concentration.

As you practice concentration, you will notice that you will pass through stages (Gunaratana, 2001). The first stage is a one-pointedness of mind that is achieved with practice. This initial stage involves applying the mind to the work of focus on an object of concentration (Bodhi, 1994). At this stage concentration can be fleeting and extends with practice (Bodhi, 1994). At the second level of concentration, there is no more thinking that disturbs the mind (Gunaratana, 2001). You feel more confident as concentration is stronger and unbroken. You may feel joy and happiness. The third level of concentration comes after you have reached the second level many times. At this stage you begin to experience an increased sense of equanimity as the joy becomes less relevant. As equanimity becomes stronger, so does concentration (Gunaratana, 2001). The fourth level of concentration comes after many repeated experiences of the third level of concentration. Equanimity is present and mindfulness is strong. The mind is completely quiet, stable, and tranquil (Gunaratana, 2001). The body, the mind, and emotions are unaffected by external triggers or influences. There are no intrusions. At this level it is believed that you have a perfectly concentrated mind and can see the object of your concentration for what it truly is. At this level, it is said that you can penetrate into the true nature of reality (Gunaratana, 2001).

Questions to Ask Your Clients
- What do you know about meditation? Tell me about your meditation experience.
- Have you practiced meditation? Describe the experience to me. What were the challenges? Benefits?
- Would you like to learn more about meditation?

For a wonderful, easy-to-read book on the Eight-Fold Path, refer to *Eight Mindful Steps to Happiness: Walking the Buddha's Path,* by Bhante Henepola Gunaratana (2001).

CONCLUSIONS

The areas of the Eight-Fold Path, the three pillars of Buddhism, the Dharma Seals, and the Four Noble Truths each provide an aspect of the pathway toward health and well-being. Many of the patients I see have spent years reacting to complicated family experiences and other challenging risks (see Chapter 2). They have adopted seemingly effective ways of coping with these stresses. That is, they engaged in self-destructive behaviors that were modeled for them, or perhaps what seemed to be the only tactic to escape intolerable physical and emotional conditions. Without knowing or having other tools, they had done the best that they could to make it to see another day. Now in therapy, they have a chance to learn a healthy and effective set of ways of seeing themselves, their environments, and the world. This new mindful conceptual platform can set the stage for embodied practices that promote well-being and neurological integration, as well as connection, attunement, and community with others. These mindful conceptualizations have been refined, practiced, and passed down for thousands of years. They offer a set of healthy techniques for understanding and coping. Referring back to the quote at the beginning of this chapter, they offer a chance at a new way of being present in the present hour so that we can perceive the worth of any life in any hour (Smith, 1965).

REFERENCES

Allen, J. (2014). *The Eight Fold Path.* Buddhanet: Basic Buddhism Guide. Retrieved from http://www.buddhanet.net/e-learning/8foldpath.htm
Bien, T. (2006). *Mindful therapy: A guide for therapists and helping professionals.* Boston, MA: Wisdom Publications.

Bodhi, B. (1994). *The noble Eightfold Path: Way to the end of suffering*. Onalaska, WA: Buddhist Publication Society of Pariyatti Publishing.

Brown, K. W., & Kasser, T. (2005). Are psychological and ecological well-being compatible? The role of values, mindfulness, and lifestyle. *Social Indicators Research, 74,* 349–368.

Brown, K. W., & Ryan, R. M. (2003). The benefits of being present: Mindfulness and its role in psychological well-being. *Journal of Personality and Psychological Well-Being, 84,* 822–848.

Brown, K. W., Ryan, R. M., & Creswell, J. D. (2007). Addressing fundamental questions about mindfulness. *Psychological Inquiry: An International Journal for the Advancement of Psychological Theory, 18,* 272–281.

Duckworth, A. L., Grant, H., Loew, B., Oettingen, G., & Gollwitzer, P. M. (2011). Self-regulation strategies improve self-discipline in adolescents: Benefits of mental contrasting and implementation intentions. *Educational Psychology: An International Journal of Experimental Educational Psychology, 31,* 17–26.

Grabovac, A. D., Lau, M. A., & Willett, B. R. (2011). Mechanisms of mindfulness: A Buddhist psychological model. *Mindfulness.* doi: 10.1007/s12671-011-0054-5

Gunaratana, B. H. (2001). *Eight mindful steps to happiness: Walking the Buddha's path.* Boston, MA: Wisdom Publications.

Hanson, R., & Mendius, R. (2009). *Buddha's brain: The practical neuroscience of happiness, love, and wisdom.* Oakland, CA: New Harbinger Publications.

Kabat-Zinn, J. (2013). *Full catastrophe living, revised edition: How to cope with stress, pain and illness using mindfulness meditation.* New York, NY: Bantam Books.

Linehan, M. M. (1993). *Cognitive-behavioral treatment of borderline personality disorder.* New York, NY: Guilford Press.

McCown, D., Reibel, D., & Micozzi, M. S. (2010). *Teaching mindfulness: A practical guide for clinicians and educators.* New York, NY: Springer.

Olendzki, A. (2012). Wisdom in Buddhist psychology. In C. K. Germer & R. D. Siegel (Eds.), *Wisdom and compassion in psychotherapy: Deepening mindfulness in clinical practice.* New York, NY: Guilford Press.

Rosenberg, E. L. (2004). Mindfulness and consumerism. In T. Kasser & A. D. Kanner (Eds.), *Psychology and consumer culture: The struggle for a good life in a materialistic world* (pp. 107–125). Washington, DC: American Psychological Association.

Said, E. (1978). *Orientalism.* New York, NY: Vintage.

Shapiro, S. L., & Carlson, L. E. (2009). *The art and science of mindfulness: Integrating mindfulness into psychology and the helping professions.* Washington, DC: American Psychological Association.

Siegel, D. (2010). *The mindful therapist: A clinician's guide to mindsight and neural integration.* New York, NY: W. W. Norton.

Smith, H. (1965). Foreword. In P. Kapleau (Ed.), *The three pillars of Zen.* Boston, MA: Beacon Press.

Sternberg, R. J. (2012). The science of wisdom: Implications for psychotherapy. In C. K. Germer & R. D. Siegel (Eds.), *Wisdom and compassion in psychotherapy: Deepening mindfulness in clinical practice.* New York, NY: Guilford Press.

Vygotsky, L. S. (1978). *Mind in society.* Cambridge, MA: Harvard University Press.

Wallace, B. A. (2011). *Minding closely: The four applications of mindfulness.* Ithaca, NY: Snow Lion Publications.

On the Cushion
Formal Mindfulness Practices

Do not believe in anything simply because you have heard it.
Do not believe in anything simply because
it is spoken and rumored by many [....]
But after observation and analysis, when you find
that anything agrees with reason and is
conducive to the good and benefit of one and all, accept it and live up to it.
(EXCERPT FROM THE BUDDHA, N.D., p. 173)

FINDING THE RIGHT TOOLS

This chapter offers a review of formal mindfulness-based practices that can help you and your clients embody self-regulation. The term *formal* refers to the "on-the-cushion" nature of the practices. A formal mindful practice is a systematic meditation practice with the specific aim of cultivating mindfulness (Shapiro & Carlson, 2009; Stahl & Goldstein, 2010). As daily practices, they involve active engagement for a discrete period of time (e.g., 5 to 60 minutes). Extended practices can be quite lengthy (Shapiro & Carlson, 2009). For example, meditation retreats can involve silent meditation that spans 7 to 14 days. Formal practices provide a structure, a format for practice. They can be practiced in session and offered as homework. Although mindfulness-based techniques have been finding their way into mainstream practice for decades, some patients may be reluctant to engage in what they perceive as odd or ineffective practices. Acceptability of an intervention is critical. It can be helpful for patients to know that research provides support for these practices. I explain that for some patients who struggle with self-regulation, mindfulness can make a difference, and research bears that out (e.g., Hanson & Mendius, 2009; Wanden-Berghe, Sanz-Valero, & Wanden-Berghe, 2011; Williams & Grisham, 2012; Witkiewitz & Bowen, 2010; see Chapter 11 for a review of mindful and yogic interventions).

For example, in a study of 49 compulsive buyers, Williams and Grisham (2012) found that mindful, attentional focus was inversely related to compulsive buying. In another study, Witkiewitz and Bowen (2010) studied 168 individuals with substance use disorder, finding that a mindfulness-based relapse prevention program helped participants negotiate cognitive and behavioral responses to depressive symptoms, explaining reductions in postintervention substance use. Moreover, in a systematic review of mindfulness-based interventions and eating disorders, Wanden-Berghe and colleagues (2011) found evidence supporting their effectiveness, with cited reductions in eating-disordered behavior in general, binge eating in response to emotions, emotional reactivity, eating concern, and self-harming behavior, as well as improvements in emotional regulation, self-awareness, positive coping skills, mindfulness, awareness of hunger and satiety, and perceived control of eating. Although there are methodological weaknesses across studies (i.e., small sample sizes) and some unexpected outcomes (e.g., an increase in subjective binges that decreased in 6 months), there appears to be emerging evidence that mindfulness-based interventions may be effective in the treatment of eating disorders. There are many more studies that address self-regulation across self-regulatory disorders such as self-injury, gambling, compulsive buying, eating disorders, and substance use (see Chapter 11).

How does this look in practice? Claire is 16 years old. Her parents got divorced when she was 9 years old. She is their only child. Her mom works long hours and has been dating. Her father remarried and Claire now has three stepsiblings ranging from 6 months old to 5 years old. Her life can feel very chaotic. When she was 15, the year her stepbrother was born, she experimented with cutting her arm. She never thought it would become a problem. Now at 16, she thinks about cutting herself all of the time. If her dad and stepmom start fighting or things get chaotic with the kids, she sneaks off to her room and takes a safety pin to her forearm. In the summer, when her arms show, she takes the safety pin to her thighs, so that her shorts will conceal the cuts. She rationalizes that things are not that bad because she does not use a razor blade or knife. She feels like she has no other options. Cutting feels like something she can control. She says, "I know you think this is hell, my cutting. But this hell I can control. It is much better than the hell I can't. So, I cut." Her parents have taken Claire to therapy since she was 15 years old. Claire has been diagnosed with borderline personality disorder (BPD), a mental disorder characterized by long-standing instability in emotions, trouble with interpersonal relationships, struggles with identify, and a set of severe and harmful dysregulated behaviors (Wupperman, Fickling, Klemanski, Berking, & Whitman, 2013). For people such as Claire who struggle, emotional experiences, even mildly uncomfortable situations, feel very distressing and intolerable (Wupperman et al., 2013). Without other tools, they often rely on self-destructive behaviors to cope. They are looking for self-regulation and contentment in the wrong place. Mark Epstein (2001) tells an old story of a seeker looking in the wrong places. Instructional Story 5.1 was inspired by his story.

INSTRUCTIONAL STORY 5.1: Seeking in the Wrong Places

A long, long time ago, a group of graduate students was walking after a research team dinner. It was a dark night, after a long meeting at the research lab. They kept to the lighted campus path to find their way. Ahead of them on the walkway they noticed an older professor crawling on the ground underneath a lamppost. The professor was on his hands and knees, his face close to the walkway. They were concerned about him. He continued to crawl as they approached. The students saw that the professor was well and seemed to be looking for something. Stepping forward, one of the students asked the professor, "Sir, it is late. The campus is closing down for the night. You seem to be looking for something. What are you looking for? Might we help?"

"I am looking for the key to my office. I have lost it," the professor explained to them.

Despite their tight schedules and deadlines, the graduate students began to help. They looked on the pathway. They looked in the plants that lined the walkway. Some of the graduate students searched the street, with undergraduates zooming by in their cars after night class. The students looked for quite a while with no success. Tired from work and full from dinner, with still quite a walk to their cars, they were becoming weary.

Looking for a better strategy, one of the graduate students asked, "Where do you think you first lost the key? We can focus our search there."

"I lost it in my office," he said. "Over there," and he pointed to a large campus building hundreds of feet away.

Confused, one of the graduate students asked, "Then for what logical or methodological reason are you searching here, under the lamppost?"

"Because the light is better here," the old professor replied.

Source: Inspired by a story told in Epstein, 2001.

Epstein (2001) explains that the story of the lost key is not quite as dismaying as it may seem. In the same way, neither is Claire's behavior. The seekers' activity may not have been in vain after all. You see, "*Looking* is the key" (p. 20). We often get lost in the fixing of the thing and lose a sense of the process. Claire has a sense that she needs tools to negotiate her stressors and her own sensitivity. She is seeking. I honor this seeking in my patients. I validate their awareness of the painful experiences in their lives and their efforts to address them. Things that have happened to us and our challenges are important. Yet, it is also critical to learn how to be with these memories and challenges and secure empowering, effective skills that can be utilized as needed (McCown, Reibel, & Micozzi, 2010).

Research corresponds to this logic—mindfulness may help Claire. In a study of 70 individuals placed in inpatient psychiatric care, Wupperman et al. (2013) found that mindfulness statistically mediated the relation of borderline personality disorder (BPD) features to reported acts of self-injury and overall harmful dysregulated behaviors. They found that difficulties in the ability to be aware, manifest attention, and accept ongoing experiences appear to play a role in the relation to harmful dysregulated behaviors. Wupperman and colleagues (2013) hypothesize that mindfulness may disrupt and prevent the cycles of distress and self-harm. Mindfulness may help develop de-centering or the ability to step back from automatic reactions and judgments, to create a space for choice (Wupperman et al., 2013). With this space, Claire can become aware of her urges to engage in dysregulated behaviors. She can choose a healthier response rather than injuring herself. Claire can also learn to prevent these cycles from occurring in the first place. As she becomes increasingly aware of the processes in her mind and her body, she will be more effective at noticing when negative affect is arising and address it before it evolves into a distressful or seemingly unmanageable feeling (Wupperman et al., 2013). In fact, Wupperman and colleagues cite research suggesting that continued mindfulness practices may help develop more functional neural pathways that enhance affect and behavioral regulation.

MINDFUL PRACTICE

Mindful practice cultivates an empowered sense of self that can negotiate both internal and external challenges (Figure 5.1). Claire first became interested in learning more about mindfulness when she heard this quote: "The mind takes on the quality it dwells on" (Bien, 2006). As patients like Claire learn to notice and allow internal and external experiences, they will gain valuable insights and the ability to be more

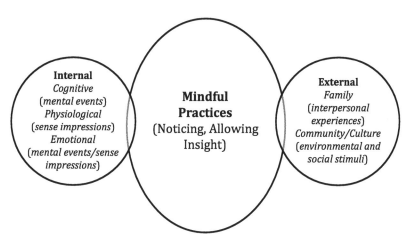

FIGURE 5.1 Mindful practices.

intentional and effective in their behavioral choices. Through these embodied practices, they experience a very different sense of self. In this chapter are several detailed, structured practices that can be used with your patients and on your own mindful path. Each of the practices is linked to the associated embodied practice (see Chapter 3). Case examples are provided to illustrate the utility of these practices with specific struggles and disorders.

What Is Meditation?

Stahl and Goldstein (2010) explain that there are two forms of meditation: insight and concentration. Insight meditation is practiced in a manner that brings full attention and awareness to the present moment and to both mind and body (Stahl & Goldstein, 2010). Further, it involves a simple noticing of experience without an effort to change anything (Hanh, 1975; Kabat-Zinn, 2013). The insight comes from what you notice as you practice. The practice is to observe without distraction, grasping, or aversion (Wallace, 2011). You will notice sense impressions such as sight, sounds, tastes, and sensations of the skin. You will notice the working of your mind and mental events such as thoughts, memories, and cognitive reactions. You will also notice emotions that tend to cross body and mind (Kabat-Zinn, 2013).

For example, as Claire began to practice meditation she noticed that thoughts of her parents' divorce kept arising. She noticed that memories of Christmas and her birthday were accompanied by deep feelings. Claire noticed grief, which is often filled with visual memories and a deep ache in the chest and belly. In the past, she would shove these feelings away, isolate herself, and reach for a safety pin in order to self-harm. In her meditation practice, she gains a powerful insight. She notices patterns of thoughts and feelings and her ability to experience them. She notices her deep emotional capacity and she observes an arising of pride in her ability to just be. This is the insight. As you practice you will learn about yourself and your patterns. For these reasons, mindfulness meditation is considered to be an insight meditation (Stahl & Goldstein, 2010).

Concentration meditation involves a focus on an object of meditation (Hanh, 1975; Kabat-Zinn, 2013; Stahl & Goldstein, 2010). This could be a mantra, a concept, an object, the flame of a candle, or the picture of a deity or loved one. I started here, as I found mindfulness meditation very challenging. I have found that many of my patients have comparable experiences. That is, they experience more tranquility as beginners when they have an object upon which to focus. In concentration meditation, awareness is brought to a single point (i.e., one-pointedness; Stahl & Goldstein, 2010). For instance, Claire began her meditation practice using a candle. Being 16 years old, she made sure that it was okay with her parents to light a candle. They helped her set up a safe place for the candle and her meditation cushion. Claire loved the ritual of setting up her special meditation area and lighting her candle. As she sat, she brought her eyes to the flame on the candle. She breathed with steady, even breath. She was able to notice when her attention, or focus, shifted. Her practice was to notice and bring her mind back to the flame of the candle. She explained that, over time, it was as if she had become one with the candle (Stahl & Goldstein, 2010). She noticed how she judged herself when her attention waned and how she clung to the times when she felt complete absorption. In these ways, concentration meditation can also lead to insights (Stahl & Goldstein, 2010). See also the discussion of embodied practice 1, be mindfully aware, and embodied practice 3, live in inquiry, in Chapter 3.

Establishing a Meditation Practice

As a mindful and yoga-informed practitioner, you may already have an established meditation practice. Use your experience to inform your mindfulness and meditation instruction to your patients. Think back to when you were first starting. Did you have a mentor or did you find your way through books and CDs? What were your questions? What did you wonder about getting right? Many beginners share questions and insecurities. In the following sections are a few guidelines for helping your patients get started with a mindfulness and meditation practice.

Beginner's Mind

No matter how long you have been practicing, begin with a beginner's mind. Beginner's mind is a quality of awareness that allows you to see things as if you have never seen them before. You notice your experience with openness and curiosity (Kabat-Zinn, 2013; Stahl & Goldstein, 2010). In this way, as actual beginners your patients have an advantage. It is important to maintain a beginner's mind, no matter how practiced or experienced you or your clients become (Marlatt, Bowen, & Lustyk, 2012). This is especially important in the treatment of self-regulation disorders. Relapses can happen when a patient begins to take for granted the ease of routines, practices, and daily functioning. Upon relapse, patients will explain how they lost their sense of mindful awareness to the challenges, stressors, and triggers in everyday life. They report feeling like they were suddenly using or engaging in the exact behavior they had worked so hard to overcome, without having a solid sense of how they got there. With a beginner's mind, your patients stay very present to each nuance of their internal and external worlds so that when risk is headed their way, they clearly see it (Marlatt et al., 2012).

Creating a Space and Tools

One of the benefits of mindfulness is that you need few supplies. In truth, you need nothing to meditate. However, like Claire, some patients and practitioners find it comforting, relaxing, and fun to set up their meditation space. At our house we have a room dedicated to yoga and meditation, with mats, meditation benches, pillows, candles, and various artifacts that we find centering. Most important, the area should be a space that is quiet, is free from distractions, and cultivates a sense of peacefulness. Wallace (2011) encourages use of a dedicated space for meditation that is not used for sleep, work, or entertainment. During my early days of meditation, my children were much younger. To ensure quiet and no interruption, I created a space in the far corner of our basement. It was not ideal in many ways. Critically, I was able to complete my meditation without interruption.

Here are some things you can consider including in your meditation area/room:

- A meditation bench or cushion (zafu, a round cushion used for seated meditation)
- A meditation candle
- A singing bowl (typically a metal bowl with a wooden dowel to signal the start and end of meditation)
- A speaker for recorded meditations
- Japa or mala beads (a set of beads used to count the number of times a mantra has been recited)

- One or two heavy blankets that can be folded and placed for comfort under your sitting bones or knees
- A meditation app for your phone. There are several wonderful meditation apps for smartphones that offer options such as setting an interval timer and an end timer. The Insight Timer (insighttimer.com) is my favorite, with options that are available for free download.

Getting Seated

Finding a good seat is important for meditation practice. If you are not comfortable, your seat becomes an obstacle to your practice (Wallace, 2011). Thich Nhat Hanh (1975) suggests sitting in the lotus position (i.e., left foot placed on the right thigh and right foot placed on the left thigh), half lotus (i.e., only one foot on one thigh), knees bent resting on your two legs or a small bench, or sitting on a cushion (Zabutan). People with back pain or difficulty getting up from a low seated position should consider a comfortable chair. Wallace (2011) notes that many people simply do not feel comfortable sitting on the floor. In a firm, supportive chair, keep your back straight (Hanh, 1975). The head and neck should be aligned with the spine (Hanh, 1975). Sit with your knees hip-distance apart and feet on the floor (Davis, Eshelman, & McKay, 2008).

Eyes can be open, partially closed, or closed (Stahl & Goldstein, 2010). If open, eyes should be focused a yard or two in front of you (Hanh, 1975). If sleepiness is present, it can be helpful to keep the eyes open or slightly open (Stahl & Goldstein, 2010). Maintain a soft smile (Hanh, 1975). A soft smile helps you relax the "worry-tightening" muscles in your face (Hanh, 1975, p. 34). Hanh (1975) says the meditation half smile is the same smile that you see on the face of the Buddha. Place the left hand with the palm side up, in your right palm (Hanh, 1975). You can also place your hands on your thighs (Stahl & Goldstein, 2010). The position that is ultimately selected should allow for alertness and comfort (Stahl & Goldstein, 2010).

Practice Script 5.1 should be read for each of the seated meditations. It helps the patient get settled and prepared for the meditation. Accordingly, each meditation scripted in this chapter begins with the words, "Start with the Getting Seated for Meditation Script."

PRACTICE SCRIPT 5.1: Getting Seated for Meditation Script
Approximate Timing: 2 Minutes for Practice

Find a comfortable place to sit. Be sure that you are well grounded (e.g., your feet are touching the floor if in a chair, or your sitting bones and legs provide a stable base if seated on the floor or kneeling). Roll your shoulders back, draw your naval in, and extend and straighten your spine as you reach the crown of your head toward the ceiling. Make any adjustments needed to help you maintain this posture (e.g., roll a blanket and place it under the back edge of your sitting bones, place supports under your knees if in an easy, cross-legged pose). If it feels okay for you, close your eyes. If you leave your eyes open, choose a focal point a few feet in front of you and rest your eyes there. Place your left hand, palm facing up, within the palm of your right hand and rest your hands. Let a half smile come to your face. Take a few moments to bring your awareness to your body becoming present, from the soles of your feet to the crown of your head. How do you feel? Notice your heart rate and any tensions in the body. Breathe into any tensions you may feel and exhale to release them. With each exhalation, release tension and soften through your body. Let go of everything. Hold on to nothing but your breath and your half smile.

Source: Hanh, 1975; Kabat-Zinn, 2013; McCown et al., 2010; Wallace, 2011.

The Meditation Practice

Hanh (1975) says that as you begin practice, you should let go of everything. He says, "Hold onto nothing but your breath and the half smile" (p. 35). Wallace (2011) recommends a dedicated time for your daily practice. He suggests the early morning hours, as you are rested and not as likely to be interrupted (Wallace, 2011). For beginners, it is best to begin with short meditation practices (Wallace, 2011). I recommend 2 to 5 minutes. Hanh (1975) says that beginners should sit no longer than 20 to 30 minutes. The length of time matters less than your attitude toward the length of time you choose. You should finish when you still feel present and have a sense that you could easily continue (Wallace, 2011). To illustrate, when Claire first started meditating, she wanted to exert 100% effort. She got her space ready, had mala beads, lit her candle, and set her meditation timer for 30 minutes. She was 100% miserable. She reported that sitting for 30 minutes was one of the hardest things she had ever done. For a week she woke up in the morning and tried to sit for her meditation for 30 minutes. Resistance grew and she began to put off her practice until after she ate breakfast. Then she started to check her e-mail before she practiced. By the end of the week she was skipping her practice and feeling guilty and stressed. With encouragement, she scaled her practice back to 5 minutes, setting her meditation timer to ring a bell every minute and a final bell at the end. At the end of the week, she felt confident and pleased, and reported that she looked forward to her practice. Small, accomplishable steps can be much more effective than big, lofty goals and unmanageable dictates. Encourage your patients to start slowly and work up. I like to use the metaphor of how ridiculous it would be to run a marathon without training. Meditation is like this. It requires practice to build competence and strength.

The meditation process is simple to describe and, as Claire knows, more challenging to practice. Hanh (1975) describes it as achieving total rest. He states that in order to achieve total rest you must accomplish two things: (a) watching your breath, and (b) letting go of everything else. It is a continual watching and letting go, watching and letting go, and watching and letting go. During this process allow yourself to release every muscle in your body (Hanh, 1975). According to Hanh (1975), relaxation is a necessary point to commence meditation. Instructional Story 5.2 was inspired by Hanh (1975).

INSTRUCTIONAL STORY 5.2: The Pebble

Imagine that you are a pebble. You were found by a little girl, cherished and polished until you were smooth. In order to make a wish, the little girl throws you into a river. Softly, you sink down through the water without effort. As a pebble, you are free from everything. You feel no attachment to the little girl and are thankful for her good care. Detached, you fall the shortest distance possible. At the bottom of the river, you are at the point of perfect rest. You can see the little girl as she looks down into the river, her heart full of promise and hope. This separation serves you both. You let go of everything. At your very center is your being. You are at the point of complete rest there on the bed of the river. It does not matter how long it took you to fall or how far you fell to get there on the riverbed. Once you reach the riverbed, you have found your own resting spot. Here, nestled in the sandy bottom of the river, you no longer are pushed or pulled by the water or anything else.

The river flows by you. As a pebble on the bottom of the riverbed, the only moment that matters is the current moment. You have let go of the little girl, her caring for you, her wish. You have felt your gratitude and now you rest. You are here, now. The only place that joy, peace, and contentment are possible is in your current spot. If you try to see the girl as she walks away, you have missed the moment. Similarly, if you look to the water that has flown by (i.e., the past), again you miss this moment. If you wonder if another child will find you and cherish you, you will miss the moment. In the same way, if you look at the water to flow your way (i.e., the future), you miss this moment. The only place to find peace, joy, and contentment is in your current spot. What has been and what will be do not matter. It is here—in this moment—where you can find enlightenment, only here in your spot.

Source: Inspired by a story told by Hanh, 1975.

The breath is used as an anchor for your mind. It is not meant to be used to chase thoughts and feelings away (Hanh, 1975; Kabat-Zinn, 2013). Breath is the methodology for uniting the mind and the body (Hanh, 1975; Kabat-Zinn, 2013). When you feel a thought or feeling arise, do not chase it with your attention. Acknowledge the presence of the thought or feeling and bring your attention back to your breath (Hanh, 1975). Hanh (1975) provides an example. He says that if a feeling of sadness arises, you should immediately recognize it. You think, "A feeling of sadness has just arisen in me" (p. 38). If the feeling of sadness continues you say, "A feeling of sadness is still in me" (p. 38). If you have a thought such as "It is very late and the dog next door is still barking," you notice, "I am thinking." If the thought persists, you say, "I am still thinking." Hanh (1975) says that what is essential is to not allow a thought or feeling to arise without noticing it in mindfulness. See the discussion of embodied practice 1, be mindfully aware, in Chapter 3.

It is important to simply notice thoughts and feelings and to forego judgment of them. If the thought that you have is wholesome (e.g., "I should donate some money to a charity tomorrow"), notice, "A wholesome thought has just arisen" (Hanh, 1975, p. 39). If an unwholesome thought arises (e.g., "I am resentful of her success"), notice, "An unwholesome thought has just arisen" (Hanh, 1975, p. 39). Do not attach to the wholesome and avoid the unwholesome; simply notice. Grabovac, Lau, and Willett (2011), Bien (2006), and Thich Nhat Hanh (1998) distilled the essence of what is to be learned in meditation practice to these three ideas (i.e., impermanence, suffering, and not-self):

1. Sense impressions and mental events arise and pass away
   (i.e., *impermanence*).
2. Habitual reactions (i.e., attachment and aversion) to the feeling tones accompanying sense impressions or mental events are the source of *suffering*.
3. Sense impressions and mental events are *not-self*.

Siegel (2010) suggests that, over time, meditation practices can help us neurologically enhance the ability to notice and discriminate various incoming sensations and mental events from our narrative-based sense of self. See the discussion in Chapter 3 of embodied practice 4, accept impermanence; embodied practice 5, cultivate nonattachment; embodied practice 6, discern what is not-self; and embodied practice 7, allow what is with nonjudgment.

FORMAL MEDITATION PRACTICES

Formal meditation cultivates the space between stimulus and response (see Chapter 4; Wallace, 2011). As you sit in meditation, you notice the stimuli (i.e., mental events or sense impressions; Grabovac et al., 2011). It may be a mental event or a thought (as Hanh [1975] describes) or it may be a sense impression, information coming from one of your senses or your body. You simply notice. Each stimulus is automatically and immediately tagged by the brain with a feeling tone: pleasant, neutral, or unpleasant (Grabovac et al., 2011; Hanson & Mendius, 2009). Research suggests that there is an added challenge. That is, due to biological mechanisms of self-protection, "Negative trumps positive" (Hanson & Mendius, 2009). These things we cannot control. However, it is at exactly this point in the process that you have a choice (Figure 5.2).

In meditation we dig into this space, the space right after the stimulus and feeling tone. This is the space in which lives can be changed. As you sit in meditation you notice stimuli and feeling tones, then you choose to attach, avoid, or allow. This is not an easy practice, as the natural tendency is to attach to and build on the feeling tone, cultivating concepts, emotions, and maybe even a line of thinking or ruminating (Grabovac et al., 2011). Many times, we have a default script we fall into in which we are the victim, everything is out of control, or we have no power. Often these stories are activated when we attach to the unpleasant feeling tone. This is identification. We experience things as if these experiences are in fact who we are (Wallace, 2011; see embodied practice 6, discern what is not-self). Other times, the feeling tone is so unpleasant that we move into aversion. We want to avoid this feeling.

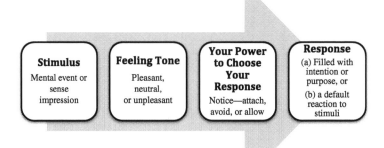

FIGURE 5.2 The space between in meditation.

This creates good soil for many problems with dysregulation. Shopping compulsively, bingeing and purging, self-harming, gambling, playing hours of video games, and using drugs or alcohol all help us avoid unpleasant feeling tones. By staying present, moving your awareness to your breath or object of concentration (mala beads, mantra, candle, concept, etc.), you bring yourself to allowing the stimuli to run its course. Any behavior you choose after this can be unencumbered, full of freedom, and full of your intentions.

As a patient practices, he or she notices the space, the choice, and the competence that comes from allowing and being present with what is. This can change the way a patient experiences his or her struggles. For example, before Claire began her meditation practice, her thinking process looked like this: stimuli (i.e., parents fighting and feeling overwhelmed), feeling tone (i.e., unpleasant), choice (i.e., aversion), and response (i.e., cutting; Figure 5.3).

Claire focused her meditation on the noticing of the arising and passing away of her awareness of mental events and sensations and on the way her brain tagged mental events and sense impressions as pleasant, unpleasant, and neutral. She watched the nearly automatic tendency to attach to the feeling tone, the mental event, or the sense impression. She noticed how simply sitting for meditation could trigger her personal narrative, "I am overwhelmed and I can't handle this." Before she began to work in this way, she had no awareness of mental events or sense impressions arising and passing away. She did not know that they were tagged to a feeling tone. Most troublesome is that she believed her story that she was always overwhelmed and that she could not handle anything.

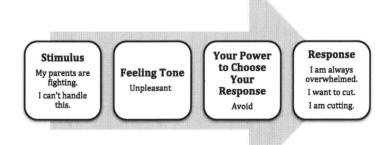

FIGURE 5.3 Claire's default reaction to stimuli.

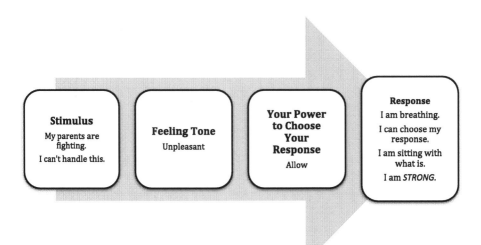

FIGURE 5.4 Claire's new choices.

Her meditation gave her insight to this path of events and she began to question her old narrative. She began to find space, choice, and power (Figure 5.4). See also the discussions in Chapter 3 of embodied practice 1, be mindfully aware; embodied practice 3, live in inquiry; embodied practice 5, cultivate nonattachment; and embodied practice 7, allow what is with nonjudgment.

The practices described next provide several structured ways to dig into the space between stimuli and response. These include the first sitting meditation script unique to this text, designed to bring awareness and competence to cultivate the space between stimulus and response. The following scripts support breath awareness, the five aggregates, a body scan, mindful eating, a walking meditation, loving-kindness, and a day of mindfulness. As you and your clients practice, use Figure 5.5 to record your experience and growing awareness (Figure 5.5).

The Space Between: Formal Sitting Meditation

The Space Between formal sitting meditation, Practice Script 5.2, is intended to bring awareness and insight. The script will help you and your clients bring awareness to stimuli, which include sense impressions and mental events, the accompanying feeling tones, the choice to notice and then attach or allow, and finally the active choice of a response (Grabovac et al., 2011; Wallace, 2011).

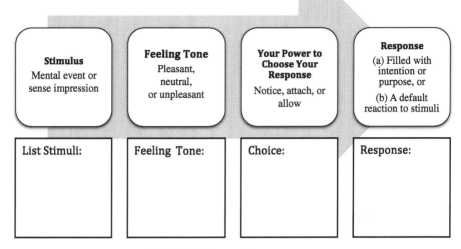

FIGURE 5.5 Your growing awareness.

PRACTICE SCRIPT 5.2: The Space Between

Approximate Timing: 2 Minutes for Introduction; 20 Minutes for Practice

Start with the Getting Seated for Meditation Script. Take a few moments to bring your awareness to your body. How do you feel? Pause and be present here in this moment. Take a deep breath in and exhale.

Bring your awareness to your breath. Notice if it is even, regular, and smooth. Your breath will be your object of concentration for this meditation. You will continually bring yourself back to your breath as an anchor. Do not try to change your breath. Simply be present to it. Notice it.

As you breathe, you will become aware of sense impressions. This can be something that you see, smell, taste, hear, or feel on your skin or inside of your body. You may hear children outside, birds chirping, a lawn mower or snow blower going. You may have a candle lit and notice a flicker in the flame and feel a slight breeze on your skin. Your stomach may grumble or your muscles may tighten. These are sense impressions. Notice them as they arise. As they arise into your awareness, say to yourself, "I am hearing the chirping of the birds," or "I am feeling the grumbling of my stomach." Notice that these sense impressions arise and pass away and that your breath is a constant. Notice this and bring your awareness back to your breath.

As your sense impressions arise, you will also notice that they feel pleasant, neutral, or unpleasant. Notice this. Notice how your brain tends to automatically label your sense impressions. Perhaps you heard the birds chirping and you feel a feeling tone, a pleasant feeling tone. Or maybe you hear a lawn mower and you feel an unpleasant feeling tone. Notice this. Notice that the feeling tones arise and pass away as well. The feeling tone comes to your awareness, it peaks, and then it softens and passes away. As you notice the sense impressions and the feeling tones, allow them to be and bring your awareness back to your breath.

As you are sitting, breathing, and attending to the nature and quality of your breath, you may notice mental events. These are thoughts, memories, concepts, and ideas. These can also be feelings tied to ideas and memories. When mental events arise as feelings, you will notice that there are sense impressions that may go with them. You might feel sadness in your belly and heaviness as you think about the dog you loved when you were little. You notice these mental events, memories, ideas, stories, as they arise. As you notice, bring your awareness back to your breath. Your breath is your anchor. Notice that the mental events arise in your consciousness, gain a stronger presence, and then pass away, getting softer as they move out of your awareness. Notice this pattern. Notice that as mental events arise and pass away, your breath is a constant cycle of inhalation and exhalation. As you sit and breathe, you may notice that your mental events also have an associated feeling tone. You notice that your brain labels them as pleasant, neutral, or unpleasant. Notice that you think and the feeling tone is seemingly connected to the thought. As you see these feeling tones, you notice that they arise and pass away just as your sense impressions and mental events arise and pass away. Notice this and bring your breath back to your awareness.

As you practice, sitting and breathing, you may notice that some sense impressions and feeling tones pull for your attention. They snag, like Velcro, on your thinking self. As you sit, you hear the lawn mower (sense impression) and you notice that the feeling tone that goes with that sense impression is unpleasant. "It is early," you think. "It is too early for mowing," you think. You start to become angry as the whole story of your neighbor's thoughtlessness comes to mind. You think about her dog that barks late into the night; how she fails to weed her garden, making the neighborhood look bad; you think about how someone who never mows the lawn is highly inconsiderate to do it before 9 a.m. when you are trying to meditate. You notice that as your mind works and works, your breath and your choice are lost.

Your power is in your anchor, your breath. The moment that you notice that you have left your breath, go back to it. It does not matter if you brought your awareness back at your first sense impression or mental event or if you were well into a long story. Bring yourself back to your breath. The growth is in your noticing. As you sit, you will see the habits of the mind. You will get to know them. As you see them, notice them. "Ah, there it is. I notice my 'neighbor story.'

I notice it and I will bring myself to my breath." Perhaps it is different, pleasant. "Ah, there are the birds chirping, I notice them. I notice the pleasant feeling tone. I bring myself back to breathing." Breathe.

As you are sitting, bring your awareness wholly to your breath. Notice the qualities of your breath. Is it even, smooth, does it move in and out without pause? Breathe and notice (pause here for 60 seconds). When it is your time to finish, cultivate gratitude for your practice, your ability to sit and notice, and for your insights gained during your practice today.

Source: Grabovac et al., 2011; Wallace, 2011.

Breath Awareness

Breath awareness and control are critical aspects of the physiological components of self-regulation. As well explicated by Davis and colleagues (2008), breathing exercises have been found to be effective in the relief of many triggering symptoms, such as anxiety and mood symptoms, irritability, muscle tension, headaches, and fatigue. Breath awareness is a wonderful place to begin a meditation practice. Thich Nhat Hanh (1975) begins his instruction on meditation with instruction on the breath:

> *"He who half breathes, half lives."*
> ANCIENT PROVERB, AUTHOR UNKNOWN

There are several ways to utilize the breath in meditation. You can follow the length of the breath (Hanh, 1975). You can notice the role the body—specifically, the diaphragm, stomach, and rib cage—plays in the extension of breath (Hanh, 1975). Hanh (1975) suggests that beginners lie down. In a clinical setting you can have your patient lie on the couch or shift down in a chair so that he or she has more access to the stomach and chest. Extension of the length of the breath can help anchor awareness on breathing. If your patient begins with four-count inhalations and exhalations, have the patient move to a six- or seven-count breath (Hanh, 1975). Hanh (1975) suggests 20 breaths is a sufficient practice of noticing and lengthening the breath.

To introduce this practice, explain to your client that you will be teaching a meditation to develop breath awareness and skills at modifying the breath that can be very helpful in reducing feelings of anxiety, increasing distress tolerance, and helping to tolerate the urge to engage in self-destructive behaviors (e.g., shop excessively, binge eat, drink or use drugs, or self-harm). For example, John, the 20-year-old male struggling with excessive alcohol use introduced earlier, explained that he frequently was not able to calm down without a drink. He said that he just gets overwhelmed and has no way to get a handle on what he is feeling. Breath awareness is a good place to start in order to help John have a sense of the power of his breath to calm and relax. This practice, shown in Practice Script 5.3, will help you and your patients develop embodied practice 2, honor your breath and physical experience (see Chapter 3).

PRACTICE SCRIPT 5.3: Breath Awareness

Approximate Timing: 2 Minutes for Introduction; 20 Minutes for Practice

Start with the Getting Seated for Meditation Script. Take a few moments to bring your awareness to your body. Breathe here. Now, bring your awareness to your breath. If possible, close your mouth and breathe through your nose. Do not try to change your breathing. Notice the qualities of your breath. Is it smooth? Is your inhalation the same length as your exhalation? Can you feel your heart beat as you breathe? What is the pace of your breathing? Is it fast, slow, moderate? Suspend judgment and action. Simply notice. As you are being aware of your breathing, you may notice that other objects enter your awareness. Simply notice that they are there and then bring your attention directly back to your breath. Do this as often as needed as you practice breath awareness.

Bring your awareness to the muscles of the face. Breathe into these muscles. As you breathe out, release any tension. You want your face to feel as soft and relaxed as the face of a sleeping baby. Bring your awareness to the very tip of your nose. Notice the air as it passes just underneath the tip of your nose. Breathe here. Now, bring your awareness to your nostrils. Notice the quality of the air, the warmth as the air leaves your body and the comparative coolness of the air as it enters. Notice if the air is dry or moist as it enters and leaves your body. As you breathe, remain aware of the focus of your mind. Continuously bring it back to your breath, your nose and your nostrils, the quality of the air, the pace of your breath. There is so much to notice right here in your present moment.

Begin to notice how the air feels as it enters your nose. See if you can feel it enter your body, move from your nose, to your throat, and into each of your lungs. Notice the pathway, how the breath feels as it moves from your nose to your throat and then from your throat to your lungs. Can you feel the breath divide as half enters one lung and half enters the other? Notice how your rib cage rises and falls as you inhale and exhale. You may begin to notice that your rib cage expands from front to back and from side to side as you inhale. You may notice that the ribs and the side of the body gently soften as you exhale. Continue breathing here. As before, notice the contents of your awareness and, as needed, bring your focus back to your breath.

Now, bring your awareness to the qualities of your breath. Notice the length of the exhalations and the inhalations. Bring awareness to the fullness of your breath. Is it shallow and in your chest? Does it go deep into your body, expanding both your chest and your belly? Is your breath smooth as it moves in and out of your body? Are there pauses at the transition from inhalation to exhalation? Do you smoothly roll from inhaling to exhaling? Slowly begin to deepen your breath. Count to four as you inhale—one, two, three, four—and then count to four as you exhale—one, two, three, four. Continue this for four breaths. (Note: Pause here and allow time for breath.) Now, continuing with deep breath, notice the transition from inhalation to exhalation. Once you feel as if you cannot inhale any further, allow your body to move, without effort, to exhalations. As you feel you cannot exhale any further, allow your body to shift to inhalation. Continue this for four breaths. (Note: Pause here and allow time for four breaths.) As Buddha taught, think, "I breathe in a long breath" and "I breathe out a long breath."

Now, allow your breath to return to normal breathing. When breathing shorter breaths, become aware. As Buddha taught, think, "I breathe in a short breath," and "I breathe out a short breath." Notice the qualities of your normal breathing. Describe them to yourself as you breathe. You might think, "My breathing is smooth, even, and without pause." Breathe and notice the qualities of your breath.

Now, expand your awareness from your breath to your chest and head and then to your entire body. Breathe as if you could breathe into your entire body. Inhale a big, whole-body inhale and exhale a big, whole-body exhale. Notice your body again. Notice any shifts or changes in the experience of your body. Slowly bring your palms together and rub them, palm to palm, generating a little warmth. Then, take the palms of your hands to your eyes, softly cupping them. Slowly open your eyes into the palms of your hands and spread your fingers slightly to allow light in. Slowly withdraw your hands from your eyes, breathing normally.

Source: Bien, 2006; Davis et al., 2008; Kabat-Zinn, 2013; Stahl and Goldstein, 2010; Wallace, 2011.

The Five Aggregates

When you sit in meditation you can direct your attention, concentration, and contemplation to the *interdependent* nature of objects and knowing (Hanh, 1975, 1998). This practice hinges on the ancient precept, "The subject of knowledge cannot exist independently from the object of knowledge" (Hanh, 1975, p. 45). In other words, to see is to see something. Similarly, to hear is to hear something (Hanh, 1975). To be angry is to be angry about something. When we hope, we hope for something (Hanh, 1975). Thinking is the same. When you think, you think about something

(Hanh, 1975). When you practice, the interdependence is present there as well. "Every object of the mind is itself the mind" (Hanh, 1975, p. 46). In Buddhism, objects of the mind are called *dharmas* (Hanh, 1975). There are five categories: bodily and physical forms, feelings, perceptions, mental functions, and consciousness (Hanh, 1975, 1998). The last category, consciousness, is believed to contain the other five categories (Hanh, 1975). To contemplate interdependence, you look deeply into all of the dharmas to see their real nature, their role in the body of reality, and the indivisibly of the great body of reality (Hanh, 1975). Practice Script 5.4 is a script for a meditation on the five aggregates.

PRACTICE SCRIPT 5.4: Meditation on the Five Aggregates

Approximate Timing: 2 Minutes for Introduction; 20 Minutes for Practice

Start with the Getting Seated for Meditation Script. Become aware of your body. The first of the five aggregates is your bodily and physical form. Bring your awareness there. Notice your connection with each aspect of your body. Contemplate your bodily form. Begin at your base and consider your feet. As you are mindful of your feet, you are considering your feet. The contents of the mind and the object you are minding are interdependent. Consider this interdependence as you move through your body. Notice your legs, your sitting bones, and pelvis. Bring your mind to your lower back and your belly. Let your awareness move up your spine and feel your shoulder blades as they rest on your midback. Feel your heart and your lungs as you breathe. Bring your awareness up through the neck, the place where your spine meets your skull. Feel your jaw, your cheeks, your tongue, your nose, your eyes, and then move your awareness to your scalp and your hair. Rest your awareness on the center of your forehead. Notice that your awareness and the object of your awareness are interdependent.

Now, notice what you are feeling. Notice the physical contents of the feeling as they manifest in your body, breath, and heartbeat. Notice how you perceive your experience, the images, sensations, and other sensory experiences as they come into your perceptual mind. Notice how the mind works with these perceptions, wanting to categorize, order, judge, evaluate, connect, and place in an order. Notice the cognitive content and processes as they arise in the content of your thoughts. Become aware of the interdependence of your feelings and your noticing of your feelings. As you become aware of various aspects of the aggregates, notice the interdependence of your perceptions and the noticing of your perceptions. Notice the connection between your mental operations and the noticing of your mental operations. To have one without the other is like clapping with one hand. It cannot happen. Consider this connectedness.

Consider a tree. Bring an image of a tree to your mind. Consider that the tree's existence is possible due to the existence of everything that is not this tree. These things include the soil from which the tree has grown, the mother tree from which this tree's seed fell, the nutrients in the soil that feed the tree, the air that provides oxygen to the tree, the rain that falls from the sky hydrating the tree, and the sun that provides the energy for photosynthesis. Notice that if you grasp the tree's reality, you also see that the tree itself is present in all of the things that are not the tree. If all of the things that have made the tree possible were to have never come together to make this tree, the tree would not be in existence. It is all interconnected, interdependent.

In the same way you have looked at the tree, look at yourself. Consider the assembly of the mind. Consider the presence of reality and the oneness into your own experience, your own self. Consider the connection between your self and the whole universe. Ask, "If the five aggregates return to their sources, does the self no longer exist?" (Hanh, 1975). The self and the assembly of the five aggregates are no different. The assembly and all that there is in the universe are not different. Contemplate the interconnectedness of all things. Consider that you are not a distinct thing. Consider that you are life, and that life is limitless (Hanh, 1975).

Source: Hanh, 1975; Wallace, 2011.

Body Scan

The body scan (Practice Script 5.5) is a good practice for integrating mind and body (Davis et al., 2008; Stahl & Goldstein, 2010). It is also a practice of embodiment and an antidote of self-objectification (McCown et al., 2010). As with the other practices, this should be done in a location in which you can be free from distractions. The body scan meditation is typically done lying down. However, in practice, you can ask your patient to lean back into the chair or lie back on the couch. You want the patient to feel grounded and comfortable in the position that he or she selects. If the meditation is done in a yoga room with supports, blankets, and pillows, a rolled blanket can be placed under the knees and a small pillow under the head. See the discussions in Chapter 3 of embodied practice 1, be mindfully aware, and embodied practice 2, honor your breath and physical experience.

PRACTICE SCRIPT 5.5: Body Scan

Approximate Timing: 1 Minute for Introduction; 20 Minutes for Practice

---

Once you are in a comfortable position, close your eyes and bring your awareness to your breathing. Notice the rise and fall of your chest and belly as you breathe.

Slowly begin to extend your breath, lengthening each inhalation and exhalation, pausing slightly at the turn of the breath. Inhale. Hold. Exhale. Hold. Do this for five complete breath cycles.

Now, bring your awareness all the way down to your feet. Notice your toes, your big toes, second toes, third, fourth, and baby toes. Breathe as if you can breathe down into your toes. Notice any tension or holding you might feel in your toes. Notice where your toes connect to your feet, notice the balls of your feet, and move your awareness to the arches of your feet. If your feet are bare, notice the feeling of the air on your skin, the muscles beneath this skin. Notice your heels, the skin, the muscle and bone. Feel your heels resting on the floor, in shoes, or on the mat. Notice the tops of your feet. Breathe as if you can breathe into your feet, noticing any sensations you may feel.

Move your awareness to your ankles. Feel the connection of your ankles to your feet. Feel the space in your ankle joints. Next, notice the muscles and the skin. Can you feel the air or socks around your ankles? Are your ankles warm or cold? Breathe as if you can breathe right into your ankles.

Next, move your awareness into your lower legs. Move your attention from your heels through your Achilles tendons and into your calf muscles. Notice the feeling of your calf muscles touching the floor or the chair. Feel any tension or relaxation that is there. Just notice and breathe into your calves. Now, move your awareness to your shins. Focus on the area where the top of your feet meet your shins and then let your awareness move up your shin bones to your knees. Breathe as if you can breathe into your shins, noticing the bones, the muscles, and skin. Notice any sensations you feel on the inside and the air or your clothes as they meet the skin on your shins.

Move your awareness, your attention to the tops of your knees. Notice the patellae as they cover the knee joints. Bring your awareness to all of the muscles and tendons that meet the joint of your knees, some under the patellae, some at the sides of the knee. Feel what you feel. Feel the space within the joint and the air or clothes around your knee. Move your awareness up your thighs. Feel the quadriceps, the large muscles on the tops of your legs spanning the length of your thighs. Notice if they are holding tension or relaxed. Have a sense of the skin, the muscles, and the bones. Feel your clothing as it meets the skin on your thighs. Breathe as if you can breathe into your quadriceps. Next, move your awareness to the undersides of your knees and up the backs of your thighs. Feel your thighs as they rest on the floor or a chair. Feel the skin as it meets the clothes on your body. Breathe as if you can breathe into your hamstrings.

Next, move your awareness up into your gluteus muscles. Feel the connection of your gluteus muscles with the chair or the floor as you rest, gently supported. Bring your awareness to your pelvis and the connection of your legs to your torso at your hips. Notice if you feel space, tension, or softness. Breathe as if you can breathe into your pelvis, your hips, and your glutes. Slowly, bring your awareness into your belly. Notice your belly rise and fall as you breathe. Is your belly soft or holding? Does it rise and fall easily with your breath? Breathe as if you can breathe directly into your belly.

Now, bring your awareness back to your gluteus muscles and then to the very base of your spine. Notice your tailbone; is it tucked, neutral, soft? Notice your lower back. Does your lower back feel supported or is there tension? Notice the connection of the lower back to your whole back, the sides of your body, and the upper sections of your spine. Breathe as if you can breathe into your lower back and up into your entire spine. Let your awareness travel up your spine to your midback, the space between your shoulder blades. Notice if you feel supported by the floor or the chair. Is your midback soft or tense? Bring your awareness across your upper back, spanning your awareness wide to reach the backs of your shoulders, the shoulder blades, and into the very base of the neck. Notice any tension or softness. Breathe as if you can breathe across your whole upper back. Feel the support of the back as it meets the chair or the floor.

Move your awareness to the center of your midback, between the shoulder blades just under your heart. Bring your awareness to your lungs, noticing them fill with air as you inhale and empty as you exhale. Become very aware of your heart, your heartbeat, and the rhythm with your breath. Notice how your heart is supported by your midback, your shoulder blades, and your lungs. Your heart is held by your body. Notice your breath and breathe as if you could breathe directly into your heart. Keep your attention here and breathe.

Bring your attention to your chest. Notice the muscles on top of the rib cage and those that span to the heads of your shoulders. Notice your skin as it meets your clothing. Bring your attention to your shoulders, to the tops of your arms, your biceps and your triceps. Notice the upper arms as they are supported by the chair or the floor. What sensations do you feel? Breathe as if you can breathe into your upper arms. Next, move your awareness to your elbows. Notice the muscles that come from the upper arms and the lower arms to your elbow joints. Breathe into the center of the elbow. Next, let your awareness travel down your forearms. Notice the skin, the muscles, and the bone. What sensations do you feel? Notice your wrists and the connections to your hands. Do you feel space here? Do you feel tension or softness? Notice what you are feeling here. Breathe as if you can breathe into your wrists. Now, notice your hands. Notice your thumbs, your first, second, third, and pinky fingers on each hand. Notice how your fingers feel. Are they straight, bent, slightly curled? Do you feel lightness or tension in your fingers? Just notice. Move your awareness to the palms of your hands. What sensations do you feel? Breathe as if you can breathe into the palms of your hands and notice what you notice. Keep your awareness here and breathe.

Bring your awareness back to your chest. Notice your chest as you breathe in and out. Become aware of any movements in your chest. Let your awareness travel to your throat. Can you feel the air pass through your throat as you *breathe? Let your awareness move to the back of your neck and then to the base of the skull. Notice the connection of the neck to the skull. Notice space, tension, or softness. Breathe as if you can breathe into the area where your neck meets the base of your skull. Keep your awareness here and breathe.*

Move your attention around to the front of your neck and up into your jaw. Feel your jaw. Are you holding, clenching, or soft in your holding of your jaw? Breathe as if you can breathe into your jaw. Next, allow your awareness to flow around to the back of your head, to the back of your skull. Notice the muscles that cover your skull moving up the back of your head around the crown of your head. Feel the muscles that extend up and across the sides of your head. Notice your head resting on the chair or your mat. Notice the support offered to your head by the floor or the chair. Breathe here. Bring your awareness to your temples, your cheeks, your mouth, your lips. Notice any sensations here. Notice your nose. Feel the air as it moves past your nostrils as you breathe. Maybe you can feel the air move through your sinuses. Breathe here and notice. Next, bring your awareness to your eyes. Do they feel soft, tense? Breathe as if you can breathe into your eyes. Keep your awareness here and breathe.

Slowly move your awareness to your eyebrows and your forehead. Notice the skin, the muscles underneath the skin, and the bone. Breathe as if you can breathe into your forehead and notice what you feel. Now, bring your awareness to the very center of your forehead. Notice the skin, the muscles, the bone. Bring your awareness to the center of your forehead to the area that some call the mind's eye. Breathe here. With your eyes closed and your awareness at the very center of your forehead, what do you see? What do you feel? Notice and breathe as if you can breathe into the very center of your forehead. Hold your awareness here and breathe. (Note: Long pause of at least 60 seconds.)

Now, bring your awareness to your whole body. Extend your awareness to the soles of your feet, the palms of your hands, and the crown of your head. Breathe as if you can breathe into your whole body, the soles of your feet, the palms of your hands, and the crown of your head. Take a big inhale, one, two, three, four, five, and a big exhale, one, two, three, four, five. Take another big inhale, one, two, three, four, five, and another big exhale, one, two, three, four, five. Slowly allow your breath to return to normal.

When you are ready, begin to wiggle your fingertips and your toes. If you are laying down, bend your elbows and your knees and slowly roll to your right side. Gently come to a seated position, ankles crossed and hands on your thighs. Bring your hands together and rub them together gently, bringing warmth into your hands. Place your hands over your eyes, and open your eyes into the palms of your hands. Open your fingers slowly to let in light and gently withdraw your hands from your face.

Source: Davis et al., 2008; Kabat-Zinn, 2013; McCown et al., 2010; Shapiro and Carlson, 2009; Stahl and Goldstein, 2010; Wallace, 2011.

Mindful Eating

Mindful eating is both a formal and informal practice. As a formal practice, the food is the object of concentration in a concentration meditation. Although we eat every day, few of us attend to what we eat, how we are eating, and the process of eating (Davis et al., 2008; Kabat-Zinn, 2013). In Chapter 6, mindful eating is described as an informal practice. Mindful eating is often done at the beginning of mindfulness-based stress reduction (MBSR) classes (see Chapter 11 for a full description of MBSR; Kabat-Zinn, 2013; Stahl & Goldstein, 2010). I use this as the first introduction to mindfulness in my course at the University at Buffalo, "The Mindful Therapist." Typically this activity, shown in Practice Script 5.6, is done with raisins. I offer a choice between a raisin and a dark chocolate chip. The practice is intended to be done in a setting that allows practitioners to be free from distractions (Kabat-Zinn, 2013; Stahl & Goldstein, 2010).

PRACTICE SCRIPT 5.6: Mindful Eating

Approximate Timing: 1 Minute for Introduction; 10 Minutes for Practice

Preparation: Provide a bowl of raisins, a bowl of dark chocolate chips, and napkins—enough for your group.

Find a comfortable seat. Be sure your feet can rest on the floor or a stable surface. As the bowls of raisins and dark chocolate chips and napkins are passed around, select from the bowls a few raisins or chips and place them on your napkin.

Now, settle into a steady even breath and relax. Begin by simply looking at your raisin or chip. Pretend that you have never seen a raisin or a chocolate chip before. This is your first time. Notice the color, texture, shape, ridges, contours, and how it is resting on your napkin. See the raisin or chip as it is right there on your napkin. Shift the raisin or chip on your napkin. What do you see now? Does the light fall in new ways on your raisin or chip? Do you see new contours or shades of color? As you practice concentration on your object, you will also notice your mind and body as thoughts and sense impressions arise and fall away. Try to simply notice any thoughts, judgments, cravings, and bodily sensations and then bring your awareness back to your object.

Next, pick up your raisin or chip with your fingers. Lift it closer to your eyes so you can see it in yet another new way. Bring your attention to what your object feels like. Is it soft or hard, smooth or rough, does it melt or get softer, is it cold? As you explore the touch sensation of your raisin or chip, you will also notice the sense impressions coming from your body in other areas. Maybe the room is cold or your chair is hard. Maybe your legs are tingling as you sit very still. Work on just noticing the sense impressions that come to mind. You will also notice mental events, such as thoughts. Perhaps you are wondering how this activity might help someone who struggles or you wonder where the raisins or chips were purchased. Simply notice these mental events and bring your attention back to your raisin or chip.

Bring your raisin or chip to your nose. Smell. What do you smell? Do you smell the earthy, fruitiness of the raisin, an essence of grapes? Do you smell chocolate? What if you had never smelled these smells before? How would you describe the smell you are smelling right now? Remember, you can't say, "I smell chocolate" or "I smell raisins." Without these words, how would you describe what you are smelling right now? As before, notice any other sense impressions or mental events as they arise and fall away.

Now, bring the raisin or chip to your mouth. Let it touch your lips so that you can feel the texture and smell the essence. Slowly place the object in your mouth without chewing. Let the object rest on your tongue. What do you taste? Find the words to describe the taste without using the words raisin or chocolate. What comes up for you? Slowly move the raisin or chocolate around in your mouth. Experience the taste and sensations. When you are ready, chew your raisin or chocolate. Has the taste changed? Did the texture change? Be aware of how your body, your mouth, your saliva respond to the raisin or chocolate in your mouth. Once you are ready to swallow, notice any shifts in awareness in your presence. With intention, swallow your raisin or chip. Notice your mouth, your nose, your hands now. What do you notice?

Take a moment to offer gratitude for the raisin or chip, for your awareness, and for the opportunity to explore mindful eating.

Source: Davis et al., 2008; Kabat-Zinn, 2013; Stahl and Goldstein, 2010.

Walking Meditation

Walking meditation (see Practice Script 5.7), involves a moment-by-moment presence with each step (Davis et al., 2008; Hanson & Mendius, 2009; Stahl & Goldstein, 2010). It involves noticing each foot as you lift it and move it forward and place it down on the ground (Kabat-Zinn, 2013; Stahl & Goldstein, 2010). Walking meditation is not about reaching a certain destination. It is the bare awareness of each aspect of the act of walking. It can be done indoors or outdoors (Davis et al., 2008). You need a space about 10 to 20 feet in length (Shapiro & Carlson, 2009). To complete a walking meditation, you and your patients should choose a quiet and pleasant space, although this is not completely necessary. To illustrate, when I teach walking meditation at the University at Buffalo, we meet late in the evening. The building is quiet and the class walks together throughout the building. I lead and the students need simply to follow the person in front of them. We walk past classrooms with instruction ongoing, up and down stairs, through the quiet hallways, and across more crowded meeting places. The focus is on the walking and the noticing. Students find it compelling to explore what they noticed as they walked the same hallways they walk every day. The shift is substantial. The choice is yours and your patients'. Gardens and labyrinths can be beautiful places for walking meditation. You can also simply walk back and forth from one spot to another, keeping your path simple and clear. It can be helpful to set a timer on your phone so that you know when it is time to stop.

PRACTICE SCRIPT 5.7: Walking Meditation

Approximate Timing: 1 Minute for Introduction; 20+ Minutes for Practice

Begin your walking meditation by standing with your feet hip-distance apart, hands at your sides, shoulders soft, and tailbone neutral. With your eyes open and chin neutral, look around. See what you see. Take in the external. Do you see people? Are there trees or grass? Are you inside and see the floor and furniture? Take it all in. Check in on what you are experiencing inside as well. How do your feet feel on the ground? Is the surface hard or soft? Do you feel supported? Scan your body from your feet to the crown of your head, across your shoulders and down your arms to your fingertips. Do you feel tension? Are you relaxed? Can you breathe into any tension you are feeling and let it go? Take a big breath in and hold for a count of four and then release your breath, slowly returning to regular breath.

Take your gaze about 5 feet in front of you. You will feel as if you have a gentle downward gaze. From grounded feet, lift your right foot off of the ground, bending at the knee, and then move your foot forward. Notice how your leg feels when you lift your foot. Notice how your foot lands on the ground. Do all four corners of your foot connect to the ground below at once, or does the heel meet the ground followed by the ball of the foot and then the toes? Place your weight on your right foot and lift your left foot. Now that you are in motion, how does the action of lifting your left foot differ from the action of initiating movement with the lifting of your right foot? How does lifting your left foot feel in your leg, your core? Place your left foot on the ground and notice the nature of the contact of your foot on the ground.

Commence a slow and steady pace that allows you to notice each and every step as you lift, propel, and place each foot. For a period of time, keep your awareness on the stepping aspects of walking. Be very curious about any changes in your steps. Perhaps you turn a corner or avoid a small rock. What does that feel like in your body? Does your pace change? Does your breath stop? Notice your feet in your shoes and the sensation of the foot, to shoe, to ground. How does the wearing of shoes feel as you walk? Do you notice qualities of the shoe?

As you walk, bring your awareness to your breath. Your body is a system. Your breath fuels your walking as oxygen is sent to the muscles in your body to propel you. Notice the rhythm of your steps, your breath, your heartbeat. Notice the synchrony of your body as it moves step by step. Expand your awareness to your whole body. Feel your body move through space as you breathe and take step after step. Feel the air on your skin as you move forward.

Be mindfully aware of any thoughts or feelings that may be arising as mental events. Simply notice them and bring your awareness back to your feet and the aspects of each step, the lifting, the moving the foot forward, and the placing to your foot on the ground.

Once you have reached your allotted time for walking meditation, return to your point of origin. Place your feet hip-distance apart, with your hands at your sides, soften your shoulders, and neutralize your chin. Take a moment to offer gratitude for your feet, your body, your breath, and your heart. Offer gratitude for your awareness during your walking meditation and the insight brought to you by your practice.

Source: Davis et al., 2008; Hanson and Mendius, 2009; Kabat-Zinn, 2013; Shapiro and Carlson, 2009; Stahl and Goldstein, 2010.

Loving-Kindness Meditation

Practice Script 5.8, Loving-Kindness Meditation, or Metta, brings a focus to loving-kindness, helps reduce resistance, and enhances presence, especially with difficult people in our lives and in the lives of our patients. It helps us dissolve barriers that can build up in our minds, such as self-centeredness, resentment, bitterness, and anger (Stahl & Goldstein, 2010). Neurologically, practice of the Loving-Kindness Meditation can help activate our social and self-engagement system, bringing a valance of compassion and kindness toward self and others into our choices and actions (Siegel, 2010). Instructional Story 5.3 highlights the history of the Loving-Kindness Meditation.

INSTRUCTIONAL STORY 5.3: The Monks and the Haunted Forest

Stahl and Goldstein (2010) explain that the history of the Loving-Kindness Meditation goes back more than 2,500 years. They tell a story of several monks who left the Buddha on a spiritual quest (Stahl & Goldstein, 2010). This story is inspired by their story.

In the middle of a beautiful, clear summer, a group of mindfulness students, inspired by the tales of the past, traveled together toward a remote forest location in Western New York. Encouraged by their teacher, they intended to practice for a period of time in order to deepen their insights. Far into a Western New York forest, the students set up camp and began to practice. They had state-of-the-art tents, canteens for their water, sitting pillows, and mala beads. They were settled in and ready for a long, fruitful practice. However, all was not peaceful. The mindfulness students began to notice strange sounds and hear scary noises. They had been told of the spiritual history of Western New York. There are vast stretches of land called the burned-over district, an area known for the Second Great Awakening and connections to the great reform movements in abolition, women's rights, and utopian society. This is why they chose this spot for their spiritual awakening. Perhaps this place was haunted in some way.

When they were not looking, their supplies and belongings were rummaged through, scattered, and some things went missing. At first students thought, "Maybe this is someone playing a trick, a scary prank?" Yet, the sounds and disturbance of their things continued with seemingly no explanation. One student thought she saw a great blue heron flying off with some of their food clutched in his feet. She told the others that he seemed angry. Concerned, they began to realize that perhaps they had disturbed the forest or the spirits somehow. Maybe they were not even safe. With an aggregated sense of worry that had evolved into fear, they folded up camp and rushed back to their spiritual teacher. Their teacher reminded them of the old story of Buddha and the monks. She explained how the monks had experienced the same fearful disruptions on their spiritual quest.

She explained that upon the return of the rattled and fearful monks, the Buddha asked them, "Why have you returned? Have you finished your quest for insight so soon?" The monks told their teacher that the forest was haunted and that they believed that the evil spirits were out to get them. They told the Buddha that there was simply no way they could meditate with that level of disturbance. The Buddha knew that what they needed was an antidote to fear. Accordingly, he taught them the Loving-Kindness Meditation. The monks practiced the meditation on their cushions. When they were ready, they headed back to the forest, returning to their quest for insight and facing their fears with loving-kindness. During their journey and upon arrival they continued the Loving-Kindness Meditation, sending loving-kindness to the spirits.

When they arrived at the destination, the spirits were there—transformed. It seems as though the loving-kindness the monks offered had a transformative influence. The sprits were of light, beauty, and support for the monks. The spirits welcomed the monks. They even washed their feet after the long journey. Then, with joy and warmth, the spirits made a feast and the monks and the spirits dined together. The monks were able to practice their meditation and the forest, once scary, was now the ideal setting for practice. A welcoming retreat, the forest became the monks' new home. And so it was, the spirits and the monks shared the forest and loving-kindness with each other. They found the Loving-Kindness Meditation so powerful that they practiced for all those who lived in the forest, all who lived beyond the forest, and all living things everywhere. Time passed and they practiced. More time passed and they practiced. Surrounded by the overwhelming beauty of their practice, enlightenment came to the monks and the spirits and love and kindness radiated gloriously from the forest.

The mindfulness students were inspired by their teacher's story of Buddha and the monks. Cars still packed, they headed back to the deep woods of Western New York. They set their tents up and meditated on loving-kindness for the rich spiritual history of the area, for the animals that thrived there, and especially for the herons. They were never sure exactly what changed; yet, for the rest of their trip they were visited by great blue herons, black-crowned night herons, little blue herons, and even a green heron. The herons dropped gifts of flowers, clumps of moss, and small branches near their tents as if to help the students build nests. Each day, one or two herons stood quietly at watch at the edge of the water near the camping grounds. In turn the students left small fish in a basin near the water for the herons to eat. In this way, the herons and the students took care of each other. The mindfulness students felt safe and protected as they meditated for many peaceful nights. With their loving-kindness practice, things seemed to have changed. Where there was fear, now there was love.

Source: Siegel, 2010; Stahl and Goldstein, 2010; Wallace, 2011.

Many of my patients have difficult people in their lives. Linehan (1993) theorizes that dysregulation, in part, comes from an invalidating environment (see Chapter 2). That is, there are important people in a person's life who neglect, ignore, or otherwise invalidate the person's emotional experience, talent, or sense of self. Much time and energy can be ineffectively spent in reaction to people in our lives who don't behave in the ways in which we would like them to behave (Wallace, 2011). The Loving-Kindness Meditation helps to shift the focus away from the unproductive, or triggering, feeling states and allow a return to present-moment awareness and experience (Wallace, 2011). It can bring people toward a sense of connectedness. Hutcherson, Seppala, and Gross (2008) found that a brief practice of the Loving-Kindness Meditation, compared with a closely matched control task, significantly increased feelings of social connection and positivity toward novel individuals on both explicit and implicit levels. Claire likes to use the meditation when she is thinking about her father, stepmother, and their deference toward what Claire calls "the new family." It helps her move out of feeling states that used to be a trigger for her self-harm.

PRACTICE SCRIPT 5.8: Loving-Kindness Meditation

Approximate Timing: 2 Minutes for Introduction; 20 Minutes for Practice

Start with the Getting Seated for Meditation Script. Cultivate the qualities of relaxation, stillness, and vigilance. Grounded in your seat, bring your awareness to your breath. Breathe deeply, inhaling and exhaling. Cultivate a sense of bare attention, passive awareness, and simple attentiveness. Begin to expand your awareness to encompass your whole body. Imagine that you are surrounded by a sphere of loving-kindness and you are at the very center. Imagine that the sphere is like a mother holding a beloved infant with care, warmth, and abounding love. This is the nature of the sphere that is around you now. As you sit within the sphere of loving-kindness, say these words:

May I be happy.
May I be well.
May I be safe.
May I be peaceful and at ease.

Once you have finished, bring your awareness back to your breath, to your whole body, and then out to the sphere. Breathe easily.

Now, bring to mind a dear friend or someone who has shown you great love and kindness. Imagine that the sphere of loving-kindness that surrounds you now is expanding to include your friend or loved one. Breathe and visualize, you, your loved one, and the sphere of loving-kindness. Repeat these words:

May you be happy.
May you be well.
May you be safe.
May you be peaceful and at ease.

Now bring to mind a friend or neighbor, somebody whom you feel a warmth and kindness toward. This can be someone from your daily travels, the person who lives next door to you, or your yoga teacher. It can be anyone you choose. Breathe and visualize, you, your loved one, and your friend or neighbor within the sphere of loving-kindness. Repeat these words:

May you be happy.
May you be well.
May you be safe.
May you be peaceful and at ease.

Now, think of someone whom you feel very neutral about. It may be someone in your life with whom you interact, yet have no feelings, good or bad, associated with this person. Maybe it is the person who serves your coffee or tea at the shop in your town or city. Maybe it is someone at the bus stop some mornings. Hold this person in your awareness. Breathe and visualize, you, your loved one, your friend or neighbor, and the neutral person within the sphere of loving-kindness. Repeat these words:

> *May you be happy.*
> *May you be well.*
> *May you be safe.*
> *May you be peaceful and at ease.*

Now, bring to mind someone with whom you struggle. Perhaps it is someone close to you, in your family, or someone at work. Bring that person to mind. Breathe and visualize, you, your loved one, your friend or neighbor, the neutral person, and the difficult person within the sphere of loving-kindness. Repeat these words:

> *May you be happy.*
> *May you be well.*
> *May you be safe.*
> *May you be peaceful and at ease.*

Now, as the monks did in the time of Buddha, it is time to expand your loving-kindness to all beings everywhere. Bring to mind those who are hungry, cold, tired, and impoverished, as well as those who have great wealth and abundance. Bring to mind beings that are sick and those who have great health. Bring to mind all beings in your town, city, state, and nation. Bring to mind all beings across the world, those who are here, those yet to be born, and those who have passed. Bring to mind all beings everywhere. Breathe and visualize, you, your loved one, your friend or neighbor, the neutral person, the difficult person, and all beings everywhere within the sphere of loving-kindness. Repeat these words:

> *May all beings be happy.*
> *May all beings be well.*
> *May all beings be safe.*
> *May all beings be peaceful and at ease.*

Feel the radiating love and kindness as you breathe. Feel the expansiveness of your sphere and the possible connections with all beings. Slowly bring your awareness back to your breath and your body. When you are ready, rub your hands together, warming them gently. Raise your hands to your eyes and slowly open your eyes into the palms of your hands. When you are ready, rest your hands on your thighs, eyes open, breath steady.

Source: Hanson and Mendius, 2009; Metta Institute, 2015; Shapiro and Carlson, 2009; Siegel, 2010; Stahl and Goldstein, 2010; Wallace, 2011.

The Five Remembrances

In his book, *Understanding Our Mind,* Thich Nhat Hanh (2006) describes the Five Remembrances, one of the Buddha's teachings. These are to be practiced each day, to center and ground your mindfulness. I use the Five Remembrances with patients who experience significant anxiety, emotional sensitivity, tendency toward escape or avoidance, and trouble with distress tolerance. The Five Remembrances ask you to be present to the truths of living as a human being. In this way, the day begins by honoring acceptance, truth, and uncomfortable feelings. Especially for those with addictive, self-regulatory challenges, the Five Remembrances (Practice Script 5.8) meditation begins the day with bare awareness and presence to those things that, as humans, we all want to avoid. Hence, this practice is an antidote to avoidance and aversion. See also the discussions in Chapter 3 of embodied practice 1, be mindfully aware; embodied practice 2, honor your breath and your physical experience; embodied practice 4, accept impermanence; and embodied practice 5, cultivate nonattachment.

PRACTICE SCRIPT 5.8: The Five Remembrances
Approximate Timing: 1 Minute for Introduction; 5 Minutes for Practice

---

Begin with the Getting Seated for Meditation Script. Steady your breath and become present to your breathing. This is your baseline breath. When you are ready, recite these phrases, one at a time, to yourself. Notice sensations, thoughts, and feelings as they arise. If thoughts, sensations, and feelings become intense, pause and breathe until you feel you have returned to your baseline breath.

- *I am of the nature to grow old. There is no way to escape growing old.*

Notice any sensations, thoughts, and feelings as they arise and pass away. If thoughts, sensations, and feelings become intense, pause and breathe until you feel you have returned to your baseline breath. When you are ready, move to the next remembrance.

- *I am of the nature to have ill health. There is no way to escape having ill health.*

Again, notice sensations, thoughts, and feeling as they arise and pass away. If any of these thoughts, sensations, and feelings becomes too intense, pause and breathe until you feel you have returned to your baseline breath.

- *I am of the nature to die. There is no way to escape death.*

Now, be present to any sensations, thoughts, and feelings. Notice the arising and passing away. If thoughts, sensations, or feelings become intense, pause and breathe until you feel you have returned to your baseline breath.

- *All that is dear to me and everyone I love are of the nature to change. There is no way to escape being separated from them.*

Notice sensations, thoughts, and feelings as they arise. If thoughts, sensations, and feelings become intense, pause and breathe until you feel you have returned to your baseline breath and your mind has stilled.

- *My actions are my only true belongings. I cannot escape the consequences of my actions. My actions are the ground on which I stand.*

Become present to any sensations, thoughts, and feelings as they arise and pass away. Breathe here, continuously bringing your awareness back to your breath. Once you have returned to your baseline breath, bring your palms together in front of your heart. Cultivate gratitude for your strength, awareness, breath, and any insights this practice has given you. When you are ready, slowly bring your hands together and rub your palms together to warm them. Bring the palms of your hands to your eyes; open your eyes into the palms of your hands, slowly bringing your hands to your lap.

A Day of Mindfulness

I chose to end this chapter with a practice that was described by Thich Nhat Hanh (1975) in his book *The Miracle of Mindfulness: An Introduction to the Practice of Meditation*. It falls somewhere between on-the-cushion (i.e., formal) and off-the-cushion (informal) practices. As such, it makes for a nice transition from this chapter to Chapter 6, Off the Cushion: Informal Mindfulness Practices.

Begin by selecting your day of mindfulness in advance. Choose a day that you can be free of commitments from the time you awake until the time you go to sleep. You may need to travel. For some it may be necessary to stay away from your home in order to be free of responsibilities. I encourage patients who do not have money for a hotel room or retreat to offer their services house sitting for a friend. In this way, you get a novel location and time alone to cultivate your practice. The night before your day of mindfulness, straighten the house and prepare for your day. You may choose to prepare whole, light foods in advance, or gather the food needed to make healthy blender drinks or juices. Go to bed well hydrated and free of alcohol or other substances.

Wake up naturally when your body is ready. Do not set an alarm. When you awake, begin by setting an intention to engage in every movement during the day at least two times slower than usual. Your first task is to take a slow-motion bath (see Chapter 6). After your bath, prepare and drink tea. During this time, engage in the reading of spiritual texts or write letters to loved ones. Take this time to cultivate a sense of tranquil reflection and contemplation. Hanh (1975) guides that when maintaining mindfulness during reading of texts and writing of letters, "Don't let the text or letter pull you away to somewhere else" (p. 88). Be present to what you are reading. Approach your reading as if it was meditation, noticing what is arising and passing away as you read. Similarly, approach your writing as if it was meditation, noticing any sense impressions, mental events, or feeling tones that arise and pass away as you write.

Next, take a mindful walk, practicing awareness of breath. Choose a peaceful location where you can be free from distractions. Walk for 45 to 60 minutes. You can follow your walk with a meditation practice. Sit for 5 to 30 minutes. Then, mindfully prepare a meal. When you eat your meal, practice informal mindful eating (see Chapter 6). After your meal you may choose to take a light rest or read.

In the late afternoon, take another walk for 45 to 60 minutes. As before, be aware of your breath. If you'd like you can make this walk a Walking Meditation (discussed earlier in the chapter). Follow your walk with another meditation practice for 5 to 30 minutes. Then, mindfully prepare a light meal and eat with mindfulness. As you prepare for bed, practice a body scan. You may wish to use a recorded relaxation. End your day with gratitude. You may choose to write your feelings of gratitude in a journal (see Chapter 6). As you prepare for sleep, feel your body in your bed, feel the covers on your body, and bring your awareness to your breath.

SUMMARY

On-the-cushion mindfulness practices offer a structured way to cultivate insight. There are both insight- and concentration-based meditations. All meditations have the capacity to bring insight through practice. Specifically, mindfulness practices can help cultivate self-regulation. Through practice we become aware that both internal and external experiences affect us. The awareness of sense impressions, mental events, and the associated feeling tones provides an opportunity to shift *out* of habitual ways of thinking and acting and *into* choice. That is, as your patients notice the ways in which they are triggered and practice allowing these sensations and mental events to arise and pass away without attaching to or avoiding them, they are empowered to choose a response that serves their emotional and relational health. These steps are laid out, as are several scripts and instructional stories for practice. Finally, Figure 5.5 is provided as a means for helping you and your patients explore and track growth and insight. For those of you who would like to read a very accessible book on the Buddha's teachings, I recommend *The Heart of Buddha's Teachings: Transforming Suffering into Peace, Joy, and Liberation* by Thich Nhat Hanh (1998).

REFERENCES

Bien, T. (2006). *Mindful therapy: A guide for therapists and helping professionals.* Boston, MA: Wisdom Productions.

Buddha. (n.d.). Anguttara Nikaya: The further-factored discourses. In Access to Insight (Ed.), *Access to Insight (Legacy Edition),* December 21, 2013. Retrieved from http://www.accesstoinsight.org/tipitaka/an/index.html

Davis, M., Eshelman, E. R., & McKay, M. (2008). *The relaxation and stress reduction workbook* (6th ed.). Oakland, CA: The Harbinger Publications.

Epstein, M. (2001). *Going on being—Buddhism and the way of change: A positive psychology for the West.* New York, NY: Harmony/The Crown Publishing Group.

Grabovac, A. D., Lau, M. A., & Willett, B. R. (2011). Mechanisms of mindfulness: A Buddhist psychological model. *Mindfulness.* doi: 10.1007/s12671-011-0054-5

Hanh, T. N. (1975). *The miracle of mindfulness: An introduction to the practice of meditation.* Boston, MA: Beacon Press.

Hanh, T. N. (1998). *The heart of Buddha's teaching: Transforming suffering into peace, joy, and liberation.* New York, NY: Broadway Books.

Hanh, T. N. (2006) *Understanding our mind.* Berkeley, CA: Parallax.

Hanson, R., & Mendius, R. (2009). *Buddha's brain: The practical neuroscience of happiness, love, and wisdom.* Oakland, CA: New Harbinger Publications.

Hutcherson, C. A., Seppala, E. M., & Gross, J. J. (2008). Loving-kindness meditation increases social connectedness. *Emotion, 8,* 720–724.

Kabat-Zinn, J. (2013). *Full catastrophe living, revised edition: How to cope with stress, pain and illness using mindfulness meditation.* New York, NY: Bantam Books.

Linehan, M. M. (1993). *Cognitive-behavioral treatment of borderline personality disorder.* New York, NY: Guilford Press.

Marlatt, G. A., Bower, S., & Lustyk, M. K. B. (2012). Substance abuse and relapse prevention. In C. K. Germer & R. D. Siegel (Eds.), *Wisdom and compassion in psychotherapy: Deepening mindfulness in clinical practice.* New York: NY: Guilford Press.

McCown, D., Reibel, D., & Micozzi, M. S. (2010). *Teaching mindfulness: A practical guide for clinicians and educators.* New York, NY: Springer.

Metta Institute. (2015). *Metta meditation.* Retrieved from www.mettainstitute.org/mettameditation.html

Shapiro, S. L., & Carlson, L. E. (2009). *The art and science of mindfulness: Integrating mindfulness into psychology and the helping professions.* Washington, DC: American Psychological Association.

Siegel, D. J. (2010). *The mindful therapist: A clinician's guide to mindsight and neural integration.* New York, NY: W. W. Norton.

Stahl, B., & Goldstein, E. (2010). *A mindfulness-based stress reduction workbook.* Oakland, CA: New Harbinger Press.

The Buddha. (n.d.). Adapted from *The book of the gradual sayings (Anguttara-Nikaya): or, More-numbered suttas.* (2001). Oxford, UK: Pali Text Society.

Wallace, B. A. (2011). *Minding closely: The four applications of mindfulness.* Ithaca, NY: Snow Lion Publications.

Wanden-Berghe, R. G., Sanz-Valero, J., & Wanden-Berghe, C. (2011). The application of mindfulness to eating disorders treatment: A systematic review. *Eating Disorders: The Journal of Treatment and Prevention, 19,* 34–48.

Williams, A. D., & Grisham, J. R. (2012). Impulsivity, emotional regulation, and mindful attentional focus in compulsive buying. *Cognitive Theory and Research, 36,* 451–457.

Witkiewitz, K., & Bowen, S. (2010). Depression, craving, and substance use following a randomized trial of mindfulness-based relapse prevention. *Journal of Counseling and Clinical Psychology, 78,* 362–374.

Wupperman, P., Fickling, M., Klemanski, D. H., Berking, M., & Whitman, J. B. (2013). Borderline personality features and harmful dysregulated behavior: The mediation effect of mindfulness. *Journal of Clinical Psychology, 69,* 903–911.

ᘓ 6 ᘔ

Off the Cushion
Informal Mindfulness Practices

Autobiography in Five Short Chapters

Chapter I
*I walk down the street. There is a deep hole in the sidewalk. I fall in. I am
lost . . . I am hopeless. It isn't my fault. It takes forever to find a way out.*

Chapter II
*I walk down the same street. There is a deep hole in the sidewalk. I pretend
I don't see it. I fall in again. I can't believe I am in this same place. But it isn't
my fault. It still takes a long time to get out.*

Chapter III
I walk down the same street. There is a deep hole in the sidewalk. <u>I see it
there.</u> *I still fall in . . . it's a habit . . . but, my eyes are open. I know where
I am. It is my fault. I get out immediately.*

Chapter IV
I walk down the same street. There is a deep hole in the sidewalk. <u>I walk
around it.</u>

Chapter V
I walk down another street.

—PORTIA NELSON (1993; EMPHASIS ADDED)

INFORMAL MINDFULNESS PRACTICES

Informal mindful practices are defined as the bringing of mindful awareness to daily activities (Kabat-Zinn, 2013; Stahl & Goldstein, 2010). The chapter-opening poem by Portia Nelson illustrates the power

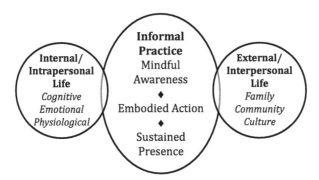

FIGURE 6.1 Informal practice as the embodied expression of self.

of awareness (i.e., "I see it there") and embodied practice (i.e., "I walk around it"). When asked, "How are we to practice mindfulness?" Thich Nhat Hanh answered, "Keep your attention focused on the work, be alert and ready to handle ably and intelligently any situation which may arise—this is mindfulness" (1975, p. 14). *Mindful awareness* comes first (Figure 6.1; see also embodied practice 1, be mindfully aware, in Chapter 3). Next, *embodied action* through formal practices begins and creates change. Embodied practice is the walking-down-another-street part of the process. Finally, informal practices create a *sustained presence* that helps to maintain the change manifest through formal practice and prevents relapse by reducing risk. Sustained presence is cultivated through the thoughts and attitudes you bring to your day as well as the way in which you complete activities.

Informal mindful practices help keep the waters of awareness clear (Bien, 2006). When we live in chaotic patterns, disconnected from our psychological and emotional selves, failing to address needs and tensions in our relationships, and disconnected from our communities, we are like rough waters in a mountain lake (Bien, 2006). If you look into the lake, you see the choppy waves and there is no clear reflection of the self and images are distorted and disjointed. When the water settles, the surface becomes as smooth as glass. Still water reflects clearly, without distortion (Bien, 2006). This is the type of sustained presence that mindfulness cultivates. In service of this intention toward stillness and clarity of mind, this chapter provides methodology for informal mindfulness techniques. The first section of this chapter addresses the cultivation of thought processes and attitudes such as being in inquiry; cultivating thoughts, feelings, and actions that serve you; and gratitude. The second section provides instruction for and examples of informal practices.

THOUGHTS AND ATTITUDES THAT CULTIVATE
AND SUPPORT MINDFUL AWARENESS

Informal mindful practices are the cultivating of a mindful way of being throughout the day. Who you and your patients are and who you and your patients are becoming depends on the daily construction and maintenance of a platform for this new way of being in the world. This platform provides the sustained presence that allows for maintenance of change and continued growth.

Inquiry

Embodied practice 3, live in inquiry (see Chapter 3), captures a critical aspect of informal mindful practices. Training in and internalization of such practices are critical. For patients with addictions, self-regulation difficulties, and compulsive behavioral struggles (e.g., eating disorders, gambling, compulsive Internet use, and shopping addiction), living in presence and inquiry can be a critical aspect of getting and staying sober and well (Marlatt, Bowen, & Lustyk, 2012). Recall the Attuned Representational Model of Self (ARMS; see Chapter 1) and the ongoing tensions and attunements that move through the internal and the external aspects of self. It can be a challenge to recover and maintain recovery without effective, daily tools. Reminiscent of the ARMS model, Figure 6.1 illustrates the experience of self through the perspective of informal practice in the embodied expression of self.

Sustaining presence and mindfulness within the context of intra- and interpersonal challenges can be difficult (Brach, 2012). Tara Brach (2012) describes RAIN, a methodology for cultivating compassion and wisdom in difficult weather. Created by Buddhist teachers, this mindfulness tool provides support for working with challenging states of mind and cultivating presence, compassion, and wisdom (Brach, 2012). It is an acronym to help trigger mindful presence and inquiry during your current situation, whatever it may be. According to Brach (2012), RAIN stands for: "Recognize what is happening, Allow life to be just as it is, Investigate inner experience with kindness, Nonidentification [and] rest in Natural awareness" (p. 40; Figure 6.2). Brach (2012) refers to steps 1 and 2 (i.e., recognizing and allowing) as the basic components of mindfulness. She describes the last two components as opportunities for deeper insight.

Asher is a 24-year-old computer programmer. He works as a software designer for a large company and makes a good living. When he was 7 years old, he was given his first hand-held video game and he loved it.

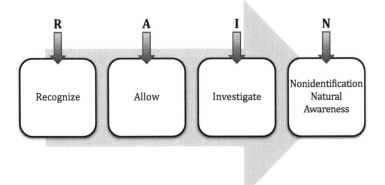

FIGURE 6.2 The RAIN process.

Each birthday, holiday, and day that involved the possibility of a gift, he asked for video game products. By the time he was in high school he had two different gaming systems and was helping his parents pay for a high-speed Internet connection for his gaming. His parents were supportive because they were very proud of his computer skills and his developing programming competency. They saw his gaming behavior as part of a larger, positive trajectory toward a career with technology.

Now at 24 years old, he is ready to admit he might have a problem. A friend of his told him about a young woman who was interested in him. Asher hasn't dated much, even through college. In fact, he has a negligible social life outside of work and gaming. He set up a date with her. The day of the date, he sat down to play a game to take the edge off of his anxiety. Three hours in, he still couldn't stop. His friend had texted him many times asking why he did not show up for the date. The young lady refused to reply to Asher's apology texts that he sent the next day. Angry and frustrated, his friend told him to get help.

Asher's difficulties include an avoidance of face-to-face interpersonal experiences. He sidesteps these experiences in an effort to avoid the anxiety he feels when interacting with others. He also has a very compulsive use of gaming motivated, in part, by the pursuit of the pleasant feelings he feels when he is winning and the avoidance of uncomfortable emotions such as loneliness, sadness, and frustration. In therapy, Asher has set goals for reducing computer gaming time, increasing interpersonal experiences, scheduling pleasant events with people, experiencing and tolerating his emotions without the need to attach or avoid, and having a better sense of when he might be at risk for what he calls, "getting lost in the game." He uses RAIN to help him notice when he is at risk.

Recognizing What Is Happening

Recognizing involves mindful awareness, presence, and attention to what is happening right now in your internal experience (i.e., mental events, sense impressions, thoughts or emotions). It involves a noticing of what is arising. This presence can be awakened by asking yourself, "What is happening inside me right now?" (Brach, 2012, p. 40). This is done without judgment and with an attitude of inquiry and curiosity. For example, Asher checks in three times a day (e.g., just before or after mealtimes as a cue to remember). He asks himself what he is experiencing inside at the present moment. When he first started he kept a RAIN journal in order to have a better sense of what his patterns might be. Beyond the three check-ins, Asher also checks in when he notices the arising of an emotion. These instances were also tracked in his journal (Figure 6.3). Asher noticed that he was often unaware of his emotions. However, when he checked in, he could feel a sense of anxiety in his belly and an ongoing script of worries running through his head.

Allowing Life to Be Just as It Is

Once you have checked in and asked yourself what is going on intrapersonally, the next task is to allow what is to simply be (Brach, 2012). This includes mental events, sense impressions, emotions, and thoughts. You ask yourself, "Can I let this be just as it is?" (Brach, 2012, p. 40). As in the work with the Buddhist Psychological Model (BPM; Grabovac, Lau, & Willett, 2011), you notice the feeling tone and any natural sense of attachment or aversion to what you are allowing to let be. Development of the

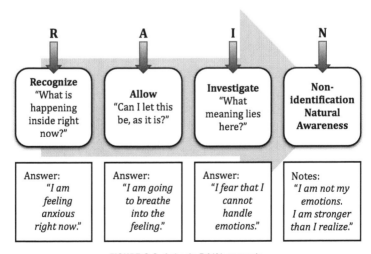

FIGURE 6.3 Asher's RAIN example.

skill, the mindful competency, to allow what is with nonjudgment (see embodied practice 7, allow what is with nonjudgment) facilitates freedom of choice and the ability to stay in your intention no matter the circumstances (Brach, 2012).

For Asher, this is one of the hardest parts of practicing RAIN. When he makes it through this step, he very often experiences success in the other two (i.e., I and N). In therapy, he has had to cultivate a solid breathing practice to help him be present to what is, especially the emotions and, principally, his anxiety. Notably, Asher finds most emotions unpleasant. He experiences emotions as being overwhelming and has tried to avoid them since he was little. In therapy, he has gained insight into the possibility that his video game interests evolved along with his efforts to not feel any feelings at all, ever. At this point, he has learned to stay with the emotions he is feeling for as long as he needs to for them to arise and pass away. He has noticed that his emotions move through him more quickly than he imagines. In fact, some feelings, the very feelings that used to drive him into 2 or 3 hours of video gaming, only last 2 or 3 minutes when he mindfully breathes into them.

Investigating With Kindness

After recognition and allowing comes the opportunity to investigate what is happening. Brach (2012) suggests that this step is especially suited for the therapeutic relationship. It involves asking questions such as "How am I experiencing this in my body?" "What does this feeling want from me?" "What am I believing about myself?" or "What does this mean for me?" (Brach, 2012, p. 42). This line of inquiry goes beyond a noticing and allowing and digs into our personal narrative, the truths or untruths that we hold about others and ourselves. Through this step, we can get ourselves and our patients closer to the truth and the authentic experience of self.

Asher came to therapy with a journal of his RAIN practice. He decided to free-associate this part of the process. That is, he asked himself, "What does this mean for me?" Then, he wrote anything and everything that came to mind. As he looked over the week of journal records, he noticed that he kept coming back to two firm beliefs. First, he held the belief that he could not handle emotions. Second, he believed that if people knew him, really knew him, they would never like him. Most certainly, they would never love him. Some of his entries documented beliefs like "I will never be able to handle my feelings," "Things are better when I feel nothing at all," and "I am afraid that if I let anyone know me, they won't like what they see." He explained that it was different when he played games. He said that he could create whatever he wanted as an avatar or image on the video games. He said that who he was in there, in the game, was a brave, strong, powerful, and aggressive man. Here, in his body, he was afraid and insecure. This was the first time he cried in therapy.

Interestingly, over the weeks and then months of this practice, his answers to this question began to change. He noticed things like "Intense anxious feelings seem to only last a few moments when I breathe into them," and "I am getting better at being with my feelings." Asher's practice was starting to shift his sense of himself. Also, his investigation of this process was bringing him an awareness of and presence to his growth. He was shifting from shame and self-aversion to self-compassion and self-love (Brach, 2012).

Realize Nonidentification: Rest in Natural Awareness

Brach (2012) explains that nonidentification means that your "self-sense is not fused with, or defined by, any limited set of emotions, sensations, or stories about who you are" (p. 44). Nonidentification leads to a natural awareness of simply being. In mindful and yogic philosophy, the self is conceptualized as the ego self (i.e., lowercase "s" self) and the soul Self (i.e., uppercase "s" Self). The ego self is interested in "I" and "I am . . .," whereas the soul Self is interested in experiencing and being. In essence, the uppercase "s" soul Self is a verb. In this step of RAIN, there is a realization of this type of being.

Asher had been so tied up in developing who he was for his games that he had an exaggerated sense of his gaming identity (i.e., ego self) and its role in his well-being. Essentially, Asher believed that if he could not be the muscle-bound conqueror of all things evil, no one would be interested in him. The truth is that Asher is a fascinating young man. He is bright, with a tremendous imagination and a wonderful sense of humor. All of these aspects of his authentic self are missed when he is "lost in the game." As he used RAIN to increase his presence, awareness, and tolerance of his feelings, and to learn a little about who he really is, he has come to recognize that he is someone with whom others would like to spend time. He jokes that he seems to be starting to like himself: "The real flesh-and-bones Asher is sort of a good guy." Arguably, RAIN is a wonderful methodology for structuring the process of living in inquiry as an attitude or intention to bring into your daily life. Associated embodied practices (see Chapter 3) are as follows: (1) be mindfully aware, (2) honor your breath and your physical experience, (3) live in inquiry, (4) accept impermanence, (5) cultivate nonattachment, (6) discern what is not-self, and (7) allow what is with nonjudgment.

Cultivating Thoughts, Feelings, and Actions That Serve You

Astrachan-Fletcher and Maslar (2009) describe Morita Therapy (see Morita, Morita, Kondo, & LeVine, 1998), in which patients are guided to act with purpose regardless of the automatic thoughts, feelings, and sensations that arise. They suggest that a good purpose is "to create a life worth being present in" (p. 22). In their workbook for patients with bulimia nervosa, they created a Modified Morita Table that I use regularly with my patients. I find it so effective that I teach it to psychologists-in-training at the University at Buffalo. The table divides experiences up into two types: controllable and uncontrollable.

Experiences that are considered uncontrollable include automatic thoughts, feelings, and sensations. Consistent with mindfulness teachings, patients are asked to accept their automatic thoughts, feelings, and sensations and the notion that they are not within their control. Additionally, I explain to patients that they can watch these automatic thoughts, feelings, and sensations arise and pass away and then let them go. There is no need or reason to keep them. Controllable experiences include conscious and deliberate thoughts (e.g., intentions and plans) and actions. Astrachan-Fletcher and Maslar (2009) encourage patients to act for their purpose (i.e., creating a life in which you would like to be present). In this clear and simple way, the thoughts, feelings, and actions that we do—or do not—want to cultivate are made distinct by this simple rule of thumb: Does this serve my life purpose? Does it help me create a life in which I wish to be present? I use a rather silly story to help patients understand the Morita Table. I believe it is the silliness of the story that helps patients see the silliness in cultivating thoughts that don't serve them. See Instructional Story 6.1, "The Ice Cream Sandwich Wrapper."

INSTRUCTIONAL STORY 6.1: The Ice Cream Sandwich Wrapper

Imagine that you are standing in a park on a hot summer day. There is a cart near you selling ice cream sandwiches. People have been eating ice cream sandwiches all day and the garbage can is full. Some of the wrappers have fallen out and are now blowing in the wind. One of the wrappers blows into your leg and sticks to your skin. Do you stand there and think, "Oh well, this is the way it is going to be. I now have an ice cream sandwich wrapper stuck to my leg for the rest of my life"? No, of course not. That would be silly. You look down. You see clearly that the ice cream sandwich wrapper is garbage and not part of what you want on your leg. Knowing this, you peel it off of your leg and throw it away. Done.

Your automatic thoughts, feelings, and sensations are this way. There are things people have told you during your life, messages you have heard in the media, perhaps even things you have told yourself, that do not serve your life purpose. There are feelings and sensations that don't serve you to cultivate. How do you know which ones are which? You ask yourself, "Does this thought, feeling, or sensation help me to create a life in which I want to be present?" If your answer is "No," see it for what it is—"garbage" or "not self"—and then let it go. Shift your energy to cultivating thoughts and actions that serve you, that work toward your life purpose.

Hanson and Mendius (2009) refer to a similar process they call "pulling weeds, planting flowers" (p. 73). They suggest that you can gradually replace negative implicit memories with positive ones by cultivating a practice of making the positive aspect of your experience prominent in your awareness. In this manner, the negative aspect of memory and experience is placed in the background and given less attention and energy. Hanson and Mendius (2009) suggest that by planting flowers (i.e., tending to the positive aspects of memory and experience) and pulling weeds (i.e., reducing focus on or cultivating an antidote for the negative), you can help shift how your brain neurologically processes information. Importantly, active effort is required, as the brain has a negative bias for reasons such as self-protection. You and your patients must actively work to heal negative experiences and to internalize the positive ones (Hanson & Mendius, 2009). Associated embodied practices (see Chapter 3) are as follows: (1) be mindfully aware, (6) discern what is not-self, and (7) allow what is with nonjudgment.

Gratitude

Both the RAIN and the Morita methods offer processes that you can apply to your daily living that can help support your mindfulness practice and your daily mindful awareness. Gratitude is one of the overarching qualities that can change the tone or tenor of your day in a positive and helpful way. According to Wood, Froh, and Geraghty (2010), gratitude is an aspect of a broader life orientation that involves noticing and appreciating the positive in the world. It is a thankfulness and an appreciation. Bringing a sense of gratitude to your daily living can help sustain presence and cultivate a positive attitude toward challenges. Wood et al. (2010) submit that gratitude has the potential of improving well-being with the practice of simple exercises. Easy-to-implement gratitude practices include pausing and noticing what one might be grateful for in the moment. For example, Asher pauses after each time he is able to resist an impulse or a trigger to turn to his video gaming rather than face his current life experience. He pauses and offers gratitude for his practice, his strength, and his willingness to stick to the path of recovery. Gratitude practice can include daily journaling, in which each evening the writer records three things for which he or she is grateful before going to sleep. It is a subtle and powerful shift from looking at life as happening to you, toward seeing life as happening for you.

Reviews by Emmons and Stern (2013) and Wood et al. (2010) suggest that gratitude has relevance for clinical practice given its strong, unique, and causal relationship with well-being. Following their review of the literature, Wood et al. (2010) identified several mechanisms that may be involved in the relation between gratitude and well-being. These include schematic biases, coping, positive affect, and broaden-and-build principles. Of note, broaden-and-build emotions (e.g., gratitude, joy, interest, contentment, pride, and love) broaden people's momentary thought-action repertoires and help build enduring resources (e.g., physical, social, and interpersonal resources; Fredrickson, 2001). The associated embodied practices (see Chapter 3) are embodied practice 1, be mindfully aware, and embodied practice 12, cultivate loving-kindness and joy.

Half Smile

The half smile is the second of the overarching qualities that can change the tenor of your day in a positive and helpful way. The half smile is an informal practice that activates the body (i.e., the muscles of the face into a smile), triggering an approach mode in the mind. The half smile is an embodiment practice. Specifically, embodiment in psychological research and theory refers to the idea that the body plays an essential role in emotional, motivational, and cognitive processes (Price, Peterson, & Harmon-Jones, 2012). Price et al.'s (2012) review suggests that there is a growing body of evidence that supports the notion that manipulated facial expressions, among other embodied practices, can influence physiological activity related to approach motivation and may play a role in the cultivation of positive affect.

Hanh (1975) suggests that you bring a half smile to your face when you first wake up. He encourages the use of a sign, a cue, to remind you to bring a half smile to your face. Upon waking, before getting out of bed, curve the corner of your lips upward and take three breaths, inhaling and exhaling gently, maintaining the half smile. Hanh (1975) suggests that when you are sitting, standing, looking at a child, noticing a leaf on a tree or a flower, cultivate a half smile. A half smile can also take the edge off of anger. Hanh (1975) recommends that you half smile the moment that you notice irritation, while inhaling and exhaling quietly.

For example, Kelsey, a 20-year-old college student, is working on her compulsive shopping behavior. As she has worked to understand the triggers for her behavior, she has realized that she has been shopping in an effort to get herself out of a negative mood state. For a year or so, she tried to simply stop shopping. She cut up all of her credit cards and stayed away from the mall and online stores. Yet, with no other tools to handle her mood, she would relapse in days or weeks. Now, she is working hard on self-care (see Chapter 12, Mindful Self-Care), nutrition, exercise, and her yoga practice to stabilize her mood, which is helping a lot. She is also incorporating informal mindfulness techniques to keep her present and moving toward a more positive mood state from the very moment she wakes up. She has placed a message on her phone alarm that tells her, "Wake up, beautiful soul, and don't forget your Buddha half smile. Today is waiting for you." Associated embodied practices (see Chapter 3) are as follows: (1) be mindfully aware and (2) honor your breath and your physical experience.

INFORMAL PRACTICES

Opportunities for informal practice of mindfulness can be found everywhere and at any time. You could be walking in a beautiful garden, taking a bath, doing dishes for over 100 monks, at home getting the children ready for school, at college angry at your roommate, or at the Department of Motor Vehicles waiting in line. These are all chances to practice. Following are a few informal practices that illustrate the opportunity to practice mindfulness anywhere and at any time.

Washing Dishes and Cleaning House

Hanh (1975) described his work doing dishes at the monastery many years ago. There were over 100 monks, cold water, no dish soap, and only ashes and rice and coconut husks to use for scrubbing. The practice was "while washing dishes, one should only be washing dishes" (Hanh, 1975, p. 3). Hahn (1975) spoke of one-mindedness, bare awareness, being in breath, and presence while washing dishes. His mind was centered and steady, and there was no way he could be "tossed around mindlessly like a bottle slapped here and there on the waves" (Hanh, 1975, p. 4).

It may seem insignificant to worry about being mindful when doing these tasks. However, shifting your relationship with these tasks can affect the quality of your life (Kabat-Zinn, 2013). It can be very powerful to intentionally bring an accepting, open, and discerning awareness to whatever you are doing (Kabat-Zinn, 2013; Shapiro & Carlson, 2009). As necessary tasks, these often consume many hours of our weekly schedule. To be ruminating, angry, frustrated, or otherwise struggling while completing these tasks is affecting quality of life. To wash dishes, clean house, or do laundry mindfully, one must do the task mindfully as if each object you are handling is an object of contemplation. Consider each bowl, each item of clothing, or each household item you are dusting as sacred. Follow your breath as you observe the item. Do not try to hurry the job (Hanh, 1975). Consider that washing dishes, doing laundry, or dusting is the most important thing in your life.

I have a personal story to illustrate this informal practice. I grew up the oldest of five children. We were all active, always in one or two sports at a time. My father was in the military and had uniforms to wash as well as his casual clothes. My mother had a 15-year battle with laundry during the peak years of our childhoods and my dad's military service. I somehow internalized her dread of laundry. Doing laundry in college, going to the laundromat, all of that made me miserable. It was that way for many years. During a short reprieve in my graduate school years, a friend and I found a laundromat next to a bar and restaurant. Somehow, those choices seemed better than addressing my discomfort. Still, when my daughters were born the laundry misery set in deep. I had to do something.

When my husband and I were able to buy a house, I decided to become very intentional about the laundry and create a process in which I could be present and at peace. I set up baskets for lights, darks, mediums, and workout-wear. I set up a basket for folding and four baskets on a table, one for each person in my family (me, my husband, and our two daughters). Almost daily, I do a load of laundry. I mindfully take the clothes from the drying machine to the folding basket. I fold each item, placing it mindfully in the appropriate basket. I stay in my breath and notice the texture of the clothes, the fabric, the shape, and the design. I stay present. I no longer experience negative feelings, drink alcohol, or eat when I do laundry. It is part of my daily ritual and brings a sense of peace and accomplishment when I am finished. Associated embodied practices (see Chapter 3) are as follows: (1) be mindfully aware and (2) honor your breath and your physical experience.

Mindful Eating

Thich Nhat Hanh (1975) recalled sharing a tangerine many years ago under a tree with a friend. As they ate they spoke, his friend describing his hopes for the future as he popped section after section of tangerine into his mouth. His friend was so distracted that even though he was vigorously eating tangerine sections, bringing the next section to his mouth before the current section was swallowed, it was as if he was not eating tangerines at all. He had no awareness. Hanh (1975) reminded his friend, "You ought to eat the tangerine section you've already taken" (p. 5).

In Chapter 5, mindful eating was explained as a formal practice that is often used in mindfulness-based stress-reduction (MBSR) programs. Mindful eating can also be an informal practice (Kabat-Zinn, 2013; Stahl & Goldstein, 2010). Because you eat at least three times a day, this practice is one that is easily implemented. Informal mindful eating involves giving your full awareness to the activity of eating. This includes sight, smell, sound, touch, and taste as well as mindful presence. To eat mindfully, meals should be taken free of distraction—no television, laptop, or phone. As with other informal practices, slow down your movement to at least two times as slow as you normally move while eating. Smell your food, look at it, notice the colors and textures, and chew slowly, tasting the food as you eat. Enjoying and contemplating food honors the process of its growth and production and the effort it took to bring the food to your table and then to your mouth. Cultivate curiosity and eat without judgment (Kabat-Zinn, 2013; Stahl & Goldstein, 2010).

Mindful eating practice may be helpful for those in later stages of eating disorder recovery or individuals who are not eating disordered and struggle with food cravings. For example, in a clinical trial Mason et al. (2014) found that increases in mindful eating predicted reductions in consumption of sweets and desserts. Of note, in a preliminary study of mindfulness eating with patients with clinical eating disorders (i.e., anorexia nervosa and bulimia nervosa), researchers found that the eating disorder group reported a significant increase in negative affect after the mindfulness intervention as compared to the distraction intervention (Marek, Ben-Porath, Federici, Wisniewski, & Warren, 2013). Conversely, the nonclinical group reported a significant decrease in negative affect after the mindfulness intervention as compared to the distraction intervention. These preliminary findings suggest that clinicians may want to proceed cautiously when using mindful eating in those with severe eating disorders during the early stages of food exposure (Marek et al., 2013). Mindful eating may be something to work toward or paired with tools for distress tolerance. For more on mindful eating, see *Intuitive Eating: A Revolutionary Program That Works* by Tribole and Resch (2012) and *Eating Mindfully: How to End Mindless Eating and Enjoy a Balanced Relationship with Food* by Albers (2012). I use both of these books with my patients. When working with clients with self-regulation challenges associated with eating, I encourage use of the Intuitive Eating Scale–2 for assessment (Tylka & Kroon Van Diest, 2013). Associated embodied practices (see Chapter 3) are as follows: (1) be mindfully aware, and (2) honor your breath and your physical experience.

Measuring Your Breath by Your Footsteps

Measuring your breathing by your footsteps is similar to a more traditional walking meditation (Hanh, 1975; Kabat-Zinn, 2013; Shapiro &
Carlson, 2009). However, this informal practice can be done any time you
or your patients are walking. Hanh (1975) suggests taking a nice garden
walk; however, you can do this walking to class, on your way into the
office, or going into a shop. Walk slowly and breathe normally. Calculate
the length of your breath by counting the number of steps it takes for you
to inhale completely. Then, count the number of breaths it takes for you
to exhale completely. Continue walking and counting this way for a few
minutes. Do not force or manipulate your breath. Let it be. Next, lengthen
your exhalation by one breath. Do not force your inhalation to change;
just observe it. Notice if it feels as if there is a desire to lengthen it. Continue this way for 10 breaths (Hanh, 1975). Finally, lengthen the exhalation for one more step. Only lengthen the inhalation if it feels like that
will make you happy. Continue this way for 20 breaths. After 20 breaths,
return to normal breathing and walking. Hanh (1975) reports that upon
practice, your breaths will naturally move to even lengths. Associated
embodied practices (see Chapter 3) are as follows: (1) be mindfully aware,
and (2) honor your breath and your physical experience.

Following the Breath

Following the breath is an informal mindful practice that you can do anywhere, at any time. You begin by inhaling and exhaling normally. Notice
the qualities of the breath. On your next inhalation, inhale gently and
normally, being aware and saying to yourself, "I am inhaling normally"
(Hanh, 1975, p. 83). As you exhale mindfully, say to yourself, "I am exhaling normally" (Hanh, 1975, p. 83). Continue this process for three to
four breaths. On the next breath, extend the inhalation with awareness
and intention. Say to yourself, "I am breathing in a long inhalation"
(Hanh, 1975, p. 83). Exhale a long and mindful exhale and say to yourself, "I am breathing out a long exhalation" (Hanh, 1975, p. 83). Continue
this process for three or four breaths. The next step is to begin to follow
your breath from inhalation to exhalation. Be present to the movement
of your body, the rib cage, the lungs, the stomach, the passage of the air
through your nostrils moving in and out. Say to yourself, "I am inhaling and following the inhaling from its beginning to its end. I am exhaling following the exhalation from the beginning to its end" (Hanh, 1975,
p. 83). Continue this for at least 20 breaths. Using your half smile, repeat
as often as you'd like. Associated embodied practices (see Chapter 3) are

as follows: (1) be mindfully aware, and (2) honor your breath and your physical experience.

Mindfulness in Making Tea

Preparing food and drink is an opportunity to be mindful. Abby, a 15-year-old high school student, has adopted this informal practice. She uses her computer as a companion to regulate her mood and manage her anxiety. She struggles to stay focused on her goals and often forgets to do, or avoids doing, her homework. She binge watches movies and YouTube videos, plays in virtual communities, and searches for exotic vacations she can't afford to take. She loses her sense of control, feeling compelled to stay engaged. Her computer behavior has further disconnected her from her family and friends. She spends hours curled up in her bed, unable to stop. She explained that there have been times when she completely forgets about everything else, her body, food, going to the bathroom, friends, her family—everything.

Seems that her homework has piled up to unmanageable levels, her friends are mad at her or have counted her out, and she is afraid that if her parents find out about school they will be very angry. When she is on her computer she doesn't worry about any of that. Of course, all of this has become unbearable and at one point she considered suicide because she was feeling so overwhelmed. She didn't really have a plan. Still, the reality that she had considered it scared her enough that she asked her parents to take her to get help. In therapy, she is working on several strategies to help reduce her computer time and increase her homework, friend, and family time. Finding informal mindful practices that she can integrate throughout her day has helped her to stay in her body and out of the fantasy life she has created on the computer.

Instead of heading right to her room after school and turning on her computer, Abby now carefully and mindfully makes a pot of tea. She puts the boiling water on the stove and gets out the beautiful teapot her parents bought her for her birthday. Abby takes time to notice the filigree on the pot and the texture of the pot as she sets it up. As Hanh (1975) recommends, Abby does each movement slowly, in mindfulness. She does not let one detail in her movement go by without being mindful of it (Hanh, 1975). When she lifts the pot by its handle she notices the bamboo on the handle and how it feels in her fingers. She notices the weight of the cast iron pot. She observes her tea container and the crinkle of the bag as she opens it up. She notices the crunch of the tea leaves and the sound of the spoon as she digs into the tea to take a portion out. She does not feel these sensations when she is on the computer. When she is on her computer, she has left herself. Distinctly, these sounds, touch sensations, visual inputs, and smells are here in her embodied experience.

The water comes to a boil and Abby notices the gradual climbing of the tone of the tea whistle, the instant change in the boil of the water as she lifts the kettle off the stove. She hears the sound of the water as it rushes through the tea filter and into her beautiful teapot. She smells the aroma of her tea, the chai, the green, and pumpkin spice of that day. She watches the steam and comes to her breath as the tea steeps. As Hanh (1975) recommends, she breathes more gently and deeply than she normally breathes. Associated embodied practices (see Chapter 3) are as follows: (1) be mindfully aware, and (2) honor your breath and your physical experience.

Slow-Motion Bath

This informal practice was recommended and described by Hanh (1975). Set aside at least 1 hour to prepare for and take your bath. First, prepare your bath area. Mindfully clean the bathing tub; set up towels and a washcloth. I like to set up a candle or two and play soft meditation music. Do not rush. Move slowly, three times as slow as you normally move (Hanh, 1975). Run your water, being mindfully aware. Notice the water, the shape of the water as it leaves the faucet. Notice the water as it meets the water now collecting in the bath. Listen to the sound of the water as it fills the tub. Smell the water. Maybe you can smell your candle. If you are using bath salts, place those in the water and stir them with your hand and notice the feeling of the water on your fingers. Slowly lower your body into the water, feeling the sensations of the water on your body. Be attentive to each and every movement (Hanh, 1975). Take your bath, using the washcloth, and then soak. "Think of yourself as being in a clean and fragrant lotus pond in the summer" (Hanh, 1975, p. 87). Once you have finished, your mind will feel as peaceful and light as your body (Hanh, 1975). As you dress, follow your breath. Associated embodied practices (see Chapter 3) are as follows: (1) be mindfully aware, and (2) honor your breath and your physical experience.

Addressing Struggles With Distraction

Within the mindfulness tradition, mindful awareness is the primary intention for practice and for daily living. Hanh (1975) described this as the essential discipline. In Buddhist scripture it is said that when you are walking, you must be conscious—"I am walking." When you are sitting, you must be conscious—"I am sitting." When lying down, you must be conscious—"I am lying down." In this manner, one is always aware of the body. However, there are times when it seems as if you cannot focus your mind. You have the desire to be mindfully aware and you know the skills, but still you struggle. As Asher was working to reduce his video game playing, he experienced this struggle often.

Gunaratana (2001) suggests that there are several steps you can take to remedy the mind. First, attempt to ignore the obstacle or distraction. For example, when Asher felt preoccupied with gaming, ignoring simply did not work. He was able to use ignoring for other things, such as a thought about what he was supposed to do later in the day or the dog barking next door during his meditation. Gunaratana (2001) recommends that when ignoring does not work, move to the next step. The second option is to divert the mind to another thing. This might be an object of attention. For example, if you are doing laundry, bring your full awareness to the texture of the clothes. If you are running, bring your awareness to the sound of your feet landing on the road. This worked for Asher sometimes. If the activity was intense in nature, such as running or playing handball, he could bring his focus to the game or to his breath. However, if he was eating dinner or resting, he found that shifting his focus away from gaming to another object of attention was very hard.

If shifting your attention to another object of attention does not work, Gunaratana (2001) suggests that you try reflection on the fact that hindrances arise from many causes and conditions, and these hindrances are in flux. This worked for Asher. His urges, drives, and impulses to play video games did vary. Further, his use of RAIN had helped him to gain competency in watching these fluctuations. He simply watched and breathed into them. Still, for some this option does not work. Gunaratana (2001) offered one last step if this one did not work. He suggested that you clench your teeth, press your tongue against your upper palate, and apply all of your energy toward overcoming the obstacle. Although Asher did not often need to do this, he found it to be a very good way to handle the distress that came along with his desire to play video games as well as with his difficulty tolerating the sensations that went along with some emotions. Associated embodied practices (see Chapter 3) are as follows: (1) be mindfully aware, (2) honor your breath and your physical experience, (4) accept impermanence, and (7) allow what is with nonjudgment.

SUMMARY

This chapter provided a review of informal mindfulness practices as a key support for sustained presence in mindfulness work. Cultivation of supportive thought processes such as RAIN and the Morita method were reviewed as ways to work through daily cognitive and mental challenges and cultivate a mindful attentional set. Gratitude practice and the half smile were reviewed as ways of cultivating a positive attitude, an approach mental set, and broaden-and-build emotions to challenges and daily events. Finally, several specific informal mindful practices were reviewed that can help your clients practice informal mindfulness daily.

REFERENCES

Albers, S. (2012). *Eating mindfully: How to end mindless eating and enjoy a balanced relationship with food* (2nd ed.). Oakland, CA: New Harbinger Press.

Astrachan-Fletcher, E., & Maslar, M. (2009). *The dialectic behavior therapy skills workbook for bulimia: Using DBT to break the cycle and regain control of your life*. Oakland, CA: New Harbinger Publications.

Bien, T. (2006). *Mindful therapy: A guide for therapists and helping professionals*. Boston, MA: Wisdom Productions.

Brach, T. (2012). Mindful presence: A foundation for compassion and wisdom. In C. K. Germer & R. D. Siegel (Eds.), *Wisdom and compassion: Deepening mindfulness in clinical practice* (pp. 35–47). New York, NY: Guilford Press.

Emmons, R. A., & Stern, R. (2013). Gratitude as a psychotherapeutic intervention. *Journal of Clinical Psychology, 69*, 846–855.

Fredrickson, B. L. (2001). The role of positive emotions in positive psychology: The broaden-and-build theory of positive emotions. *American Psychologist, 56*, 218–226.

Grabovac, A. D., Lau, M. A., & Willett, B. R. (2011). Mechanisms of mindfulness: A Buddhist psychological model. *Mindfulness*. doi: 10.1007/s12671-011-0054-5.

Gunaratana, B. H. (2001). *Eight mindful steps to happiness: Walking the Buddha's path*. Somerville, MA: Wisdom Publications.

Hanh, T. N. (1975). *The miracle of mindfulness: An introduction to the practice of meditation*. Boston, MA: Beacon Press.

Hanson, R., & Mendius, R. (2009). *Buddha's brain: The practical neuroscience of happiness, love, and wisdom*. Oakland, CA: New Harbinger Publications.

Kabat-Zinn, J. (2013). *Full catastrophe living: Using the wisdom of your body and mind to face stress, pain, and illness*. New York, NY: Bantam Books.

Marek, R. J., Ben-Porath, D. D., Federici, A., Wisniewski, L., & Warren, M. (2013). Targeting premeal anxiety in eating disordered clients and normal controls: A preliminary investigation into the use of mindful eating vs. distraction during food exposure. *International Journal of Eating Disorders, 46*, 582–585.

Marlatt, G. A., Bowen, S., & Lustyk, M. K. B. (2012). Substance abuse and relapse prevention. In C. K. Germer & R. D. Siegel (Eds.), *Wisdom and compassion: Deepening mindfulness in clinical practice* (pp. 221–233). New York, NY: Guilford Press.

Mason, A. E., Daubenmier, J., Moran, P. J., Kristeller, J., Dallman, M., Lustig, R. H., . . . & Hecht, F. M. (2014). Increases in mindful eating predict reductions in consumption of sweets and desserts: Data from the Supporting Health by Integrating Nutrition and Exercise (SHINE) clinical trial [abstract]. *The Journal of Alternative and Complementary Medicine, 20*, A17.

Morita, S., Morita, M., Kondo, A., & LeVine, P. (1998). *Morita therapy and the true nature of anxiety-based disorders (Shinkeishitsu)*. New York, NY: SUNY Press.

Nelson, P. (1993). *There is a hole in my sidewalk*. Hillsboro, OR: Beyond Word Publishing.

Price, T. F., Peterson, C. K., & Harmon-Jones, E. (2012). The emotive neuroscience of embodiment. *Motivation and Emotion, 36*, 27–37.

Shapiro, S. L., & Carlson, L. E. (2009). *The art and science of mindfulness: Integrating mindfulness into psychology and the helping professions*. Washington, DC: American Psychological Association.

Stahl, B., & Goldstein, E. (2010). *A mindfulness-based stress reduction workbook*. Oakland, CA: New Harbinger Press.

Tribole, E., & Resch, E. (2012). *Intuitive eating: A revolutionary program that works*. New York, NY: St. Martin's Griffin.

Tylka, T. L., & Kroon Van Diest, A. M. (2013). The Intuitive Eating Scale–2: Item refinement and psychometric evaluation with college women and men. *Journal of Counseling Psychology, 60*, 137.

Wood, A. M., Froh, J. J., & Geraghty, A. W. A. (2010). Gratitude and well-being: A review and theoretical integration. *Clinical Psychology Review, 30*, 890–905.

The Yogic Self

C⅞ 7 ⅔

Yoga
The Basic Principles

In practice, yoga approaches the job of restoring health and harmony
in two ways: by removing obstacles that block our path,
and by revealing the unshakeable presence of peace, awareness,
and joy within.—SANDRA ANDERSON AND ROLF SOVIK (2000, p. 2)

YOGA IS FOR EVERYONE

Yoga philosophy views the experience of self as dwelling in two worlds: an inner world of thoughts, emotions, and sensations, and an outer world with which we interact (Anderson & Sovik, 2000). The yogic view of self is one of the root underpinnings of the Attuned Representational Model of Self (ARMS; see Chapter 1). Successful functioning is contingent on the ability to live capably in both worlds (Anderson & Sovik, 2000). Symbolic of the process, the term *yoga* is derived from the Sanskrit verb *yuj*, which means "to join or unite" (Anderson & Sovik, 2000; Iyengar, 1996). Through practice, it is believed that we are yoked to our higher nature—the pure nature of the self (Anderson & Sovik, 2000; Iyengar, 1996). The essential goals of yoga involve these three aspects: (a) integration of the inner world (b) harmony with the outer world and (c) union with the true nature of the *Self* (see Figure 7.1). As you read about the different types and schools of yoga in this chapter, you will see that although they vary in content and process, they all hold to these three major foci.

As therapists and counselors, we frequently ask our clients to link their attention to their thoughts, sensations, emotions, and behaviors

167

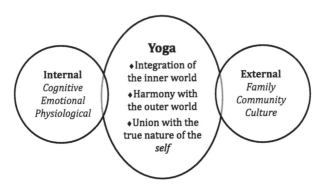

FIGURE 7.1 The essential goals of yoga.

(Simpkins & Simpkins, 2011). Some of our patients simply do not have the tools to effectively do this (Simpkins & Simpkins, 2011). They experience challenge with obstacles such as a lack of objectivity, an inability to still their bodies and minds, and trouble focusing attention (Simpkins & Simpkins, 2011). Yoga is a method designed to help develop self-awareness and show how to create harmony within the context of the external world (Anderson & Sovik, 2000). Recent findings in the field of neuroscience support use of yoga to foster a healthy, natural rebalancing and integration of the mind–brain system (Simpkins & Simpkins, 2011).

The yogic method is informed by knowledge passed down through oral transmission through the ages, ancient texts, modern books, and lineages of guru-to-student teachings that continue today (Stephens, 2010). The tradition of yoga is that true knowledge must be garnered through one's own experience (Anderson & Sovik, 2000). Yoga practices work like a mirror. They provide a methodology for examining the self, *your self,* directly (Anderson & Sovik, 2000). When the yogic method is followed in a systematic manner, it allows you to behave in alignment with your needs, intentions, and values. Further, it provides a structure of strengthening the body, relaxing the nervous and emotional systems, and bringing one-pointed, bare awareness to the mind (Anderson & Sovik, 2000).

Perhaps the most compelling aspect of yoga is the belief that within every human being is a self that is inherently balanced and whole (Anderson & Sovik, 2000). Yoga is seen as a process, or methodology, for increasing awareness of the inner self, our true nature (Anderson & Sovik, 2000). Often described as an inward journey, yoga philosophy holds that practice moves you through five layers (i.e., *koshas*) that surround the self (Anderson & Sovik, 2000; Stephens, 2010). The five layers exist in three manifestations of the body. The outermost layer comprises the physical body. Next, the subtle body comprises energy, sensations, and wisdom. At the innermost layer, the causal body, is the true nature of the self, or bliss (Stephens, 2010). Specifically, the five layers, or sheaths, consist of the physical body (i.e., *annamaya kosha*), internal energy of the subtle body (i.e., *pranamaya kosha*), the conscious mind of the subtle body (i.e., *manomaya*), the inner wisdom of the subtle body (i.e., *vijñanamaya*), and the causal body, or bliss, happiness, wholeness, and contentment (i.e., *anandamaya*). Yoga is an awareness of the interwoven fabric of these bodies and layers (Stephens, 2010). At times, these layers can function like clouds around the sun shrouding awareness of self, our inner light. The path inward moves through each layer toward the true self and one-pointed concentration (Anderson & Sovik, 2000). Anderson and Sovik (2000) say that the innermost self is beyond the reach of the mind and words. When sages are asked to describe it, silence is their reply (Anderson & Sovik, 2000).

Christina Sell (2003) wrote of her journey through body image issues, eating-disordered behavior, substance use, and sexually acting out toward a sense of inner peace in her book *Yoga From the Inside Out: Making Peace With Your Body Through Yoga*. She describes the story of a little girl sexually abused by her best friend's brother and an eager young gymnast pushed to her limits who begins a long battle with her body, trying to overpower all that she saw as deficient and broken (Sell, 2003). In her yoga practice she began to see a new way of being with her body: "I saw that every time I had ignored my pain I had basically ignored myself. I saw that I had been training throughout my life to perpetuate the war against my body that had also pushed me to ignore my very being" (Sell, 2003, p. 12). She realized that if she continued to practice ignoring her pain and criticizing and reprimanding herself with an intense inner dialogue, she would continue this war her entire life. Sell describes how her yoga evolved, over time, from what was another external physical practice into a true yoga practice that served her soul, her true self. This new embodiment she described as practicing yoga from the inside out (Sell, 2003).

Yoga is for everyone (Kraftsow, 1999). I first practiced yoga when I was 35 years old because I had a mistaken belief that yoga was not for people like me. I was a swimmer and a runner challenged to touch my toes. I had experienced exclusion in dance classes due to my lack of ability and I assumed that yoga class would be much the same. That is, the talented, physiologically gifted, and flexible people would be encouraged to take their places in the front of the room and people like me would be met with a lukewarm welcome and asked to stand in the back row, far from the front of the stage. As it turns out, that was not the way it should have been in dance class. Most important for the trajectory of my life, I was wrong about yoga. When I read Christina Sell's book, there were sections that felt very much like my own autobiography. Yoga is for me, you, your patients, for everyone.

THE STUDY AND HISTORY OF YOGA
AS AN INTERVENTION

There is comparatively less research on yoga interventions as compared to the body of research on mindfulness. Chapter 10 reviews the state of yoga research, specifically detailing several of the yoga interventions that have been studied. Also, contraindications, research gaps and challenges, as well as recommendations for future directions in research are covered. This chapter is intended to provide a brief overview of the basic tenets of yoga. The challenge lies in writing about yoga as an intervention in a way that honors the extensive history of yoga practice, yoga culture, and mentorship, as well as the philosophical foundations and ancient texts, and then to somehow look at this complex practice with a rich history within the confines of the scientific method and empiricism (McCall, 2007). There are innumerable sources, including ancient texts, modern interpretations of ancient texts, how-to texts written by yoga teachers and experienced yogis, and focused books written by mental health professionals and yogis, addressing yoga for a particular disorder or challenge (e.g., yoga for depression, anxiety, or trauma). The texts vary in how they balance empirical or academic rigor and practice guidance. I teach courses on mindfulness and yoga interventions at the University at Buffalo. When reflecting on a text we used for one of the courses, a doctoral student noted, "That text is nothing more than an extensive literature review. I can do that on my own. I want to understand the process, get the big picture, and learn what to do." That is the intention of this text.

Since ancient times, yoga has been evolving, adapted to meet the needs of individuals with different challenges, cultures, and traditions (Kraftsow, 1999; McCall, 2007; Simpkins & Simpkins, 2011). It is believed that yoga has been practiced in India for more than 40 centuries, since before recorded history (Anderson & Sovik, 2000; Simpkins & Simpkins, 2011; Stephens, 2010; Weintraub, 2004). There is no convergence of evidence to definitively confirm how old yoga practice actually is (McCall, 2007). Yoga was originally developed as a methodology for improving physical and mental clarity in service of transcendence to the true self (see Chapter 3; Douglass, 2007). Elements of yoga philosophy can be found in Hinduism, Jainism, and Buddhism (Simpkins & Simpkins, 2011; Stephens, 2010). Yoga's integration of focused concentration, deliberate body positioning (i.e., asana), and control of the breath provides an enduring practical system that is not limited to any particular philosophical system (Simpkins & Simpkins, 2011). Approximately 2,000 years ago, the Yoga Sutras were organized by a sage named Patanjali (Anderson & Sovik, 2000).

Yoga scholars have identified several ancient texts that are believed to be the early foundations of today's yoga. These include the Vedas (i.e., Rig, Yajur, Sama, and Atharva), Upanishads, Bhagavad Gita, Vedanta, and Yoga Sutras (Simpkins & Simpkins, 2011; Stephens, 2010). The Vedas, written around 1200 BCE, are ancient texts that vaguely express yoga's root themes. They are believed to be the earliest known writings on yoga (Stephens, 2010). The Upanishads, written between 800 and 600 BCE during the later end of the Vedic period, were the first Indian texts to include philosophy. They teach key yogic concepts, such as that we are all part of something greater, that answers lie within, and that the knowledge of the true self can be found through consciousness (Simpkins & Simpkins, 2011; Stephens, 2010). Written sometime between the fifth and second centuries BCE, the Bhagavad Gita is the sixth book in a larger Indian text (i.e., the Mahabharata). It is a lovely read of the dialogue between a great warrior named Arjuna and the god Krishna, Arjuna's charioteer (Simpkins & Simpkins, 2011; Stephens, 2010). I think of this text as the yoga of the self within the context of the external world. Krishna guides Arjuna through battles, teaching him yoga philosophy and skills as Arjuna faces the dilemmas of battle (Gandhi, 2011). The version interpreted by Gandhi is especially easy to understand and can be a good start for your study of the Bhagavad Gita (see *The Bhagavad Gita According to Gandhi* [Gandhi, 2011]).

This text will focus on the Yoga Sutras, the text most fundamental to modern yoga philosophy (Iyengar, 1996; Simpkins & Simpkins, 2011; Stephens, 2010). Believed to be written between the second century BCE and the fourth century CE, the Yoga Sutras are a series of concise sentences, or aphorisms, conveying the essential concepts of yoga theory and practice, and were originally written in Sanskrit (Anderson & Sovik, 2000; Iyengar, 1996; Simpkins & Simpkins, 2011; Weintraub, 2004). Originating as an oral tradition, the passages were passed down from teacher to student over many, many years. Patanjali is the personified author, described as person or entity tasked to write the Yoga Sutras down for record (Simpkins & Simpkins, 2011). It is important to note that there are yoga scholars who believe that Patanjali was a professor of grammar and linguistics and that he wrote the Yoga Sutras much later; however, there is no consensus for this claim (Simpkins & Simpkins, 2011). Patanjali presented yoga practice in eight limbs (Anderson & Sovik, 2000; Stephens, 2010; Weintraub, 2004).

Far from its philosophical roots, today's Western yoga is focused primarily on hatha yoga, the yoga of postures. The historical path of yoga from the East to the West is over 200 years old. Understanding the nature of the origins of yoga is important, as current manifestations and applications are considerably different than early forms. In order to be able to effectively field inquiries, mental health professionals should have a sense of the history, religious tensions, and concerns over authenticity.

Yoga was introduced to Europe via a translation of the Bhagavad Gita from Sanskrit to English in 1785, which eventually made its way to America by 1845 (Douglass, 2007). At first, the interest was intellectual and academic. Ralph Waldo Emerson enthusiastically embraced the translation, inspiring serious inquiry into Hinduism and yoga (Douglass, 2007). In the 1850s, the first signs of a critical shift were emerging. That is, oriental religions were being conceptualized as potential forms of practice rather than mere objects of study (De Michelis, 2008). Emerson's student, Henry David Thoreau, was the first to transition from the intellectual study of yoga to active practice. In a letter, Thoreau described himself to a friend as a *yogin* (Douglass, 2007).

Tensions developed as academic scholars struggled with their interest in yoga and Asian religions and the Christian belief that there is a single path to God (Douglass, 2007). Thoreau's continued practice of yoga begged the question, "Does the study and practice of yoga lead the practitioner away from Christianity?" (Douglass, 2007). Max Muller nearly personified the tensions with his scholarship on ancient texts such as the *Rig Veda* (Singleton, 2010). The negative tenor of his writings, which approached disgust, inspired a Hindu boycott of his lecture series in India (Douglass, 2007). Reports suggest that perhaps Muller saw the early roots of yoga as acceptable, as they were more philosophical in nature (Singleton, 2010). However, he described later forms of yoga (e.g., hatha) as part of the degeneration of yoga toward coarse practical applications.

Throughout the 1800s and 1900s, Hindus were profoundly affected by the critical perspective that Christian scholars applied to the analysis of yoga and Hinduism (Douglass, 2007). As a result, some Hindus converted to Christianity; others downplayed religious aspects of their beliefs and emphasized more practical aspects (Douglass, 2007). The 19th century also witnessed a rise in the phenomenon of the performing yogi (Singleton, 2010). In some cases yogis panhandled and performed advanced asanas in sideshows. This echoed European contortionism, which was held as a vulgar form of popular entertainment (Singleton, 2010). Some argue that present-day Instagram and Facebook posting of asanas is a reverberation of this voyeuristic and perhaps exclusive trend, instigating thoughts such as, "Only thin, athletic, and beautiful people do yoga," "Yoga is an art form to be observed and not practiced," or "I could never do that. Yoga is not for me." Others argue that these photos and videos, including the historical photos, are inspiring.

In 1893, Swami Vivekananda, well versed in both Western philosophy and Indian traditions including yoga, spoke at the World Parliament of Religions (De Michelis, 2008; Douglass, 2007). Although not embraced by academics, Vivekananda's framing of yoga as an approach to physical health accessible to everyone helped defuse tension around Christian commitment, opened the door to yoga as a subject for all Americans, and stimulated a genuine interest in the health benefits of yoga (Douglass, 2007). Overnight, Vivekananda became a popular icon of spirituality (De Michelis, 2008). As they were with Thoreau, scholars were critical of Vivekananda's reinterpretations of yoga and seemingly reckless blending of Eastern and Western religions and popular Western culture (Douglass, 2007). In 1898, William Flagg's book echoed Vivekananda's cultural inclusivity and emphasized yoga as a way to enhance one's own spiritual beliefs (Douglass, 2007). By the end of the 1880s, most American students of yoga circumvented religious conflict, adapting a view of yoga as a method for enhancing physical and mental health (Douglass, 2007).

From 1900 to 1940 the exploration of yoga took divergent paths in academia and popular culture. Notably, this period was marked by the substantially disruptive and intellectually unsettling influences of World War I and World War II as well as surges and intellectual debates in the field of psychology (De Michelis, 2008). In the growing field of psychology there was a movement away from laboratory experiments and toward practical applications in the field of mental health. These included the rise of behaviorism with John Watson, Ivan Pavlov, and later B. F. Skinner as well as the growing popularity of Freud and psychoanalysis. Later, Neo-Freudians emerged, such as Melanie Klein. Karen Horney introduced a more feminist approach to psychology. In the 1930s and 1940s intellectual assessment was taking hold, and Wechsler introduced his IQ scales. In the late 1940s neuropsychological research surfaced with the work of Donald Hebb.

In the field of yoga, academic literature highlighted exotic, magical, and occult aspects of classical yogic texts, perhaps discounting its potential to enhance personal growth (Douglass, 2007). Despite the direction of academics in yoga, popular culture continued to embrace the health aspects (Douglass, 2007). In 1932, marking a point of integration, Carl Jung wrote a piece on the psychology of Kundalini yoga, making comparisons across West and East (Douglass, 2007). In the 1950s, the idea that there was a single East and single West was softening and academics began to talk about the way cultures mutually benefited from an exchange of ideas and practices (Douglass, 2007). English translations of yoga texts were becoming increasingly available. For example, in 1966 B. K. S. Iyengar's 544-page *Light on Yoga* was published, with complete descriptions and illustrations of yoga postures and breathing techniques. Americans were studying yoga in India in growing numbers. A stage was set for the personal exploration of yoga (Douglas, 2007).

Throughout the 1960s and 1970s, yoga was becoming popular and being practiced by rock stars like the Beatles. In fact, Swami Satchidananda opened the legendary Woodstock music festival (Douglass, 2007). It was around this time that the history of yoga took another interesting turn. The practice and study of yoga became intertwined with the infamous LSD studies conducted by Harvard psychologists Richard Alpert and Timothy Leary. These studies and the behavior of the professors inspired ethical concerns across the country. Ultimately, the two left Harvard. Alpert departed to study Buddhist meditation in India, returning as Ram Dass to propagate new ideas on consciousness (Douglass, 2007). I saw him speak at University at Buffalo when I was a doctoral student. With the charisma of a practiced storyteller, he spoke of his journey from the LSD experiments to a life-long practice of meditation. Leary took a different path, urging the youth of America to "Turn on, tune in, and drop out" (Douglass, 2007, p. 40). For some, yoga's association with drugs and rock music solidified the practice as another problematic activity on a long list of deviant behaviors (Douglass, 2007). In the 1970s, yoga conceptually evolved to include exploration of sexuality and gender, wholeness, freedom from oppression, as well as a pathway to a more perfect uppercase "S" *Self* (Douglass, 2007). It was at this point that the concept of yoga as a complement to Western psychology emerged (Douglass, 2007). A body of research began and the gradual adoption of yoga as a pathway to health and well-being grew across the country to what it is today. We see yoga studios in nearly every city. Yoga is practiced in gyms, prisons, treatment centers, and schools. *(Note that the Self, written with a capital "S," refers to the yogic understanding of the integrated Self. This aspect of Self is seen as one with the universe and having no concern with issues of personal identity, success, or achievement. In brief, the Self can be thought of the as soul Self, and the lowercase "s" self as the ego self.)*

Many had thought the tensions surrounding religion were to continue to slowly dissipate the remaining part of the history of yoga. In Encinitas, a coastal beach city in San Diego County, California, the religion debate resurfaced and went to the court systems. The lawsuit emerged from a set of concerned parents within the Encinitas Union School District in California (Baird, 2014). The district had received a grant from the Jois Foundation to offer Ashtanga yoga practice to the students. In an effort to accommodate concerned parents, the yoga was presented free of Sanskrit terms and Hindu references. For example, postures were given different names (e.g., sukhasana was called crisscross applesauce). Nevertheless, a group of parents moved forward with the lawsuit, demanding that the school district suspend its unconstitutional religion-based physical education program. The school district argued that it was offering a contemporary physical education program that included stretching, breathing techniques, and relaxation strategies for children, and that is was *not offering* a religious program. On July 1, 2013, the court system agreed with the school district, ruling that the practice of yoga in schools neither endorses nor inhibits any religion (Baird, 2014). The case went before the appellate court in March 2015.

Finally, as yoga has evolved in Western culture, there are both scholars and practitioners who raise concerns over its *authenticity*. In their text, Singleton and Byrne (2008) address apprehension over the authenticity, explicating the continued tension. Specifically, they describe the school of thought that posits the existence of an authentic Indian practice that should be held as a standard with which all yoga should be compared and contrasted. Further, they explain that there are others who suggest that contemporary practices of yoga should "not be dismissed or condemned simply on account of their dislocation from perceived tradition" (Singleton & Byrne, 2008, p. 6). In his chapter, Liberman (2008) argues that there never was a pure yoga as some imagine and that the concept of pure yoga is a social construction. He argues that asana practice, as we know it now, did not manifest until the 10th to 12th centuries (Liberman, 2008). Liberman (2008) describes the earliest forms of yoga as consisting primarily of contemplation and mantra. In his piece, Liberman (2008) traces the roots of yoga in order to illustrate that modern, or contemporary, yoga is derived from a tradition that "was itself a derivative and syncretic form of spiritual practice" (p. 104). Liberman (2008) guides the interested practitioner, specifically the seeker of authenticity, to explore the guru-teacher lineage of practice, the oral tradition from which the roots might extend. He says that this is where a sense of authenticity might be found. As the early yogis advise, true knowledge comes from experience and not from texts (Liberman, 2008).

Today's yoga as researched and practiced continues to be complex, multifaceted, and heterogeneous. To know one type of yoga is *not* to know all types. The medicalization of yoga, which advocates the practice of yoga for health, somewhat relieved religious and cultural tensions, providing validity of the practice from another source—the field of medicine (De Michelis, 2008). Scholars are calling for a way to standardize or describe yoga interventions in order to effectively study outcomes (see Chapter 10). Generally, there is a movement toward academic and popular acceptance of yoga as a method for improving well-being, reducing stress, and enhancing mental and physical health, as evidenced by insurance companies reimbursing members for classes in many states and the addition of federal funding streams supporting research on yoga and other complementary approaches to health.

As I review the history of yoga and the changes in form and substance over thousands of years, Yoga Sutra II.21 comes to mind: rad-artha eva drsyasyatma (Bryant, 2009). In English, this translates to "The essential nature of that which is seen is exclusively for the sake of the seer" (Bryant, 2009). Bryant (2009) explains that this means that all that is knowable, which in this case we are speaking of knowing yoga, exists only for the growth of the seer. In this way, yoga has changed in form and substance to serve the growth of those who seek. Perhaps thousands of years ago, yoga was in the exact form the yogis and culture needed. As years pass, needs change, and cultures evolve, the goal of yoga stays the same—to integrate mind and body and bring growth to the soul Self. In this way, what is known as yoga today may look different, be different, from yoga in the past; yet, it is in the exact form that we need. History also tells us this—it is quite likely that as we continue to study and practice yoga, it will continue to evolve in both form and content. Moreover, we will continue debating and exploring issues like authenticity, religious content, and efficacy. For a more detailed review of the history of yoga, see Singleton (2010) and Douglass (2007).

THE EIGHT LIMBS OF YOGA

The eight limbs of yoga (see Table 7.1) are described in the Yoga Sutras. My three favorite interpretations of the Yoga Sutras are listed here in order of complexity of the interpretation, from most basic to extensive: *The Essential Yoga Sutra: Ancient Wisdom for Your Yoga* by Geshe Michael Roach and Christine McNally (2005), *How to Know God: The Yoga Aphorisms of Patanjali* by Swami Prabhavananda and Christopher Isherwood (2007), and *The Yoga Sutras of Patanjali* by Edwin F. Bryant (2009). They are all adequately indexed for ease of use. Reading the Yoga Sutras is a very helpful contemplative practice (see discussion of self-study later in this chapter). I often read the interpretations from each of the three of these texts as I work to come to an understanding of the aphorism and its meaning for my life at the time of the reading.

The overview of the basic tenets that follows presents concepts and ideas that may not fit into traditional scientific paradigms. McCall (2007), in his text *Yoga as Medicine: The Yogic Prescription for Health and Healing*, suggests that it can be helpful to think of yoga terms like metaphors in the same way psychoanalysts use terms like *id*, *ego*, and *superego* to understand the dynamics of the mind. I use yoga concepts to help patients consider their challenges and growth in new ways. Yoga provides a positive, growth-oriented framework for emotional regulation, thinking, and

TABLE 7.1 The Eight Limbs of Yoga

Foundational, External Limbs (Daily practices for coping, centering, and self-awareness)

Limb 1	*Yama (Conduct of self in society)*	*The Five Restraints*
	Ahimsa	Nonharming
	Satya	Truthfulness
	Asteya	Nonstealing
	Brahmacharya	Moderation of the senses
	Aparigraha	Nonpossessiveness
Limb 2	*Niyama (Conduct of self)*	*The Five Observances*
	Shaucha	Purity
	Santosha	Contentment
	Tapas	Self-discipline
	Svadhyaya	Self-study
	Ishvara pranidhana	Self-surrender
Limb 3	*Asana*	*Posture*
Limb 4	*Pranayama*	*Control and Expansion of Energy (Breath work)*
Limb 5	*Pratyahara*	*Sense Withdrawal*

Meditative, Internal Limbs (Daily practices cultivating awareness of the true self)

Limb 6	*Dharana*	*Concentration*
Limb 7	*Dhyana*	*Meditation*
Limb 8	*Samadhi*	*Self-realization*

Source: Anderson and Sovik, 2000; Bryant, 2009; Iyengar, 1996; McCall, 2007; Prabhavananda and Isherwood, 2007; Roach and McNally, 2005; Simpkins and Simpkins, 2011; Stephens, 2010; Weintraub, 2004.

behavioral choices. That is, it provides a supportive structure for embodied self-regulation.

The eight-limbed path is a sequential pathway to contentment, happiness, and the true, or soul, Self (Bryant, 2009; Prabhavananda & Isherwood, 2007; Roach & McNally, 2005). Anyone who follows this path is a yogi or yogin (Iyengar, 1996). The first five limbs are considered the external limbs of yoga. They are practices associated with the outer world, the external aspects of the self (Anderson & Sovik, 2000). They are intended to serve as the preliminary steps to strengthen the mind and body in preparation for the three later steps of meditation (Anderson & Sovik, 2000; Weintraub, 2004). The external pathway provides guidance on negotiating people in our lives, navigating decisions and challenges, and care and conditioning of the physical body. Interestingly, yoga as a methodology does integrate the physical asana practice as a critical aspect of the pathway to knowing the true, or soul, Self. The body is viewed as the temple of the soul and the vehicle for overcoming obstacles to enlightenment (Simpkins & Simpkins, 2011). However, asanas (i.e., the yoga postures) are often the only limb of yoga Westerners think of when they bring the term *yoga* to mind. Most people have little understanding of the entire system of yoga and the role asanas play within the context of the larger methodology.

The final three limbs are considered the internal limbs and the pathway to self-awareness, or samadhi (Anderson & Sovik, 2000; Stephens, 2010). Each of them is described next. Further, as in Chapter 4, a set of guiding questions is provided to help begin discussions on these topics with your clients.

Yamas

The five yamas are the first set of ethical guidelines in yoga (Iyengar, 1996; Simpkins & Simpkins, 2011; Weintraub, 2004). Yamas help us get along in society and within our relationships with others and ourselves (Stephens, 2010). Iyengar (1996) calls them the rules of morality for society and the individual. These are restraints, abstinences, disciplines, or things that one should not do (Iyengar, 1996; McCall, 2007; Simpkins & Simpkins, 2011; Weintraub, 2004). First, ahimsa is nonviolence or non-harming toward self or others (Iyengar, 1996; Weintraub, 2004). This yama is especially practical for work with self-regulation. These types of struggles often impact the self and others substantially. For example, David has been working to overcome his difficulties with compulsive gambling for about 6 months. For a long time his focus had been on the possibility of winning and the fun he felt he was having when playing. What eventually brought him to counseling was his long-term partner James, who told David that he was ending the relationship if he did not get help. The two had hoped to get married. However, despite David's lucrative law career, he was digging himself into deeper and deeper debt, leaving James to cover the bills month after month. Fortunately, David's yoga practice, exploration of the yamas, along with James's discontent, were cultivating substantial inner conflict for David. He said, "Yoga is ruining my gambling. I used to frame James's complaining as controlling, buzz-killing. As I move toward a life of ahimsa, I can't lay in savasana [i.e., often the final pose in a yoga class in which the yogi lays in silent meditation, relaxation, or contemplation] without feeling only what I can call guilt for what I have put both James and myself through." David's story is similar to stories I have heard many times. We often joke in yoga class that yoga will ruin your addictions and your addictions will ruin your yoga. In the presence and stillness that are cultivated by a solid and consistent practice, it is very difficult to continue behaviors that manifest substantial negative consequences for yourself and others. The embodied practices (see Chapter 3) that would be discussed in this context include: (1) be mindfully aware, (2) honor your breath and physical experience, (3) live in inquiry, (6) discern what is not-self, and (9) be of your values.

The next yama is satya, or abstaining from falsehood (Simpkins & Simpkins, 2011; Stephens, 2010; Weintraub, 2004). Iyengar (1996) refers to satya, or truth, as the "highest rule of conduct or morality" (p. 33). This yama spoke to Addison, a 22-year-old young woman who has spent the last 2 years in recovery from bulimia nervosa (BN). When I was working with her on the specific goal of symptom reduction, it was not helpful to assess how many times she binged and purged each week without a more positive, skill-building, fear-facing context. When therapy becomes a reporting in on symptoms, it does not feel too much different from a shamed-filled weigh-in at a diet club meeting. Often perpetuating symptom-propagating habits, patients have fertile soil to lie to you in order to look good, be a good patient. As a result, the entire authenticity of the therapeutic relationship can be lost. Rather than ask about her symptoms, we looked at how hard it was for her to be in her truth all week.

You see, eating disorders, especially BN, are disorders of secrecy. As the patient builds up a false, seemingly highly competent, externally oriented, representational self, the inner world is consumed with a secret cycle of food restriction, uncontrollable bingeing, and compensatory purging (Cook-Cottone, 2006; see Chapter 2). Recovery requires truth. That is, the self that is functioning out there in the world must authentically, truthfully represent the inner self—body and mind (Cook-Cottone, 2006). Symptoms become obstacles to the truth (Cook-Cottone, 2006). In this manner, setting a goal of satya can be a catalyst to a reduction of symptoms. Addison, who sees herself as a good person, was very uncomfortable with the notion of herself as not truthful. Living in truth became a core motivation in her recovery. We worked on using her voice (see throat chakra in Table 7.4 later in this chapter; Anodea, 2004), honoring her own needs (see solar plexus chakra in Table 7.4 later in this chapter; Anodea, 2004), and staying present to the feelings that arose when she felt the need to misrepresent what she really needed (Cook-Cottone, 2006). By focusing on truth and self-care (see also Chapter 12 on self-care), Addison shifted into positive, healthy self-representation and out of symptoms. Associated embodied practices (see Chapter 3) include: (1) be mindfully aware, (2) honor your breath and physical experience, and (3) be of your values.

Asteya refers to abstinence from stealing anything, including property, time, attention, and aspects of another's identity (Simpkins & Simpkins, 2011; Stephens, 2010; Weintraub, 2004). Iyengar (1996) describes this yama as a managing of the desire to possess and enjoy what another person has. There are many ways to apply this yama to practice. For example, Zuri, the 13-year-old introduced in Chapter 1, is very unhappy with the state of her life. Her mom struggles with addictions and their family is poor. Without her mother as a role model, Zuri looks to Westernized images of Black women as ideals. She restricts food in an attempt to manage her feelings and to be as thin as the models and actresses she sees in magazines and on television. This is not her identity. Preventing any further development of anorexia nervosa (AN) means helping Zuri construct her own sense of identity that allows her to be strong, competent, and healthy. Associated embodied practices (see Chapter 3) include: (6) discern what is not-self, (7) allow what is with nonjudgment, (9) be of your values, and (10) observe compassion for self and others.

Brahmacharya is the yama of overall restraint (Roach & McNally, 2005; Simpkins & Simpkins, 2011). Appropriate to apply to each of the areas of dysregulation, this yama was originally specific to sexual restraint (Simpkins & Simpkins, 2011). Weintraub (2004) suggested that this yama is perhaps the most complex. Even today, many yogis continue to see this yama as speaking specifically to abstinence and sexual restraint (Weintraub, 2004). Given the long, chronicled history of the failure of compulsory celibacy, the broader interpretation may be an attempt to bring this yama to current-day relevance. See the discussion in Chapter 3 of embodied practice 9, be of your values.

Parigraha means collecting or hoarding (Iyengar, 1996). Aparigraha is the yama of greedlessness, or the abstinence from greed and cultivation of nonattachment (Bryant, 2009; Simpkins & Simpkins, 2011; Weintraub, 2004). Accumulation of, and attachment to, possessions, can lead to a fear of their loss—a clear obstacle to knowing the true, or soul, Self (Weintraub, 2004). According to Simpkins and Simpkins (2011), this yama is one of the central values of Buddhism. That is, craving and attachment are the source of all suffering (Simpkins & Simpkins, 2011). See Chapter 9 for a case study exploring the use of aparigraha in therapy, and see the discussion in Chapter 3 of the following embodied practices: (2) honor your breath and physical experience, (5) cultivate nonattachment, (6) discern what is not self, and (9) be of your values.

Questions to Ask Your Clients

- In what ways do your difficulties with self-regulation cause harm to you or the people in your life? Tell me about the feelings that arise as you answer.

- What does it feel like, in your body, when you are not truthful? What would your life look like if you were to live in complete truth? How would this affect your relationships? How would this affect your difficulties with self-regulation?
- What does your struggle with self-regulation take, or steal, from you? Are there ways you take from others, such as a sense of identity or requiring them to monitor and control your behavior? What would a life of cultivating self-regulation and identity on your own look like?
- What arises when you feel the urge, or craving, to engage in your problematic behavior? What feelings, thoughts, or needs are pushing for attention underneath your desire to engage in your behavior? What would it look like if you were to tolerate your craving and experience what was happening in your body? How would this affect your relationships?

Niyamas

The niyamas are five observances, or things we should do (Bryant, 2009; McCall, 2007; Simpkins & Simpkins, 2011). Niyamas are the guidelines for conduct that apply to the individual, our relationship with ourselves (Iyengar, 1996; Stephens, 2010). The niyamas include saucha, santosha, tapas, svadhyaya, and ishvara pranidhana.

The first is saucha, which means purity of body and mind (Iyengar, 1996; Stephens, 2010). The observance of purity ranges from practices of physiological cleanliness to refinement of speech and actions (Iyengar, 1996; Simpkins & Simpkins, 2011; Weintraub, 2004). Saucha shares a conceptual and behavioral overlap with self-care (see Chapter 12 for an assessment and description of self-care practices). It also has diagnostic importance in terms of the clinical impact of disorder on daily functioning (American Psychiatric Association [APA], 2000). In recent diagnostic manuals this was referred to as Global Assessment of Functioning. In the current *Diagnostic and Statistical Manual of Mental Disorders*, 5th edition (APA, 2013), assessment in this area includes daily washing of the whole body, getting dressed, and taking care of the household. Deficits in these aspects of basic self-care are signs that a patient is not functioning well. A good saucha and self-care practice can be the central support for the reduction of symptoms. Conversely, increased symptoms can be associated with deterioration in saucha and self-care. See the discussion in Chapter 3 of the following associated embodied practices: (8) prioritize self-care and (9) be of your values.

Santosha is the niyama referring to contentment (Bryant, 2009; Simpkins & Simpkins, 2011; Weintraub, 2004). "A mind that is not content cannot concentrate" (Iyengar, 1996, p. 37). Individuals with difficulty with self-regulation typically do not have a practice of contentment. Recall that risk factors for self-regulation problems include difficulties with reward areas of the brain, negative affect, trouble with restraint, urges to escape, impulsivity, distress intolerance, and loneliness (see Chapter 2). Contentment practice can be viewed as an antidote. That is, along with management of triggers and urges to engage in problematic behavior, patients practice seeing and appreciating the present moment. They work on the possibility of not needing to add to it or escape from it.

To illustrate, Erin is a 36-year-old female. She is a yoga teacher and a recovering alcoholic and drug addict, now 10 years sober. She explains that contentment was her biggest challenge. She explains that since the time she was a little girl, even if she was happy, she was compelled to the bigger, better happy. Watching a movie with her friends wasn't enough. They had to add candy and ice cream and have a sleepover after. As a teen, a beer party wasn't enough. She found marijuana and later cocaine, taking the parties to the next level. If people were sitting, she would get them to dance. If they were dancing, she would get them to go to a better club. When she was uncomfortable, lonely, or sad, contentment was nowhere to be found. She did all she could do to get herself "the hell out of the moment." No holds were barred, no limits set. For Erin, whether it be good times or bad, contentment did not exist.

At 10 years sober, Erin practices a moment-by-moment mindfulness of her contentment. If a behavior is assessed as meeting an escape demand, a drive to take her away from the present moment, she does not do it. She asks herself first, "What can you find in this present moment to cultivate contentment?" The answer might be found in her breath, the touch of her faithful dog, or the smile of her loving husband. She organizes her behaviors around authentic physiological, psychological, and emotional needs. For example, she practices intuitive and mindful eating every day (see Chapters 5 and 6 for a review). She works to stay present rather than let her thoughts and behaviors take her away from the present moment. In this manner, fueling of the body brings her more presence and awareness and ultimately enhances contentment. Associated embodied practices (see Chapter 3) include: (2) honor your breath and physical experience, (5) cultivate nonattachment, (7) allow what is with nonjudgment, (9) be of your values, and (11) maintain equanimity.

The observance, or niyama, tapas is an important aspect of personal growth and can be the key to whether or not a patient makes progress, or is ready to make progress, in therapy. Weintraub (2004) refers to tapas as the "fires of change" (p. 76). McCall (2007) explains that the ancient yogis saw the body like an unbaked clay pot. Yoga practice was like the kiln that strengthens the pot, making it durable enough to withstand challenge and distress. Tapas refers to a sincere commitment to personal growth and the willingness to engage in the behaviors that will help manifest growth (Bryant, 2009; Iyengar, 1996; Simpkins & Simpkins, 2011). Therapists who work with patients with self-regulation difficulties often assess the stage of change in which the patient presents (Norcross, Krebs, & Prochaska, 2011; Table 7.2). Patients who are ready to make change are beginning to have a sense of conflict, as in David's growing awareness of the problems that his gambling was creating in his life. If tapas is not present or is at emergent levels, encourage mindfulness, asana, meditation, and breath work outside of therapy sessions and engage in motivational interviewing to encourage tapas (Markland, Ryan, Tobin, & Rollnick, 2005). Associated embodied practices (see Chapter 3) include: (1) be mindfully aware, (3) live in inquiry, and (9) be of your values.

TABLE 7.2   Stages of Change and Progression of Tapas

Precontemplation (No tapas present)

- No intention to change behavior in the foreseeable future
- Lack of unawareness or underawareness of problems
- People around the patient are well aware of the patient's self-regulation problems

Contemplation (Tapas emerging as concern and internal conflict)

- Awareness that a problem exists
- Serious contemplation of overcoming difficulties
- No commitment has been made to take action
- Internal conflict between the positive evaluations of self-regulation problems and cost to overcome (i.e., effort, energy, and loss)

Preparation (Emergence of tapas in practice as intention and exploratory efforts)

- Intention to take immediate action (i.e., within the next 4 weeks)
- Reports of small behavioral changes with some reduction in dysregulated behavior
- Lack of sufficient behavioral change to meet criterion for effective action

Action (Establishing embodied tapas)

- Modification of behavior, experiences, and/or environment to overcome problems
- Overt behavioral changes present for at least 1 day to 6 months in which the patient remains free of the dysregulated behavior and engages in healthy self-regulation practice(s)
- Commitment of time and energy

Maintenance (Embodied tapas)

- Overt behavioral changes present for at least 6 months in which the patient remains free of the dysregulated behavior and engages in healthy self-regulation practice(s)
- Active prevention of relapse
- Consolidation of improvements reached during action

Source: Bryant, 2009; Norcross et al., 2011; Simpkins and Simpkins, 2011.

The niyama svadhyaya refers to self-education, or the pursuit of self-improvement via learning (Simpkins & Simpkins, 2011; Weintraub, 2012). Iyengar (1996) reminds us that the most important study is self-study. "The person practicing svadhyaya reads his own book of life, at the same time he writes and revises it" (Iyengar, 1996, p. 38). Weintraub (2012) warns that yoga asana practice without self-study is insufficient for personal growth. Especially for growth in self-regulation, one must be aware of the functions of behaviors so that the root causes can be addressed. Otherwise patients run the risk of simply shifting from one self-destructive behavior to another. Svadhyaya can include all types of study (e.g., self-study and spiritual study).

For Erin, described earlier, svadhyaya was another critical aspect of her recovery. Through self-study, she noticed that after refraining from a self-destructive behavior her cravings and triggers would often begin to lead to a new addictive behavior. I call this shape shifting. Rather than being present with the emotions, thoughts, and physical experiences that arose and passed away when a patient was refraining from behaviors, he or she would simply move to the new behavior. For example, when Erin quit drinking she started shopping, a lot. When she quit shopping, she started running excessively. It was not until she decided to begin the study and practice of yoga that she began to learn how to be with the emotions, triggers, thoughts, and cravings that were driving her to the next shape-shifting behavior. Erin's study of yoga evolved from roots of self-study to yoga teacher training and certification. To this day, she continues her pursuit of knowledge through self-study as well as through more formal educational programs. Associated embodied practices (see Chapter 3) include: (3) live in inquiry and (9) be of your values.

Ishvara pranidhana is the niyama that involves a dedication and surrender to something bigger than you (Simpkins & Simpkins, 2011; Weintraub, 2004). This might be God, the universe, Mother Nature, Daoism, or Buddhism. A critical aspect of self-care (see Chapter 12), finding a greater meaning and spiritual direction, provides support for efforts toward healthy, wholesome living and embodied self-regulation (Simpkins & Simpkins, 2011). As a reason for being, meaning can make all the difference. See the discussion in Chapter 3 of embodied practice 9, be of your values.

Questions to Ask Your Clients

- How are your daily living skills? Are you taking care of yourself every day (showering, housekeeping, and other forms of self-care; see Chapter 12 for a self-care assessment)?
- Do you practice contentment? Can you stay in the moment? Or, are you always trying to make experiences better, bigger, more intense?

- Have you made a commitment to change? Are you actively refraining from dysregulated behavioral choices? Do you have healthy, noncompulsive practices in place to meet your needs?
- Are you learning new things about yourself and the world? Tell me about your ongoing self-education and any continuing education you are doing to grow your knowledge base.
- What is your reason for being? Tell me about your beliefs and how they support you in your self-regulation.

Asana

Asanas are postures that have evolved over centuries to exercise each muscle, nerve, and gland in the body (Iyengar, 1996). Notably, the Yoga Sutras do not discuss specific postures or asanas (Stephens, 2010). There is a reference to asana in Chapter 2, aphorism 29, of the Yoga Sutras, which addresses asana as one of the eight limbs, and one in Chapter 2, aphorism 46, "II.46 sthira-sukham asanam," of the Yoga Sutras (Bryant, 2009, p. 283). *Sthira* refers to steadiness and *sukham* refers to ease and comfort (Prabhavananda & Isherwood, 2007). Thus, the Yoga Sutras instruct us to approach the yoga postures with steadiness and ease. The Sanskrit roots of the term *asana* tell us a bit more (Prabhavananda & Isherwood, 2007; Stephens, 2010). The Sanskrit root *as* connotes being or living in one's body, with the full term *asana* referring to taking one's seat (Stephens, 2010). Prabhavananda and Isherwood (2007) explain that asana means two things: "the palace on which the yogi sits, and the manner in which he sits there" (p. 168). Thus, asana refers to embodiment (see the discussion in Chapter 3 of associated embodied practice 1, honor your breath and your physical experience).

"Asana brings steadiness, health, and lightness of limb" (Iyengar, 1996, p. 40). The practice of asana is not, however, merely a physical exercise. It is intended to integrate body, mind, and breath within the context of holding postures and moving from one posture to the next. The asanas are named after natural phenomena (e.g., tree pose), animals (e.g., fish and frog poses), and sages and heroes (e.g., Hanumanasana). Iyengar (1996) describes the names of poses as intentionally reflecting the evolutionary process from plants; to more primitive animals; to more advanced animals; to the human embryo, a baby, and child; and ultimately to the sage and hero. Iyengar (1996) posits that by taking the shapes of all creatures and things, the practitioner develops empathy and compassion for all things. Depending on the type of practice or school of yoga, the postures may be linked together in a sequence or flow.

Since ancient times, yoga postures have been described in precise terms (Kraftsow, 1999). It was believed that by mastering the specific forms of each of the asanas, mastery of the basic principles of movement was demonstrated (Kraftsow, 1999). Kraftsow (1999) warns that the practice of asana should be done as it was intended—that is, based on each individual's actual condition with the asana in terms of its function rather than its form (Kraftsow, 1999). Kraftsow (1999) worries that Western interpretations of yoga have overemphasized the achievement of precise, fixed forms and preconceived, external standards of perfection. This is not the true intention of yoga. We should not practice yoga to meet or comply with external standards. If we do, we are doing nothing substantially different than what a young girl at risk of eating-disordered behavior does when she attempts to emulate airbrushed models in the magazines. If we pursue external perfection, we most certainly have lost the practice of yoga. Associated embodied practices (see Chapter 3) include: (1) be mindfully aware, (2) honor your breath and physical experience, and (9) be of your values.

Questions to Ask Your Clients
- Have you assessed the physiological, embodied aspects of your struggle with self-regulation?
- Have you noticed the association between healthy, consistent physical practices and your symptom expression?
- Do you do something to be in your body every day?
- Do you have the tools that you need to integrate your breath, body, and intentions?
- Do you feel a sense of a strong and capable physical body?
- Can you shift away from judging or controlling your body and toward sensing and experiencing your body?

Pranayama

Prana means respiration, breath, vitality, life, wind, energy, and strength (Iyengar, 1996). The term refers to the soul rather than the body (Iyengar, 1996). *Ayama* refers to expansion, stretching out, length, and restraint (Iyengar, 1996). Pranayama is the practice of breath work to calm down and energize the body (Simpkins & Simpkins, 2011). Control of breath allows for control of emotions and mood (Weintraub, 2012). Iyengar (1996) identifies three ways to control the breath (a) inhalation, inspiration, or filling up; (b) exhalation, expiration, or emptying; and (c) retention.

Advanced yogis deem the breath so powerful that in some schools of yoga, the practitioner must show competence in the first three limbs for some time before breath work is attempted (McCall, 2007). Iyengar (1996)

TABLE 7.3   The Qualities of Good Breathing

Quality	Description
Depth	Breath is deep and driven by firm, steady contractions of the diaphragm
Flow	Flow is smooth; without pause, agitation, or hesitation
Constancy	Exhalations and inhalations are equal in length
Sound	Breath is silent, without sound
Continuity	Breath is continuous with smooth transitions between exhalations and inhalations

Adapted from Sovik, 2005. Reprinted with permission.

warns of its power and importance, stating, "Pranayama is thus the science of breath. It is the hub around which the wheel of life evolves" (p. 43). Breath work typically begins with simple observation of the breath and the qualities of breath (Sovik, 2005; Table 7.3). The qualities of breath will vary depending on the breath work done and the goal of the practice. For example, ujjayi pranayama involves breathing through the nose with a slight constriction of the throat that causes a soft sound that allows a practitioner to attend more easily to the breath (Stephens, 2010). Over time and with aggregated experience, more advanced and complex techniques are introduced (Stephens, 2010). See the discussion in Chapter 3 of the following associated embodied practices: (1) be mindfully aware, and (2) honor your breath and physical experience.

Questions to Ask Your Clients
- Are you aware of the role the breath plays in emotional arousal and soothing?
- Have you incorporated any breathing techniques into your work on self-regulation?
- Are you open to learning more about the breath and how it can facilitate impulse control, self-soothing, management of triggers and cravings, presence during challenge, and emotional control?

Pratyahara

Pratyahara is the practice of turning inward (Bryant, 2009; Simpkins & Simpkins, 2011; Stephens, 2010). Pratyahara exercises prepare you for meditation by quieting the senses, withdrawing them from outward objects, so that the senses and the mind can rest (Sovik, 2005). Stephens

(2010) put it this way, "As we sense, so we think, and as we think, so we tend to act" (p. 11). By turning inward, the process of self-regulation can shift from a set of external reactions toward an internal noticing. Sounds, tactile input, smells, sights, and other sensations (described as sense impressions in Chapters 4, 5, and 6) are simply there as you focus your attention inward (Stephens, 2010). Associated embodied practices (see Chapter 3) include: (1) be mindfully aware, and (9) be of your values.

Questions to Ask Your Clients
- Are you able to intentionally bring the focus of your mind inward?
- Do you feel triggered by external stimuli, internal thoughts, and worries?
- Do you have tools that help you turn inward?

Dharana, Dhyana, and Samadhi

Dharana, dhyana, and samadhi are the three internal limbs (Bryant, 2009; Simpkins & Simpkins, 2011). The external limbs prepare the yogi for these practices. The practitioner is ready for dharana when the body has been tempered by asana, the mind has been refined by pranayama, and the senses have been brought under control by pratyahara (Iyengar, 1996). Dharana is the practice of one-pointed focus of attention (Bryant, 2009; Iyengar, 1996; Simpkins & Simpkins, 2011; Stephens, 2010). Dhyana is the practice of focusing on inner thoughts and feelings as the yogi focuses on the object of attention (Simpkins & Simpkins, 2011). "As water takes the shape of its container, the mind, when it contemplates an object is transformed to the shape of that object" (Iyengar, 1996). Stephens (2010) refers to this as a "mind-body-breath" state of mind (p. 12).

The eight limbs of yoga are conceptualized as a tree (Stephens, 2010). Iyengar saw each aspect of the eight limbs as contributing to the tree, ultimately creating the life force and structure need for samadhi (Figure 7.2).

Samadhi is the ultimate union, or joining, with the object of attention (Simpkins & Simpkins, 2011). This is direct perception of the object without the filter of the senses (Simpkins & Simpkins, 2011). There is no sense of "I" or "mine" associated with the working of the body and there is a sense of "peace that surpasses understanding" (Iyengar, 1996, p. 52). It is as if the body and the senses are asleep and the mind and reason are alert and awake (Iyengar, 1996). There is a sense of alertness, lightness, and of being fully conscious (Iyengar, 1996). Associated embodied practices (see Chapter 3) include: (1) be mindfully aware, (3) live in inquiry, (4) accept

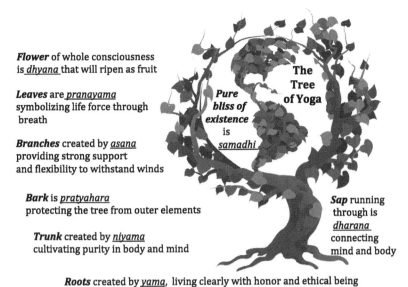

Flower of whole consciousness is _dhyana_ that will ripen as fruit

Leaves are _pranayama_ symbolizing life force through breath

Branches created by _asana_ providing strong support and flexibility to withstand winds

Bark is _pratyahara_ protecting the tree from outer elements

Trunk created by _niyama_ cultivating purity in body and mind

The Tree of Yoga

Pure bliss of existence is _samadhi_

Sap running through is _dharana_ connecting mind and body

Roots created by _yama_, living clearly with honor and ethical being

FIGURE 7.2 The tree of yoga.
Text informed by Iyengar, 1996; Stephens, 2010.

impermanence, (5) cultivate nonattachment, (6) discern what is not self, (7) allow what is with nonjudgment, and (9) be of your values.

Questions to Ask Your Clients

- Do you have a meditation practice?
- Can you see the elements of mindfulness working with the elements of yoga to help you make progress with your self-regulation struggles?
- Would you like to learn more about methods for building a meditation practice?

TRADITIONAL TYPES OF YOGA

There are many forms of yoga. Traditionally, yoga is described in older texts in terms of seven main paths (i.e., Hatha, Raja, Jnana, Mantra, Karma, Bhakti, and Tantra; Anderson & Sovik, 2000; Simpkins & Simpkins, 2011; Stephens, 2010). No path is considered entirely separate and the final goal remains the same across all paths: integration of the inner world, harmony with the outer world, and union with the true nature of the _Self_ (Anderson & Sovik, 2000). More recently evolved forms or schools of yoga, as their core, integrate the three key aspects of yoga in various proportions and emphases of these components: asana, pranayama, and meditations. The other aspects of yoga (e.g., yamas and niyamas) may or may not be included, and if they are, they are included at variable amounts in variable proportions. There is no yoga that is best or ideal. There is only the yoga that works best for you and your clients and for the needs and goals of you and your clients right now. An individual may migrate through different types of yoga over a lifetime depending on needs and goals or a person might stay with one school throughout his or her entire lifetime. Neither of these options is right or wrong. The traditional forms of yoga are described here. More recent styles of yoga are reviewed in Chapter 8, "On the Mat: Formal Yoga Practices." Note that there is no generally accepted source that delineates all types of yoga. Sources and discrepancies and similarities between and among sources are cited in this chapter's discussion.

Hatha Yoga

Hatha yoga is the yoga of health (Simpkins & Simpkins, 2011). This style integrates the postures (i.e., asanas), breath work, and meditation as a path to physical health and well-being (Simpkins & Simpkins, 2011). Some see Hatha yoga as a term that conceptualizes nearly all Western types of yoga, whereas others use it to describe a particular type of Western yoga (Simpkins & Simpkins, 2011). Associated embodied practices (see Chapter 3) include: (1) be mindfully aware, and (2) honor your breath and physical experience.

Raja Yoga

Raja yoga is focused on the mind, consciousness, and character (Simpkins & Simpkins, 2011). Some refer to Raja yoga as the royal path (*raja* means "royal" in Sanskrit). Rather than reliance on rational thought, this path is the pursuit of wisdom through the techniques of focused attention, concentration, and contemplation with the intention of discipline of the mind (Simpkins & Simpkins, 2011). Anderson and Sovik (2000) describe Raja yoga as encompassing the eight limbs of practice providing the discipline, guidance, and organization for a life of practice. Associated embodied practices (see Chapter 3) include: (1) be mindfully aware, and (3) live in inquiry.

Jnana Yoga

Jnana is referred to as the yoga of knowledge, wisdom, awareness, and discrimination (*jnana* means "knowledge" in Sanskrit; Anderson & Sovik,

2000; Simpkins & Simpkins, 2011; Stephens, 2010). This yogic path involves meditation and contemplation using conceptual, rational thought to bring the mind toward higher consciousness. Practitioners address worries and fears as they work to discover truth (Simpkins & Simpkins, 2011). Associated embodied practices (see Chapter 3) include: (1) be mindfully aware, (3) live in inquiry, and (6) discern what is not-self.

Mantra Yoga

In Mantra yoga, the practitioner uses mantra (i.e., sounds and words) on the path to high consciousness (Simpkins & Simpkins, 2011; Stephens, 2010). Sound is seen as a tool of the mind (in Sanskrit, *manas* means "mind" and *tra* means "tool"; Simpkins & Simpkins, 2011). Many mantras can be found in the Vedas (Stephens, 2010). Some mantras are used solely for meditation, whereas others are used in ritual and as tools for contemplation (Anderson & Sovik, 2000). Associated embodied practices (see Chapter 3) include: (1) be mindfully aware, and (2) honor your breath and physical experience.

Karma Yoga

Karma yoga is considered the yoga of service for everyday life (Simpkins & Simpkins, 2011; Stephens, 2010). In Sanskrit the word *karma* means "to do" or "union through action" (Simpkins & Simpkins, 2011; Stephens, 2010). Specifically, the concept of karma refers to daily actions and their relationship with fate and destiny (Simpkins & Simpkins, 2011). Karma yoga emphasizes an intentional focus on cultivating wholesome deeds in action without expectation or attachment to reward, outcome, or acknowledgment (Anderson & Sovik, 2000; Simpkins & Simpkins, 2011). Associated embodied practices (see Chapter 3) include: (1) be mindfully aware, (9) be of your values, and (12) cultivate loving-kindness and joy.

Bhakti Yoga

Bhakti yoga is the yoga of devotion (*bhakti* means "devotion" or "to adore, to love" in Sanskrit; Anderson & Sovik, 2000; Simpkins & Simpkins, 2011; Stephens, 2010). The practice involves devotion, compassion, and selfless love for a higher power (Simpkins & Simpkins, 2011). It is believed that a life of work devoted to others facilitates the journey through the personal self toward the experience of the true, or soul, Self (Simpkins & Simpkins, 2011). This practice has really worked for David, the 54-year-old introduced in Chapter 4. When he quit drinking for good, he found it extremely helpful to do what he called "Let go and let God." His devotions and commitment to a higher power have allowed him to be present in his life, trusting that God has things under control. As you recall, David's wife's cancer was a trigger for his escalation in drinking. Sober, his fear for her health can get the better of him some days. He takes that to prayer and stays present in his life. Associated embodied practices (see Chapter 3) include: (1) be mindfully aware, and (9) be of your values.

Tantra Yoga

Tantra yoga is a yoga of symbolic experiences designed to weave mind and body into one (*tantra* means weaving together, continuation; Simpkins & Simpkins, 2011). Tantra has a long history, with roots in Hinduism and Tibetan Buddhism (e.g., vajrayana), and is a formative root of modern Hatha yoga (Simpkins & Simpkins, 2011; Stephens, 2010). Essentially, the central theme of tantric yoga is that every single thing in the entire universe is an expression and source of divine being (Stephens, 2010). There are many tantric practices, such as Tantra yoga, a method that combines tantric ritual and the use of mandalas (a mandala is a spiritual symbol in Hinduism and Buddhism, often representing the universe; Simpkins & Simpkins, 2011). Perhaps the most controversial of yoga techniques, tantra extends to sensual and emotional practices within relationships (Simpkins & Simpkins, 2011). McCall (2007) cautions that much of the bad reputation that tantra has acquired is based largely on misunderstandings and the practices of a few fringe tantric cults, which do not reflect mainstream practices. Associated embodied practices (see Chapter 3) include: (2) honor your breath and physical experience, and (9) be of your values.

Kundalini Yoga

Kundalini yoga involves awakening and assimilation of the energy of consciousness (Anderson & Sovik, 2000). Kundalini yoga targets mind–body–spirit integration through cultivation and regulation of the spiraling flow of prana, or life energy (*kundalini* in Sanskrit means coil, spiral, ring; Simpkins & Simpkins, 2011). A tantric method, Kundalini yoga philosophy posits that there are three primary channels of life: energy flow in the body, or *ida* (i.e., "moon" in Sanksrit; energy flowing on the left side of the body); *pingala* (i.e., "sun" in Sanskrit; energy flowing on the right side of the body); and *sushumna* (i.e., meaning "most gracious" in Sanskrit; the central channel for balanced energy within the spine; Simpkins & Simpkins, 2011). For Kundalini yogis, sushumna represents life force, universal light, and higher consciousness (Simpkins & Simp-kins, 2011). Practice is believed to help life-force energy move up from the base of the spine to the crown of the head through a series of channels. Some of you may have heard of the term *kundalini rising,* which refers to this process.

It is believed that the three energy channels integrate at *chakras* (*chakra* means "spinning wheel" in Sanskrit; *chakras* refers to centers of integra-tion within the body; Simpkins & Simpkins, 2011). The methods include breath work (i.e., pranayama), meditations, asana (i.e., postures), and work with the chakras (see Table 7.4 for a brief overview of the charkas). Each chakra has a location in the body, symbol, color, and meaning (Ano-dea, 2004). The integration of movement and breath is believed to affect the pranic or energetic body (McCall, 2007). Often, practice is devoted to a center of energy or chakra with the intention of moving through the channels of energy, bringing the energy and connection toward higher consciousness (Simpkins & Simpkins, 2011).

In this area of practice, truth is held as one of the highest values. Note that some Kundalini practitioners are devoted to a form of Sikhism, a tra-dition of guru teachings, in which top teachers wear white turbans, dress in white, and take the last name Khalsa, which means "pure" (McCall,

TABLE 7.4 The Chakras

Chakra (Sanskrit)	Body Location	Symbol (Color/Element)	Meaning
Crown Chakra (Sahasrara)	Crown of the head	Thousand-petal lotus (violet/space and thought)	Pure consciousness, spiritual understanding, selfless devotion, inspiration
Third Eye Chakra (Ajna)	Above the nose, between the eyebrows	Two-petal lotus (indigo blue/time and light)	Intelligence, intuition, trust of inner wisdom, mood
Throat Chakra (Vishuddha)	Throat	Sixteen-petal lotus (light turquoise/sound)	Communication, expression, faith, inspiration
Heart Chakra (Anahata)	Heart, center of the chest	Twelve-petal lotus (green/air)	Love, compassion, equilibrium, acceptance, trust, self-acceptance
Solar Plexus Chakra (Manipura)	Bottom of the rib cage	Ten-petal lotus (yellow/fire)	Self-esteem, ego, personal empowerment, identity
Sacral Chakra (Svadhisthana)	Lower abdomen	Six-petal lotus (orange/water)	Relationships, emotions, creativity, sexuality
Root Chakra (Muladhara)	Base of the spine	Four-petal lotus (red/earth)	Stability, security, attachment

Source: Anodea, 2004; Simpkins and Simpkins, 2011; Stephens, 2010; Weintraub, 2012.

2007). Associated embodied practices (see Chapter 3) include: (1) be mindfully aware, (2) honor your breath and physical experience, and (9) be of your values.

Questions to Ask Your Clients
- What aspect of yoga speaks to you most? Consider exploring character, working with mantras, cultivating a practice of service to others, devotion to a higher power, or work with symptoms as compelling ways to work with self-regulation.
- Which type of yoga would you like to learn more about?

THE FOUR IMMEASURABLES

The four immeasurables can be found both in the Yoga Sutras and in Buddhist texts (Bryant, 2009; Wallace, 2010). Yoga Sutra 1.33, *"maitri-karuna-muditopeksanam sukkah-dukkha-punyapuny-visayanam bhavanatas citta–prasadanam,"* is interpreted as meaning that the undisturbed calmness of the mind can be attained by cultivating friendliness (i.e., loving-kindness) toward the happy, compassion for the unhappy, delight (i.e., joy) in the virtuous, and indifference (i.e., equanimity) toward those who struggle (Bryant, 2009; Prabhavananda & Isherwood, 2007; Roach & McNally, 2005). Roach and McNally (2005) summarized Yoga Sutras 1.32 and 1.33 this way:

> And if you wish to stop these obstacles there is one, and only one crucial practice for doing so. You must use kindness, compassion, joy, and equanimity. Learn to keep your feelings in balance where something feels good or whether it hurts; whether something is enjoyable or distasteful. (p. 24)

Loving-kindness is an attitude or quality of mind that is expressed in behavior (Wallace, 2010). It is a yearning for the person who is the object of your attention to be happy and well (Wallace, 2010). The object can be yourself, an animal, a friend, or someone with whom you struggle (Wallace, 2010). The associated embodied practice is embodied practice 12, cultivate loving-kindness and joy (see Chapter 3).

Compassion refers to kindness toward self and others (Wallace, 2010). In compassion we witness suffering of our own or the suffering of another (Wallace, 2010). There is an accompanying yearning for the suffering to be relieved (Wallace, 2010). See Chapter 10, "Off the Mat: Informal

Yoga Practices," for an overview and assessment of compassion for self and others. The associated embodied practice is embodied practice 10, observe compassion for self and others (see Chapter 3).

Joy is the simple action of rejoicing in the well-being of others (Wallace, 2010). Joy is easy to cultivate for those we love. However, it can be more challenging to cultivate joy for those with whom we are in conflict or those with whom we are in competition. The current culture of the West is rich soil for competition, with long-held beliefs such as social Darwinism and ideas like survival of the fittest, pure capitalism, and market economies. These ideas are neither inherently good nor bad. I will leave it to economics professors to figure out if they are effective. However, I do have a sense of what it does to my patients to be in this culture. There is a sense that if they are not the best, winningest, prettiest, smartest, fastest, wealthiest, then, ultimately, they are not good enough. The other side of this coin is the emotions that one feels toward those who seem to be experiencing success.

For example, recall Alexandria (Alex) from Chapter 2, who felt a strong need to be effortlessly perfect. In pursuit of the illusion of perfection, she had shopped her way into over $60,000 in debt. Recently, one of her good friends landed an amazing job with a software company in San Francisco. This success was earned. Alex's friend had done all of the work to get into a good school for undergraduate training. She had worked hard to secure experience and later worked day and night to complete an MBA. Her experience, her grades, and the accomplishments at her local software company made her an ideal candidate for this six-figure job. Alex knows all of this. She also knows that the universe is not a zero-sum game. She knows that her friend's success in no way diminishes Alex. Still, she struggled to feel happy for her friend. Instead, she was bitter that it was not she. Cultivating joy for her friend and then digging into the feelings and sensations that were stirred up with the practice would be a wonderful place for Alex to engage in therapy. See the discussion of associated embodied practice 12, cultivate loving-kindness and joy, in Chapter 3.

Equanimity can also be thought of as impartiality (Wallace, 2010). Not indifference, equanimity allows us to be present with the highs and lows of life without losing a sense of our balanced inner self. For example, as Addison was working toward satya, or truthfulness, there were days that she had slips. Triggered by stress at work or an off-handed comment a coworker had made about her body, Addison would find herself halfway into a binge and in deep regret. Terrified to keep all of the food she had eaten in her stomach for fear of gaining weight, she purged. Her practice was to have a sense of equanimity at these times. Of course it was best if she stayed mindful and avoided bingeing in the first place. However, if she did slip, the moment she caught herself, she moved into a practice of equanimity. She put away or threw away the food she had not eaten and cleaned up her area while deep breathing, saying to herself, "This is neither good nor bad. It is what it is. I can breathe and stay steady."

Notice how Addison was not dissociated from or indifferent to her situation (Wallace, 2010). Dissociation and indifference are concepts distinct from equanimity, and equanimity tends to bring patients toward growth. By practicing staying present and centered after a binge, Addison felt the effects of the binge and breathed into her feelings and sensations with equanimity. The fruits of this practice were her deepened awareness of when she was stressed or triggered and her ability to abstain from binges in the future. This practice was very challenging for Addison and she was very proud of herself for cultivating equanimity during such intense feelings of distress. See the discussion in Chapter 3 of associated embodied practice 11, maintain equanimity.

Questions to Ask Your Clients
- How often do you feel warm feelings or feelings of loving-kindness toward yourself, your family, friends, and others who are in your life? What role does your struggle with self-regulation play in these relationships?
- Tell me about compassion in your life. Do you have compassion for yourself? For others? Is your compassion for others deeper than your self-compassion? What role does self-compassion play in your struggle with self-regulation?
- How often do you feel joy for the success and happiness of others? Does your struggle with self-regulation play a role in the feelings and experiences of joy for yourself and others?
- When was the last time you felt a sense of equanimity about your situation, your triggers, or aspects of your struggle? Describe this to me.

SUMMARY

This chapter reviewed the basics of yoga philosophy with an emphasis on the Yoga Sutras of Patanjali. An overall definition of yoga was provided. The three manifestations of the body and five koshas were reviewed. The key texts were identified and then the basic tenets of the practice were detailed as they are described by yoga scholars, interpretations of the sutras, master yogis, and mental health professionals who use yoga techniques to facilitate growth and wellness. These were all tied to the mindful and yogic embodied practices detailed in Chapter 3. Chapters 8, 9, and 10 provide context and methodology for on-the-mat, or formal, yoga practices and off-the-mat, informal practices that can be used in your own personal growth and to cultivate self-regulation within your patients.

REFERENCES

American Psychiatric Association. (2000). *Diagnostic and statistical manual of mental disorders* (4th ed., text rev.). Washington, DC: Author.

American Psychiatric Association. (2013). *Diagnostic and statistical manual of mental disorders* (5th ed.). Arlington, VA: American Psychiatric Publishing.

Anderson, S., & Sovik, R. (2000). *Yoga: Mastering the basics.* Honsedale, PA: The Himalayan Institute.

Anodea, J. (2004). *Eastern body, Western mind: Psychology and the chakra system as a path to the true self.* Berkeley, CA: Celestial Arts.

Baird, T. (2014). Encinitas Union School District; Yoga in the Schools Conference keynote. A keynote presentation given at the Yoga in the Schools Conference (April 23–25) at Kripalu, Lenox, MA.

Bryant, E. F. (2009). *The Yoga Sutras of Patanjali.* New York, NY: North Point Press, a division of Farrar, Straus, and Giroux.

Cook-Cottone, C. (2006), The attuned representation model for the primary prevention of eating disorders: An overview for school psychologists. *Psychology in the Schools, 43,* 223–230.

De Michelis, E. (2008). Modern yoga: History and forms. In M. Singleton & J. Byrne (Eds.), *Yoga in the modern world: Contemporary perspectives* (pp. 17–35). New York, NY: Routledge.

Douglass, L. (2007). The yoga tradition: How did we get here? A history of yoga in America, 1800–1970. *International Journal of Yoga Therapy, 17,* 35–42.

Gandhi, M. (2011). *The Bhagavad Gita according to Gandhi.* Blacksburg, VA: Wilder Publications.

Iyengar, B. K. S. (1996; rev. ed. 1977). *Light on yoga.* New York, NY: Schocken Books.

Kraftsow, G. (1999). *Yoga for wellness: Healing with the timeless teachings of Viniyoga.* New York, NY: Penguin Putnam.

Liberman, K. (2008). The reflexivity of the authenticity of Hatha yoga. In M. Singleton & J. Byrne (Eds.), *Yoga in the modern world: Contemporary perspectives* (pp. 100–116). New York, NY: Routledge.

Markland, D., Ryan, R. M., Tobin, V. J., & Rollnick, S. (2005). Motivational interviewing and self-determination theory. *Journal of Social and Clinical Psychology, 24,* 811–831.

McCall, T. (2007). *Yoga as medicine: The yogic prescription for health and healing.* New York, NY: Bantam Dell, Random House.

Norcross, J. C., Krebs, P. M., & Prochaska, J. O. (2011). Stages of change. *Journal of Clinical Psychology, 67*(2), 143–154.

Prabhavananda, S., & Isherwood, C. (2007). *How to know God: The yoga aphorisms of Patanjali.* Hollywood, CA: Vedanta Press.

Roach, G. S., & McNally, C. (2005). *The essential yoga sutras: Ancient wisdom for your yoga*. New York, NY: Three Leaves Press, Doubleday.

Sell, C. (2003). *Yoga from the inside out: Making peace with your body through yoga*. Prescott, AZ: Hohm Press.

Simpkins, A. M., & Simpkins, C. A. (2011). *Meditation and yoga in psychotherapy: Techniques for clinical practice*. New York, NY: John Wiley & Sons.

Singleton, M. (2010). *Yoga body: The origins of modern posture practice*. New York, NY: Oxford University Press.

Singleton, M., & Byrne, J. (2008). *Yoga in the modern world: Contemporary perspectives*. New York, NY: Routledge.

Sovik, R. (2005). *Moving inward: The journey to meditation*. Honesdale, PA: Himalayan Institute Press.

Stephens, M. (2010). *Teaching yoga: Essential foundations and techniques*. Berkeley, CA: North Atlantic Books.

Wallace, B. A. (2010). *The four immeasurables: Practiced to open the heart*. Ithaca, NY: Snow Lion Productions.

Weintraub, A. (2004). *Yoga for depression: A compassionate guide to relieve suffering through yoga*. New York, NY: Broadway Books.

Weintraub, A. (2012). *Yoga skills for therapists: Effective practice for mood management*. New York, NY: W. W. Norton.

CR 8 BO

On the Mat
Formal Yoga Practices

As a person acts, so he becomes in life....
You are what your deep, driving desire is.
As your desire is, so is your will.
As your will, so is your deed.
As your deed, so is your destiny.

The Upanishads
—(EKNATH & NAGLER, 2007, p. 114)

AS GOES YOUR BREATH . . .

The preceding quote is the root source of what is now often recited in yoga classes and quoted as the following:

Watch your thoughts; they become words.
Watch your words; they become actions.
Watch your actions; they become habit.
Watch your habits; they become character.
Watch your character; it becomes your destiny.
(Barwick, 1983, p. 23)

It is an example of the evolving interpretations of yoga scripture. The original version comes from an interpretation of the Upanishads by Eknath and Nagler (2007). Finding the source took some doing and the skills of a professional librarian. What we found was that as these words have been passed down from yoga teacher to student, they took on a form more consistent with current culture, perhaps reflecting the Eastern roots as well as the spirit of Western self-determination. Like interpretations of the yoga texts, the Western version of yoga has taken on many forms.

Yoga practices offered in the United States range from classes that are near neighbors to aerobics or fitness classes and those that are steeped in Eastern tradition. It makes sense that yoga is being embraced by Western culture. It is well accepted that yoga enhances overall physiological health, strength, and flexibility (McCall, 2007). And, yoga offers more. Consistent with the chapter-opening quote (i.e., "As a person acts, so he becomes in life. . ."; Eknath & Nagler, 2007, p. 114), yoga is embodied learning. It is an on-the-mat opportunity for growth. As yoga practitioners build physical health, strength, and flexibility, they learn.

This chapter conceptualizes yoga as *embodied learning*. To do this, the neurological, emotional, and behavioral implications are covered. The limbs of yoga are reviewed from the external foundational practices to the internal meditative practices. Figures, case examples, and instructional stories are used to illustrate points.

YOGA AS EMBODIED LEARNING

"As goes your breath, so goes your heart, as goes your heart, so go your thoughts." This quote comes from my own yoga teaching. I often use this quote and the Eknath and Nagler (2007) quote together, as they link the trajectory, the destiny, of your life all the way back to the union of breath and body. Living from this level of awareness and presence is a way of being that comes from the center of who you are and creates a strong, empowering sense of integration. For many years, psychology focused on the cognitive aspects of functioning and on cognitively driven or modified behaviors. This outside-in or top-down approach has deep philosophical roots in *Descartes' Error*, the philosophical separation of mind and body (Damasio, 1999; Douglass, 2011). In an effort to improve outcomes, emotions were addressed as yet another aspect of self that could be cognitively mediated from the top down. For nearly 100 years, mainstream Western psychology cognitively managed nearly everything. For some, this worked. Sorting out their thoughts, perspectives, and understanding was what they needed to get better. However, for many others it takes more than this. Our bodies are not something to control, a subordinate entity to be subdued by the mind and authorities (Douglass, 2011). In private practice, every so often parents will ask why their son or daughter

can't just use willpower to overcome eating-disordered behavior. They ask, "Why don't they just stop?" Nearly each patient I see has already tried this—to use the will to maintain *power over* the body. Use of will-power does not promote a union of body and mind. It is a continuation of the struggle and dis-integrating. Eisenstein (2003) said it well: "Reliance on willpower reveals a profound distrust of one's self" (p. 4). As advances in neuroscience have confirmed, the body is not an external entity that we train, control, reward, punish, or objectify. It is us.

Your Body, the Seat of Your Mind, Is You—Is Self

Our bodies are the vessels, some even say temples, of our existence. In health and well-being, we exist as our bodies, nourishing, nurturing, challenging, and attuning. Douglass (2011) posits that thinking is only and always embodied. She holds that yoga is an educational tool, an embodied learning in which practitioners systematically engage "in the process and action of thinking through the body" (p. 85). That is, you move from thinking about states of mind to embodying new ways of thinking (Douglass, 2011). It is a very powerful and empowering shift in how you experience your body. As explained in Chapter 2, embodiment and active practice are necessities for symptom reduction for some patients. To shift away from symptoms, our patients must see the body as an aspect of self to which they need to listen to, care for, and nurture and with which they must communicate (Douglass, 2011; Levine, 2010).

Embodiment, as seen in yoga, promotes well-being at the neurological and physiological levels in these three ways: (a) It enhances neurological integration (i.e., neurological differentiation and linkage); (b) it reduces reactivity, increases reflective engagement, and improves access to restful and restorative states; and (c) it improves emotional and behavioral regulation (Figure 8.1).

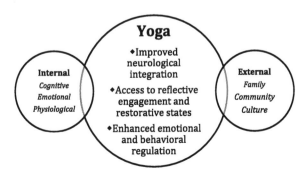

FIGURE 8.1 Neurological and physiological benefits of yoga.

Neurological Integration

First, formal yoga practices can help with self-regulation by facilitating mind–body integration. To be independently and effectively self-regulated, you and your clients need neurological integration. We may lack integration for a variety of reasons, including childhood environments and the quality of familial relationships, a genetic or physiological background (i.e., physical or emotional trauma) that has resulted in a brain that needs more practice and support for integration than most brains, or engagement in behaviors or practices that disrupted integration. When individuals get caught up in disordered eating; substance use; self-harm; or problem gambling, gaming, or shopping; repeated engagement in the behaviors can strengthen the disorder, promoting neurological connections and further priming their brains to be more easily triggered to re-engage in the behavior. These processes repeatedly strengthen neurological networks that support the problematic behavior, trigger reward areas of the brain, and disrupt healthy, engaged problem solving and well-integrated neurological networks.

For example, when Addison, the 22-year-old in recovery from bulimia nervosa introduced in an earlier chapter, binged and purged for the first time, she was 14 years old. She had a lot to deal with at home: parents with high expectations, a younger sister with a kidney disorder that needed a tremendous amount of medical attention and support from her parents, and a little brother who needed Addison a lot. She never intended to have an eating disorder. In fact, she went on a diet with her mom as something fun the two of them could do together. As Addison started to lose weight, she got compliments from the other kids at school and boys who had not paid attention to her before were asking her out. But, she was hungry all of the time and she wasn't performing well in soccer. One night after practice, she was starving. She started eating and she lost a sense of control. She didn't care. She felt like she had been holding herself back for weeks. She ate and ate and ate until her stomach felt like it might burst. Then, she panicked. She snuck to the bathroom and intentionally vomited. A tremendous sense of relief ran through her body. She felt relieved about the food, yes, and she felt a little more clear about everything—school, her parents, her sister, and all the extra work of taking care of her little brother. She swore she would never do it again.

What was supposed to be a one-time thing turned into a daily habit, sometimes twice a day. Weeks passed, months passed, and then years passed. Addison began to count on her symptoms to cope. When she had a hard day, a difficult conversation, any challenge at all, she fell into her eating disorder. She worked hard to not feel anything stressful, overperformed at school, and smiled the biggest smile at nearly all times to be sure no one would suspect what was going on in the bathroom after she ate. A very disciplined person, she swore each night that this would be her last, only to find herself bingeing and purging the next day. She planned and set goals. She tried cognitive behavioral self-help books. She reworked her thoughts. Still, she struggled. Addison's sense of self was split, disintegrated (see Chapter 2). Her strong deference to thinking rather than feeling perpetuated her struggle. Her emotional regulation and relationship with her body was tied, almost exclusively, to eating-disordered behavior. Her smile was so mechanical, automatic, and externally focused that she even smiled when she cried. Through years of splitting herself apart, she had no sense of an embodied integrated self and did not know what to do.

Yoga practice integrates. When practiced as intended, it brings all of the split-apart aspects of the self together, allowing for integration and healing. Recall the yogic view of the body as the physiological sheath (e.g., kosha) that is integrated with the subtle body (i.e., energy, mind, and intellect) and the casual body (i.e., bliss or the true self; Stephens, 2010). The sheaths are viewed as intertwined and inseparable (Rybak & Deuskar, 2010). Interpersonal neurobiologists posit a similar understanding of the mind–body system, describing mental life as an *embodied* relational flow of energy and information (Siegel, 2012). That is, the mind is not separate from the body—it both arises from and regulates it (Levine, 2010; Siegel, 2012). Hence, speaking both from a yogic and neurological point of view, self-regulation is, most certainty, an integrated, embodied experience. More specifically, neurological integration manifests as linkage of the differentiated aspects of self (Siegel, 2012).

To use a yoga asana as a metaphor, I must have a differentiated awareness of the core muscles of my hips, torso, and shoulders and activate them in an integrated, linked manner to achieve and maintain a headstand. When I first began my yoga practice, I did not have a felt sense of my body, let alone a felt sense of the various muscle groups and individual muscles. When I attempted a headstand, I struggled and had no real sense of why or what to do to fix it. Teachers had explained to me which muscles were involved. I watched videos that explained what to do. After a while I cognitively understood what I needed to do. This was not enough. One millimeter and one breath at a time, I have worked to transition to and hold a headstand. I had to map what I knew in my head onto what was happening in my body. I had to feel muscles that I had never consciously felt before and then learn how to activate and deactivate them. Now, when in a headstand, I have a felt sense and mindful coordination of my hip flexors, my abdominal muscles, and the muscles through my midback and shoulders. I can feel the areas that need more attention, energy, and effort. With this differentiated awareness, I can self-correct, coordinate, and self-regulate. Integration and yoga work like that. Research bears this out. For example, as compared to engagement in general aerobic exercise, yoga is associated with greater awareness of and responsiveness to bodily sensations (Daubenmier, 2005). See also Sheila Reindl's (2001) *Sensing the Self: Women's Recovery from Bulimia* for well-written accounts of embodied self-regulation and recovery from bulimia. In Reindl's (2001) book she describes detailed case studies of women who moved from judging the self to sensing the self as a pathway to recovery. Further, in a qualitative study of women in a 12-week yoga treatment program for binge eating, researchers found that yoga enhanced the mind–body connection, cultivated a healthier connection with food and physical self-empowerment, and showed positive symptom outcomes (McIver, McGartland, & O'Halloran, 2009).

Accessing Reflective Engagement and Restorative States

Many of my clients do not have knowledge or a felt sense of regulating themselves emotionally, psychologically, or physically. They often feel as if they are subject to their external world and any stressors that come from it, their unsettled internal world, or both. Access to reflective engagement and restorative states of being is critical to symptom reduction. Stephen Porges (2011), the author of *The Polyvagal Theory: Neurophysiological Foundations of Emotions, Attachment, Communication, and Self-Regulation*, suggests that yoga training may improve the ability to self-regulate, dampen physiological reactivity, and feel more comfortable in your body. The general physiological and neurological bases of self-regulation lie in the ability to respond to the outer world and to inner events (e.g., thoughts, memories) in a neurologically integrated (see previous discussion) and nonreactive manner (Levine, 2010; Siegel, 2010). In part, this means that we have the capacity to access the reflective and relational aspects of the nervous system even when we are triggered, threatened, or challenged (Porges, 2011). We need tools for bringing the body away from stressed, defensive reactions and toward calmness, alertness, and engagement as well as access to states of rest and restoration (Levine, 2010; Porges, 2011). To develop these skills, we need to engage in practices that require reflective engagement of the central nervous system while in action, intention, and challenge (like my headstand) and those that empower the practitioner to intentionally move from one state (e.g., activation, defensive reaction) to another (i.e., restoration and repair).

It can help patients to understand what is going on in their bodies and within their nervous systems. There are neurological systems that regulate aspects of the body critical to self-regulation (Levine, 2010; Porges, 2011). Recent research suggests that these systems are a bit more complex than originally understood and are involved in the regulation of physiological, emotional, and relational aspects of self (Porges, 2011). When working with patients, first I explain that the nervous system comprises the central nervous system (CNS; the brain and spinal cord) and the peripheral nervous system (PNS; Levine, 2010). The PNS comprises the autonomic nervous system (ANS; maintains homeostasis and regulates organs and metabolism) and the somatic nervous system (involves voluntary muscle control, touch, and proprioception; Levine, 2010). I explain that feeling triggered and in reaction involves the ANS, which is comprised of two systems: the sympathetic nervous system (SNS; fight-or-flight response) and the parasympathetic system (PS). The vagus nerve, the 10th cranial nerve, plays a substantial role in the dynamics of these systems and self-regulation (Porges, 2011). The PS functions through what is believed to be two subsystems: (a) the unmyelinated primitive vagus system associated with immobilization and shutdown, and (b) the myelinated vagus system associated with social engagement and muscles in the face, middle ears, and throat (Levine, 2010). In safety, the PS also promotes functions that are associated with rest, growth, and restoration, while the SNS promotes increases in metabolic output to negotiate challenges that come from outside of the body (Porges, 2011). It is believed that when threatened or challenged, the nervous system works in a problem-solving hierarchy (Table 8.1).

It is believed that these systems activate both in the face of real danger and perceived dangers (Levine, 2010). Individuals who have been chronically traumatized, abused, or neglected can experience a domination of the immobilization or shut-down system (Levine, 2010). Those who have experienced acute trauma or challenge may be more dominated by the fight-or-flight system (Levine, 2010). Choice is lost and self-regulation problems can follow. Sharing this neurological information with patients helps them to understand that (a) there are physiological foundations for emotional and self-regulation (see Chapter 2); (b) dysregulation of these systems can play a role in self-regulation challenges; and (c) yoga is an integrated system of tools that can support neurological integration, down-regulation of sympathetic (i.e., defensive or reactive) and immobilizing parasympathetic responses, increases in reflective engagement, and promotion of health, strength, and flexibility (Field, 2011; Levine, 2010). Yoga can help. Levine (2010) states, "Somatic approaches can be enormously useful, or even critical, in [the] healing effort" (p. 115).

TABLE 8.1   A Hierarchy of Neurologically Based Response Strategies

Problem Stage	Response and *Example*
Problem or challenge presents	Social engagement, communication, and self-soothing systems are activated. The muscles of the face and throat are stimulated and social engagement is attempted (i.e., activation of the myelinated parasympathetic nervous system).
	Zuri's mom storms into the room, obviously drunk, and seems enraged. Zuri asks, "Momma, are you okay? What happened?" Zuri says to herself, "You've got this. Everything is going to be okay."
Problem or challenge is unresolved or escalates	The body prepares for fight or flight. The nervous system activates the sympathetic nervous system, sending information and energy to the limbs and away from rest and restorative processes such as healing and digestion.
	"No, Zuri, I am not okay. I just ran over your f%##@# bicycle in the driveway." She reaches for a belt, "Get over here. Let me show you how many hours I worked to pay for the %%#% bike."
	Zuri runs upstairs, slams her door, and pushes a chair against it. She tries to open the window. It's stuck. She hears her mom coming. Her mother beats her horribly when she's drunk. Zuri can't escape.
Problem or challenge is unresolved or escalates	The body is immobilized or freezes. The nervous system activates the vagus nerve and dorsal vagal systems.
	Her mom gets through the door. She has the belt and she is enraged. Zuri has dropped to the floor. Unable to escape, she is immobilized, frozen.

Source: Levine, 2010.

Embodied practices help move patients through immobilization and re-action and toward equilibrium and social engagement (Levine, 2010). For example, yoga is believed to enhance vagal activity and reduce cortisol as compared to general aerobic activity (Field, 2011). For a review of interpersonal neurobiology, see Siegel (2012); for an extensive review of the research on the vagus nerve, see Porges (2011); and for an exploration of trauma and the body, see Levine (2010).

Feeling Your Feelings

Yoga practice provides opportunities to experience your feelings as embodied. Understanding what is happening in your body and how it affects your behavior is critical to recovery and maintenance of healthy behavior. Within the field of research on emotions, it is generally accepted that emotions coordinate behavior and physiological states during survival-salient events and pleasurable interactions (Nummenmaa, Glerean, Hari, & Hietanen, 2014).

The process is intricate, involving regions across and within the brain. A recent functional magnetic resonance imaging (fMRI) study supports yogic and mindful theory and explicates the processing of feelings as they occur in the brain. Specifically, Oosterwijk et al. (2012) reported on a study testing a constructionist model of the mind in which participants generated three kinds of mental states (emotions, body feelings, or thoughts) while they measured activity within large-scale distributed brain networks using fMRI. First, they identified a *salience network* in the brain. Both sense impressions and mental events are processed by the salience network, in which areas of the brain work together to rate the importance, the salience, of incoming stimuli. Next, the authors identified a neurological process in which information is tagged as pleasant or unpleasant, further supporting components of the Buddhist Psychological Model (BPM; Grabovac, Lau, & Willett, 2011). Underscoring the importance of understanding the felt sense of experience, Oosterwijk et al.'s (2012) findings suggest that representations of body sensations play a role beyond the experience of physical sensations in the body or affective states such as emotions. Specifically, they found that in situations in which participants were presented with evocative or behaviorally relevant information, the salience network tended to guide the direction of attention based on body sensations. This finding was true irrespective of whether people were directed to experience an emotion or objectively think about the situation. Oosterwijk et al. (2012) reported that this finding was consistent with several recent suggestions in the literature that body cues are a ubiquitous component of mental life.

Nummenmaa and colleagues (2014) agree. Emotions are felt in the body. Further, somatosensory feedback may trigger conscious emotional experiences. In order to map the location of emotions in the body, Nummenmaa et al. (2014) used a unique topographical self-report method. In a set of five experiments, participants ($n = 701$) were shown two silhouettes of bodies alongside emotional words, stories, movies, or facial expressions. Nummenmaa et al. (2014) asked participants to color the bodily regions in which they felt activity increasing or decreasing while viewing each stimulus. After analysis the researchers found that different emotions were consistently associated with statistically discernable bodily sensation maps (Figure 8.2). The authors concluded that emotions are represented in the somatosensory system as categorical somatotopic maps, and that perception of emotion-triggered bodily changes may play a key role in generating consciously felt emotions.

In yoga class and in private practice, I ask yogis and patients to feel their feelings. Whether it is a yogi in class struggling with holding a basic posture or a patient who is describing something deeply emotional, I create a pause in the process and ask them to describe what they are

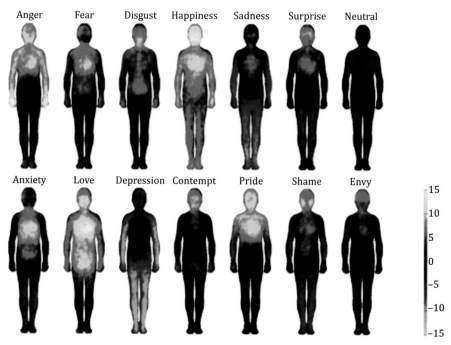

FIGURE 8.2 Topographical map of emotions in the body.
Source: Nummenmaa et al., 2014.

feeling, specifically where they are feeling the emotion in their bodies. Next, I ask them to simply breathe into the feeling and allow it. See Practice Script 8.1, Feel Your Feelings.

Some styles of yoga focus on the emotional aspects of being more than others. For example, the Trauma Informed Mind-Body (TIMBo) program created by Sue Jones (YogaHOPE, 2015) is designed to provide support for women who have experienced trauma. The manualized program helps women: (a) understand how and why their bodies feel the way they do; (b) notice their emotional sensations nonjudgmentally; and (c) take effective action in regulating the difficult sensations (YogaHOPE, 2015). Levine (2010) explains that by staying aware and tracking spontaneous physical reactions and emotions and breathing into them, we trigger our innate capacity for self-regulation. It is believed that by learning these skills to navigate emotional experience, the women who participate will be less likely to turn to drugs, alcohol, and destructive behaviors to cope. Early TIMBo research looks promising. For example, in a study conducted in Haiti, Jackson (2013) found TIMBo to support the mitigation of traumatic symptomology among women who were abuse survivors and those who experienced trauma during the Haitian earthquake.

The mindful and yogic approach to emotional regulation is explicated in Table 8.2. The table aligns this approach to Koole, van Dillen, and Sheppes's (2011) model of emotional regulation. In yogic approaches, regular focus on the yamas and niyamas along with daily practice of asana, pranayama, pratyahara, and meditation cultivate neurological integration and reduced reactivity over time. Further, these practices are down-regulating; they decrease the triggering potential of both sense impressions and mental events. Stages 2 through 4 reflect the mindful and yogic approach to negotiating emotionally salient information and behavioral choices. Ultimately, this process cultivates embodied self-regulation that honors the present-moment experience, creates balanced and sustainable self-mastery, and allows attunement within self and with others (see Chapter 1, Table 1.1).

Work with patients can be structured within this model. Rather than talk about emotional regulation, encourage and provide opportunities for patients to learn through lived experience, to embody the process.

TABLE 8.2   Mindful and Yogic Processing of Feelings

Stage	Emotional Regulation (Koole et al., 2011)	Mindful and Yogic Process (See Chapter 3)
Stage 1	• Situational triggers, encounters (e.g., situational selection, situational modification)	• *Situational shifts over time* Yamas and niyamas and daily practice shift exposure to triggers and neurological reactivity to triggers over time. • *In present time* Sense impressions Mental events
Stage 2	• Attention/inattention to emotionally relevant features (e.g., attentional deployment)	• Mindful awareness (noticing) • Selection of attachment, avoidance, or allowing • Honoring breath and physical experience
Stage 3	• Cognitive appraisal of the situation (e.g., cognitive change)	• Understanding of how and why brains and bodies feel the way they do • Impermanence, not-self, nonjudgment, and allowing • Observing compassion for self and others • Maintaining equanimity
Stage 4	• Emotions expressed in behaviors (e.g., response modulation)	• Expression of authentic self (*through intentional choice of movement or voice*) • Prioritizing self-care • Acting within values • Cultivating loving-kindness

Source: Jackson, 2013; Koole et al., 2011.

Practice Script 8.1 is designed to bring awareness to feelings and the locations of feelings in the body. I have worked with several patients using this technique. It can be especially helpful for those patients who have very little awareness of emotions and the embodied experience of emotions. Patients who struggle with negative affect, show a tendency to escape uncomfortable situations or emotional experiences, have deficits in the awareness of bodily states and awareness, have difficulty detecting triggers or cues in their bodies, self-objectify, and have experienced invalidating environments are good candidates for this activity.

Before you begin, invite your patient to participate, explaining the process and the reasons for the process. Let the patient know that you will be asking him or her to elicit four feelings: safety and happiness, sadness, anger, and anxiety or fear. You can expand on emotions depending on your patient's treatment plan. For patients who have trauma histories or little experience with emotions this can be a very challenging activity. Often, I present the idea and allow patients to choose when we do it (e.g., "Let me know when you would like to try this activity in a session"). I also develop a cue or signal with which they can notify me that they need a break or would like to stop for the day. Following the activity, it is important to engage in breath work and supportive communication in order to help the patient return to baseline physiological activation. I also encourage patients to schedule a quiet afternoon or evening with supportive family or friends if the session has been particularly challenging.

PRACTICE SCRIPT 8.1: Feel Your Feelings
(Approximate Timing: 2 Minutes for the Introduction; 30 Minutes for Practice)

[To prepare, have four photocopied sheets of a gender-neutral outline of a human figure and a box of colored pencils or crayons.]
Sit in a comfortable position. Be sure that you feel grounded, with your feet on the floor and solid support under your sitting bones and behind your back. Close your eyes and become aware of your breath. Breathe in and out, noticing the air as it enters your body and as you exhale. Feel the sensation of your chest, rib cage, and belly as they expand to take in air and contract to release air. Allow your breathing to be steady and natural.

Now, bring your awareness to a time when you were feeling very safe and happy. Picture yourself in this moment. Have a sense of where you were, maybe even what you were wearing. Were you inside or outside? Recall who was around you. Bring to mind any sights, sounds, and smells. Now, bring your awareness to your body. Feel the feelings of safety and happiness. Explore where you feel these feelings in your body. Scan your body from your feet to the crown of your head. Feel your arms and legs. Breathe into the areas of your body where you are feeling. It might help to place one or both of your hands on the place that you are feeling something. Breathe as you watch the feeling arise and slowly pass way. Notice that feelings have a point at which you become aware of them, a peak, and then a gradual lessening. Breathe and notice. Take as much time as you need. (Pause.) When you are ready, slowly open your eyes. Reflect on your experience and draw what you were feeling in your body on the figure here. Choose whatever colors you'd like to reflect what you were feeling and where you were feeling it. Use color to show intensity and how the feeling may have felt different in various parts of your body. Let me know when you are done.

When you are ready, sit back and return your focus to your breath. Next, think of a time when you were feeling very sad. As before, cultivate a sense of your surroundings, the people, the sounds, sights, and smells of the environment. As you remember, see what you see and feel what you feel. Now, bring your awareness to your body. Locate the sadness in your body. Breathe and notice. Breathe into the areas of your body where you are feeling sadness. It might help to place one or both of your hands on the place(s) that you are feeling sadness. Breathe as you watch the feeling arise and slowly pass away. Notice if the emotions seem to peak. Breathe and notice. (Pause.) Take as much time as you need. When you are ready, open your eyes. Color on this sheet where you were feeling sadness in your body. Choose whatever colors you'd like in order to best reflect what you were feeling and where you were feeling it.

When you are ready, sit back and bring your focus to your breath. Close your eyes. Bring to mind a time when you were angry. Do you remember why you were angry? Think about the anger. Who was present when you were feeling angry? Where were you? Do you recall what you were wearing, or any sights, sounds, and smells? Bring the feeling of anger to your awareness. Now, bring your attention to your body. Where do you feel the anger in your body? Scan your body from the crown of your head to your feet. Feel your arms, your torso, and your legs. Feel what you feel. Breathe into the areas of your body where you are feeling the anger. It might help to place one or both of your hands on the place that you are feeling anger. Breathe as you watch the feeling arise and slowly pass way. Breathe and notice the feeling. (Pause.) Take as much time as you need. When you are ready, open your eyes. Indicate with colors where you were feeling anger in your body. Choose whatever colors you'd like to reflect what you were feeling and where you were feeling it.

When you are ready, return to a comfortable seat and close your eyes. Bring your awareness to your breathing. This is the final emotion we will be working on today. Bring to mind a time when you were anxious or afraid. Recall the circumstances, the location, and the people who were there. Recall if it was day or night and the location. Try to recall any sights, sounds, and smells. Now, turn your attention to your body. Where do you feel the anxiety or fear in your body? Take time to scan your body from your center out to your hands and feet, to the crown of your head. Feel what you feel. Breathe into the areas of your body where you are feeling the fear or anxiety. It might help to place one or both of your hands on the area that you are feeling the fear or anxiety. Breathe as you watch the feeling arise and slowly pass way. Take as much time as you need (pause). When you are ready, open your eyes. Color on this sheet where you were feeling fear or anxiety in your body. Choose whatever colors you'd like to reflect what you were feeling and where you were feeling it.

[Label each of the drawings: safe and happy, sad, angry, and anxiety or fear. Place them one next to the other on the table. Have your patient describe the pictures to you, how the feelings showed up in his or her body, and how the feelings were similar and different. Ask your client to reflect on the process of feeling and drawing feelings. Some people will have many details and experiences to share with you and others will have fewer. There is no right or wrong, just what was experienced or not. Once the patient is done describing, comparing, and reflecting, return your patient to his or her breath.]

Find your comfortable seat. Bring your awareness to your breath. Notice your breath as you inhale and notice your breath as you exhale. Each time you inhale, have a sense of gratitude for your willingness to explore, experience, and allow your feelings. Each time you exhale silently say the words "Let go" and release any tensions that you may be experiencing. Do this for five breaths, inhaling gratitude and exhaling release. When you are ready, slowly open your eyes.

This activity can be done once or in a series. As your patient becomes increasingly aware of his or her felt sense, the drawings will change. I have found it very instructional to review the drawings that have been created over time and reflect on growth and challenges. Ultimately, feelings need to be felt, experienced, breathed through, and sometimes expressed. In a series of interviews with individuals who had recovered from bulimia nervosa (BN), Sheila Reindl (2001) found that, oftentimes, the eating disorder served as a method for processing feelings and took the place of the person's voice in his or her interpersonal world. By feeling, processing, and expressing feelings and needs, recovery was accessible (Reindl, 2001). Associated embodied practices (see Chapter 3) include: (1) be mindfully aware, (2) honor your breath and physical experience, (3) live in inquiry, (4) accept impermanence, (5) cultivate nonattachment, (6) discern what is not-self, (7) allow what is with nonjudgment, and (10) observe compassion for self and others.

Yoga and Craving and Symptoms

Yoga practice can help you and your patients regulate behavior by reducing craving and interrupting the behavioral chain from trigger to engagement in behavior. Yoga Sutra II.23, "*sva-awami-saktyoh svarupopalabdhi-hetuh samygah*," reflects the notion of yoga as a process of learning about two things: (a) the true nature of the objects of attention and (b) you as the one who sees, identifies with, or notices (Bryant, 2009, p. 229; Prabhavananda & Isherwood, 2007). In yoga you learn that all things (e.g., mental events, sense impressions, cravings, and objects) arise in intensity and pass away. You also learn that as a witness or seer you have a choice to notice, attach, or avoid. In her article on yoga practice and eating disorder recovery, Robin Boudette (2006) tells a story of a patient in her 20s who was struggling with addiction and BN. Robin noticed that the young woman, we will call her Laura, was moving through the initial postures with little enthusiasm. When Laura was able to catch Robin's eyes, she asked her if she could leave class. Robin asked Laura to stay until the postures ended and if she still wanted to leave at that time she could. What happened during that yoga class is what happens on the other side of the urge to bolt, run, avoid, and fall into old struggles or disordered ways of being (see Chapter 4 and the Buddhist Psychological Model; Grabovac et al., 2011). On the other side of the urge is choice, and in choice is freedom from triggers and movement toward recovery. Well, Laura made a choice to stay. In fact, she stayed through the entirety of the class. After class, she told Robin, "That was better than a cigarette" and then described how surprised she was to be feeling a sense of peacefulness (Boudette, 2006, p. 168). In mindfulness-based relapse prevention this is called *urge surfing*, in which you ride the wave of the urge to its peak and all the way back down (Marlatt, Bowen, & Lustyk, 2012).

B. K. S. Iyengar is often quoted as saying, "The pose begins the moment that you want to leave it." I reword this for patients: True recovery begins the moment you want to leave it. What is so powerful about yoga practice is that you can live the moments of triggers and urges in a practice of experiencing and breathing into them. You can practice noticing them and allowing them. It is an embodied practice in which your patients have confidence that they can manage an urge or trigger, because they have. In practice, the breath, posture, and awareness hold steady as the trigger, craving, or urge arises and passes away.

Figure 8.3 illustrates the intensity of a craving or reaction to a trigger. In practice, you notice that the craving or trigger peaks; it slowly increases in intensity and eventually comes to its peak. After the peak,

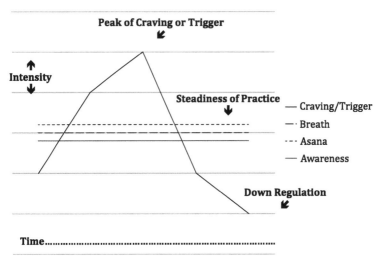

FIGURE 8.3 Arising and passing away of craving and triggers in yoga.

the intensity of the sensation drops. If you breathe, practice, and remain mindful through the noticing of the rise and fall of your craving and trigger, you can facilitate down-regulation or movement into a restful, restorative, relaxing state, as illustrated in Figure 8.3 and in the narrative by the young student Laura in Robin Boudette's class (Boudette, 2006). It is important to note that negotiation of cravings involves embodied action of empowering behaviors. Laura did not escape—nor did she freeze; she continued to move and breathe with and through her feelings. Embodiment of right action, a learning of empowered ways of being with feelings and cravings, is the key (Levine, 2010).

By learning new ways of being with triggers and cravings, your patients can effectively reduce symptoms. Research supports the notion that practice can help reduce symptoms. In a randomized controlled clinical trial of yoga in the treatment of eating disorders, Carei, Fyfe-Johnson, Breuner, and Brown (2010) found that yoga decreased eating disorder symptoms during the 12-week intervention as compared to controls. For more on yoga outcomes see Chapter 11.

What might this look like? Eli is a 16-year-old young man going into his junior year of high school. Although barely anyone knows this, he has binge-eating disorder (BED; see Chapter 2). He is a football player and solid B+ student. He works very hard at football and pretty hard at school. As part of summer conditioning, the athletic department at the high school is offering a range of activities for the kids. This includes weight lifting, interval work, and yoga. Having heard that the teams that won the Super Bowl and the World Cup integrated yoga into their workouts and about the benefits of yoga in school health class, Eli signed up for yoga. His counselor at school had been encouraging him to try it all spring. She would be happy to know that he had been taking classes nearly all summer long. He could see already how yoga was helping him improve his flexibility and mental strength.

About 6 weeks in, the instructor placed them all in a deep crescent lunge (i.e., feet in parallel tracks, one foot in front, knee bent and stacked over the ankle; one foot behind, leg straight, weight on the ball of the foot, and heel pressing back; arms high, shoulders in). Eli was getting frustrated. His hip flexors were extremely tight (i.e., the muscles in the front of the hip that help you bring your leg up toward your belly). In crescent lunge, the extension of the back leg and corresponding pulling in of the belly and neutralizing of the tailbone stretch the hip flexor. The instructor asked them to feel what they were feeling, both physically and emotionally. He asked them to stay present and just notice. He said, "Let go of your reaction to the physical sensation. Let go of your need to judge, assess, or think about what is going on. Be present with it, allow, and breathe." Eli did this. He breathed deeply and imagined that he could breathe right into his hip flexor. They held the pose for what seemed like a long time. Then, they moved to a forward fold and the tension, the stretching, passed. The instructor asked them to notice the warmth in their hip flexors and how the sensations they were feeling had passed. He said to the class, "Moments throughout your day are like this. The intensity arises and it passes away. Stay steady with your breath, awareness, notice, and allow. This is a very powerful way to be present in your life." His instructor has been saying stuff like this for weeks. Today, these words landed for Eli.

Later that day after a hard pick-up game with some teammates, Eli was frustrated again. He was worried about the guys not knowing their plays. He felt they would never be ready for fall practice and he wanted, needed, to make it to the championship game this year. His mom was talking to him about college, SATs, and grades. His dad started chiming in about the team and queries from college coaches. This moment—right here, at the peak of frustration and the out-of-control feeling of his parents talking at the same time—this is the moment when Eli typically starts to binge eat. He hates feeling this way. When moments like this show up, he eats until his stomach almost bursts. He is a big guy and thankful for it, because no one knows that he uses food for coping. He tunes people out and shoves in the food. Then, he lays on his bed, sick from everything he ate, and passes out in what he called his "food coma."

Today was different. It was as if the whole process had slowed down and he could see more clearly. He felt the frustration and it was an echo of what he felt in crescent lunge earlier that day. Yeah, he was frustrated. He felt it. Breathing slowly and deeply, he chose to be present and allow. He looked at his mom. She was talking about college and all that. Eli noticed that she seemed worried about him. He noticed that she was trying to help him feel better. Eli deepened his breath. He looked over at his dad. His dad was eating, talking, eating, and talking. "Wait," he thought. Eli noticed that his dad was bingeing. His dad was stressed, overwhelmed, and binge eating just like Eli usually does. Eli got his plate and sat down with them. He said, "Hey, I had a long day. I am not sure if the guys are ready for the season. I am stressed about them. I am worried about college, too. I could use a break. Could we talk about something else? Who is in on the trip to the Adirondacks this year?" Eli took a breath, ate, and listened as his parents shifted the conversation to the Adirondacks, his aunts and uncles, and cousins. He ate a normal dinner. For the first time in about 4 months, Eli ate a normal dinner. Yoga works like that. Associated embodied practices (see Chapter 3) include: (1) be mindfully aware, (2) honor your breath and physical experience, (3) live in inquiry, (4) accept impermanence, (5) cultivate nonattachment, (6) discern what is not-self, (7) allow what is with nonjudgment, and (10) observe compassion for self and others.

ASPECTS OF PRACTICE AND THE PATH TO EMBODIED SELF-REGULATION

In yoga, there are a variety of styles, schools, and methodologies to consider. Of critical importance is the need to match your needs and your patients' needs to the practice. In previous chapters, the mindful path has been reviewed, including a detailed explication of the processes that occur as one engages in meditation (see Chapters 4, 5, and 6). The mindful and yogic approach to self-regulation integrates aspects of mindfulness into the comprehensive practices of yoga. The foundational and external practices of yoga (i.e., yama, niyama, asana, pranayama, and pratyahara) provide a firm footing for the internal meditative practice (i.e., dharana, dhyana, and smadhi). The process of noticing sense impressions and mental events, noticing the accompanying feeling tones (i.e., pleasant, unpleasant, and neutral), considering the noticing and mindful options (i.e., attaching, avoiding, or allowing), and the final behavioral outcomes are relevant across and throughout all of the practices of yoga (see Figure 8.4). As you engage in yamas and niyamas each day you notice the mental processes that move through your mind and the choices you make. As you practice postures, engage in breath work, and

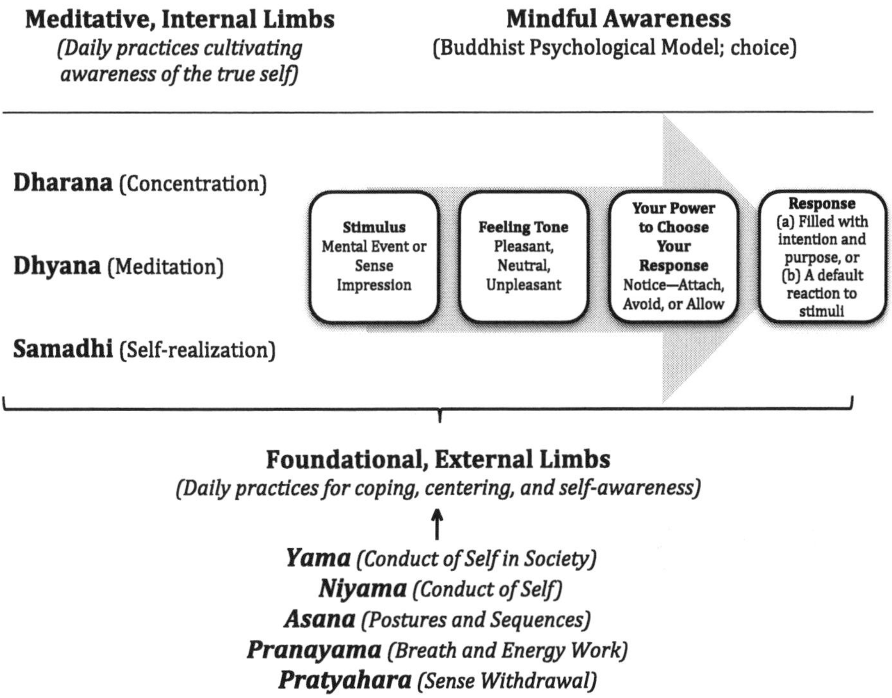

Meditative, Internal Limbs
(Daily practices cultivating awareness of the true self)

Mindful Awareness
(Buddhist Psychological Model; choice)

Dharana (Concentration)

Dhyana (Meditation)

Samadhi (Self-realization)

Stimulus Mental Event or Sense Impression	Feeling Tone Pleasant, Neutral, Unpleasant	Your Power to Choose Your Response Notice—Attach, Avoid, or Allow	Response (a) Filled with intention and purpose, or (b) A default reaction to stimuli

Foundational, External Limbs
(Daily practices for coping, centering, and self-awareness)

↑

Yama (Conduct of Self in Society)
Niyama (Conduct of Self)
Asana (Postures and Sequences)
Pranayama (Breath and Energy Work)
Pratyahara (Sense Withdrawal)

FIGURE 8.4 The integrated mindful and yogic path to self-regulation.
Source: Anderson and Sovik, 2000; Bryant, 2009; Grabovac et al., 2011; Iyengar, 1966; Stephens, 2010.

turn inward, you notice the habits of the mind and make active choices. Finally and perhaps most easily and clearly overlapping with mindfulness practice, within the meditative, internal limbs you practice the same noticing and choosing. It is this process—the noticing and choosing across daily asana, breath work, and meditation—that promotes growth.

The yamas and niyamas are the foundation for the practices (Stephens, 2010). Iyengar (1966) refers to them as prerequisites of asana. Iyengar (1966) explains, "Without firm foundations a house cannot stand. Without the practice of yama and niyama, which lay down firm foundations for building character, there cannot be an integrated personality" (p. 57). Iyengar (1966) suggests that the practice of asana without a foundation of yama and niyama is simple acrobatics. In Chapter 10 there is further discussion of the yamas and niyamas.

Asana (The Yoga Postures)

Yoga asana has many benefits, such as increased flexibility, strengthened muscles, enhanced balance, improved immune system, better posture, enhanced lung function, slower and deeper breathing, enhanced oxygenation of tissues, and relaxation of the nervous system (Anderson & Sovik, 2000; McCall, 2007; Stephens, 2010). In his book *Yoga as Medicine*, McCall (2007) lists and details over 40 benefits. There are many guides for instruction in asana practice. These include texts and videos (see Iyengar, 1966; Kraftsow, 1999; McCall, 2007; Stephens, 2010). An especially well-done book for beginners is *Yoga: Mastering the Basics*, by Sandra Anderson and Rolf Sovik (2000). This book separates beginner's sequences detailing each pose, as well as instruction on breath, relaxation, and meditation. *Yoga Journal* (www.yogajournal.com) and the Himalayan Institute's *Yoga International* (yogainternational.com) offer free access to asana, yoga, classes, and boundless information on yoga. Each offers descriptions of asana, including step-by-step instructions, tips, and contraindications for each pose. The yoga postures, or asanas, stretch and tone muscles, help keep the tissues and joints flexible, and may, in some poses, massage internal organs and glands (Field, 2011). Poses are typically done in concert with deep, diaphragmatic breath (Field, 2011). They are often grouped into these categories: standing, core, arm balances, backbends, twists, forward bends, hip openers, and inversions (Stephens, 2010).

Asana may be best learned with a teacher or mentor. Yoga is an oral tradition passed down from teacher to student through active instruction of practice. Combining individual and class instruction with personal practice and study allows for instruction on your asana, guidance during your practice, and personal opportunities at home to practice and study what you have learned.

The Lesson of Asana From Inside Out

Primarily, the lessons learned from asana practice are about you. The body is active and the mind is alert and in observations (Iyengar, 1966). As you move from pose to pose, the postures, the muscles, the challenge, the sensations, all trigger memories, thoughts, and feelings (Anderson & Sovik, 2000). Some long-held memories reside in the body. Yoga is an opportunity to rewire the postures, the sensations, the experience with even breath and a steady, loving presence. Imposing an idealized concept of what a pose is supposed to look like can create tension, a rigidity, in practice, even injury (Anderson & Sovik, 2000). See Instructional Story 8.1 for a script on the power of embodied yoga practice. Associated embodied practices (see Chapter 3) include: (1) be mindfully aware, (2) honor your breath and physical experience, (3) live in inquiry, (6) discern what is not-self, and (7) allow what is with nonjudgment.

INSTRUCTIONAL STORY 8.1: You Are Water and Asana Is Your Container

As water takes the shape of its container,
the mind, when it contemplates an object is transformed
to the shape of that object.—(Iyengar, 1966, p. 51)

If water takes on the shape of its container and you are water, what container do you choose? How do you choose your container? What aspect of you chooses? Does your ego self or your soul Self choose? It's important that you know, because these aspects of self choose differently. You see, the little ego self often accommodates the external demands of others, community, and culture. The world says, "Here is how I want you to look, act, be, and feel," and the ego self thoughtlessly reaches out and takes the container. Quite differently, the soul Self chooses carefully, mindfully. In fact, only certain containers will do. They must inspire growth, depth, and presence. Yes, these are the containers that the soul Self desires.

There once was a young woman, named Anahi, who knew only her ego self. Most of us know our ego selves pretty well. It is the self with whom you identify. When the ego self asks Anahi who she is, what she does, and what she is like, she answers, "I am Anahi. I am a nurse, a daughter, and a sister. I am always nice. I am pretty. I am a yogi. I am these things." Anahi's ego self presses hard to maintain these aspects of her identity. She would never tell anyone any of this out loud. Nevertheless, she works to be an excellent nurse, a beloved daughter and sister, and achieved at her yoga practice. She wants everyone to like her and admire her appearance. She becomes defensive about and sometimes afraid of what people think of her. She practices her yoga in the back of the room, perfecting each pose, doing just as the teacher says, pushing and driving even when she is tired. She is always proud of her discipline and discouraged by her progress. With self-talk, she yells at herself to be better, less ugly, less fat, and less stupid. These are the containers Anahi squeezes into: rigid perfection, oppressive discipline, compliance, bitterness, anger, fatigue, woundedness, and hopelessness. These containers hurt and Anahi is too afraid to let them go. Until one day in yoga class. . . .

In asana practice, the object of your attention is the body, breath, and the asana. This day, the teacher asked the students to let go of judgment and the need to get the asana right. The teacher asked the class to imagine that they were water, pure, crystal-clear water. She asked the class to imagine each asana as a container. She told them that as water, they were filling the container, transforming to the shape of the asana. As water fills from the bottom of the container up, she asked the students to fill the poses from their feet, through their legs, into their core, shoulders, then through the crown of their heads. She asked them to take the pose warrior I, a beautiful, strong, front-facing pose, with the back foot pressing down, outer edge sealed and arch lifted. In this pose, all four corners of the front foot are pressing into the mat. The knee is bent over ankle. With strong torsos, the yogis were reaching their hands toward the ceiling and drawing their shoulders into their bodies. The teacher said, "Now, fill the container of warrior. You are a warrior. From your feet to your fingers you are the warrior. You are strong, steady, ready to defend what you love."

Anahi became the warrior. She embodied the warrior. She was water and warrior was her form. Gone was the rigid perfection. Gone was her need to get it right. She wasn't being nice and she wasn't thinking about being excellent. She was a warrior. Anahi was in the present moment, feeling what she was feeling and breathing right into it all. She was, for the first time in a long time, getting a sense of her soul Self. She felt connected to her body. Her awareness and her body were one. She felt connected to the other yogis in the class. She felt warmth in her chest. She felt free and strong. And then it passed, as everything does. Anahi, having a taste, a sense, of the soul Self, began wondering about the possibility of practicing in a new way, like water. Then her teacher said, "Do you know that you are always water? You are always taking the shape of the objects of your mind. If you contemplate hate, you take that shape. If you contemplate fear, you take that shape. If you contemplate warrior, you take that shape." Anahi listened as her teacher asked, "What shapes are you taking?" Anahi was listening.

As Yoga Sutra II.21 reminds us, the object of experience, your asana, right now, exists only to serve the purpose of your soul Self. It is sometimes said this way: Life does not happen to you, it happens for you—for your soul Self. Yoga philosophy explains that the ego can drive our dysregulation. It can drive your secrets, encouraging you to hide your vulnerability and need for help. If not coached well or supported, your ego self might stick with asanas you know you can do and might worry about trying new things and facing challenges and uncomfortable feelings. Your ego self watches all the time for rules on how to look good, be successful, attract admiration. This ego self readily uses the cookie cutter handed out by cultural ideals to chop off little pieces that might not fit into the way we are supposed to be. The ego self, when left without guidance, does stuff like that.

Prananayama

Pranayama refers to breath and life force. "Without awareness of breathing, there is no yoga" (Sovik, 2005, p. 11). In yogic breathing, the breath is used to calm, purify, and strengthen the nervous system and enhance concentration (Anderson & Sovik, 2000). Breathing is also a good proxy for awareness. "Slipping from awareness, the breath usually fades" (Stephens, 2010, p. 237). The typical tempo of breath is slow, averaging about 16 breaths a minute (Anderson & Sovik, 2000). The rate of breathing varies throughout the day in service of your autonomic nervous system (ANS) as well as your intentional direction of the breath (Anderson & Sovik, 2000). It is the only function of the ANS that can be accessed in an intentional manner (Anderson & Sovik, 2000). The breath is a barometer for the nervous system changing as it experiences stress and imbalance. The breath and the nervous system create an internal feedback loop as changes in breathing perpetuate internal distress (Anderson & Sovik, 2000). Conversely, relaxed, deep, diaphragmatic breathing can restore the nervous system to a coordinated, integrated functioning (Anderson & Sovik, 2000). Reflecting its larger role in self-regulation, pranayama translates to "breath control" (Stephens, 2010, p. 237). For an overview of breath training, see Anderson and Sovik (2000).

Diaphragmatic Breathing

Due to the importance of yogic breath in self-regulation, many beginners' yoga sessions begin with instruction in diaphragmatic breathing (Anderson & Sovik, 2000). Teaching patients about diaphragmatic breathing is crucial to supporting their efforts at embodied self-regulation. Diaphragmatic breathing involves breathing deep into the belly. The lungs are not made of muscle fibers and depend on the muscles of respiration (e.g., diaphragm, intercostal muscles, pectoralis minor and major, sternocleidomastoid, serratus interior and superior, and transversospinal, scalene, and abdominal muscles; Anderson & Sovik, 2000; Stephens, 2010). Stress and the development of bad breathing habits can result in a shallow, restricted breathing (Anderson & Sovik, 2000; Stephens, 2010). In healthy, diaphragmatic breathing, the abdomen expands as one inhales (Anderson & Sovik, 2000; McCall, 2007). This expansion signifies the compression of the organs in the abdomens as the diaphragm presses down, making space for the expansion of the lungs (McCall, 2007). On exhalations, the diaphragm releases, moving back up toward the lungs, leaving more room for the organs (McCall, 2007). The belly will move back in. Notably, some patients may have what is called paradoxical breathing. In paradoxical breathing, the diaphragm and belly contract on inhalation and expand on exhalation. Often, this is noticed when you begin doing breath work. McCall (2007) indicated that this type of breathing is very arousing for the nervous system and can contribute to a feeling of chronic stress. Practice Script 8.2 can be used to guide a patient through diaphragmatic breathing.

PRACTICE SCRIPT 8.2: Diaphragmatic Breathing

(Approximate Timing: 5 Minutes for Practice)

Begin by getting comfortable in your seat. Place one hand on your chest and one hand on your belly. Bring your awareness to your breath. Soften your belly so that it is free to move. Rest the muscles connected to your rib cage. Slowly begin to breathe deeply, extending your inhalation by one count and your exhalations by one count. Continue to breathe deeply as you use your breath. Notice your hands, your chest, and your belly. Notice that your hands rise and fall with your breath. Notice, does the hand on your rib cage move more or less than the hand on your belly? To bring your breath toward deep diaphragmatic breathing, inhale so deeply that the hand on your belly lifts as the belly expands. See if you can breathe so that the hand on your chest is moving only slightly as your rib cage expands and the hand on your belly is rising and falling noticeably with each breath. Be sure to keep your breath slow, deep, smooth, and even. If you notice that you are getting lightheaded, pause at the end of each inhalation and exhalation and count to four before cycling to the next part of your breath. Continue breathing with your hands on your chest and your belly, breathing deeply into the hands on your belly for 10 more breath cycles.

Source: Anderson and Sovik, 2000; McCall, 2007; Stephens, 2010.

Opposite-Nostril Breathing (Nadi Shodhana)

Opposite-nostril breathing, or Nadi Shodhana, is believed to help balance and calm the sympathetic and parasympathetic nervous systems (Anderson & Sovik, 2000; McCall, 2007). The word *nadi* means "river" or "energy channel" (Anderson & Sovik, 2000; Weintraub, 2012). This breathing technique is thought to help balance the left and right channels of energy within the body. Some believe that this is the most complex and refined of all of the pranayamas (Stephens, 2010; Weintraub, 2012). See Practice Script 8.3, Opposite-Nostril Breathing.

PRACTICE SCRIPT 8.3: Opposite-Nostril Breathing

(Approximate Timing: 5 Minutes for Practice)

Find a comfortable seated position in which you can breathe freely. Be sure your spine is erect. On your right hand, curl your index and middle fingers toward the palm of your hand, extending your thumb, ring finger, and pinky. Place your thumb and ring finger on either side of your nose at the nostril. You will notice that you can press your thumb on your right nostril to close it or your ring finger on your left nostril to close it, simply by shifting your hand to the left or the right. Breath diaphragmatically through both nostrils for several breath cycles.

To begin the opposite-nostril breathing process, inhale through both nostrils. Next, shift your hand to the left, placing your thumb on your right nostril to close it. Slowly exhale through your left nostril completely. Then, inhale through your left nostril. Now, shift your hand to the right, releasing your thumb from the right nostril and compressing your left nostril with your ring finger. Exhale evenly and completely through your right nostril. As the exhale is complete, inhale through the right nostril. Continue to do this, alternating exhaling and inhaling through one nostril and then exhaling and inhaling through the other. Completion of an exhale and an inhale on both sides constitutes one cycle. Complete this process for six cycles. Notice your breath. Notice your thinking, continually bringing your awareness to your breath. Consider sense impressions and mental events as they arise and pass away, continuously bringing your awareness back to your breath.

Source: Anderson and Sovik, 2000; Grabovac et al., 2011; McCall, 2007; Stephens, 2010; Weintraub, 2012.

Ujjayi Breathing

Ujjayi breathing involves breathing through the nose, mouth closed, with a slightly constricted throat (Stephens, 2010). Some teach the breath by asking practitioners to first make the "ha" sound as if fogging a mirror with the mouth open. Next, they ask the practitioner to make the same "ha" sound with the mouth closed and the breath moving through the nose (McCall, 2007). Creation of the same sound and sensation while inhaling and exhaling is encouraged (Stephens. 2010). This type of breath is believed to provide additional physiological and sensory feedback regarding the breath. It has the effects of both energizing the body and bringing focus to the mind (McCall, 2007; Stephens, 2010; Weintraub, 2012). See Stephens (2010) and Weintraub (2012) for more scripts on yogic breathing techniques. Associated embodied practices (see Chapter 3) include: (1) be mindfully aware, (2) honor your breath and physical experience, and (7) allow what is with nonjudgment.

Relaxation and Meditation

Anderson and Sovik (2000) remind us, "Beneath the ups and downs of everyday life there is a profound state of balance. By resting for brief periods in that state we create a resilient and stable mind even in the face of stress" (p. 197). Relaxation exercises create a bridge from the more active, external practices of yoga to the internal, meditative practices (Anderson & Sovik, 2000; Stephens, 2010). Relaxation and meditation are part of a continuous process of depending and stilling the mind and moving toward self-awareness (Stephens, 2010; Table 8.3). Once there, the meditation process in yoga is much like meditation in mindfulness.

As in concentration meditation seen in mindfulness practice (see Chapter 5), there is a yogic meditation called one-pointed attention. In this type of yogic meditation, you concentrate on one thing. This could be your breath, a sound or phrase (e.g., mantra), candles, or an image of a deity or guru (McCall, 2007; Sovik, 2005). In yogic meditation, there is an acknowledgment of the business of the mind. The practice of meditation is the continuous bringing of the thoughts back to the one point of concentration. In yoga classes, I remind practitioners that in yoga it only matters if they try; the benefits come from trying, not in whether or not they are getting it perfect every time. McCall (2007) suggests that whether or not you think you are meditating well does not matter. That is, both those who think they are meditating well and those who think they are not benefit in terms of positive health outcomes such as reduced blood pressure, heart rate, and stress hormone levels.

Systematic Relaxation
In systematic relaxation (see Practice Script 8.4), your awareness moves across the length of your body from the head to the toes and back to the

TABLE 8.3   Deepening Awareness Toward Self-Awareness

Step in the Process	Practice
Pratyahara	Turn inward and cultivate withdrawal of the senses.
Finding stillness	Find a quiet place, sitting or lying down, and begin the process of mindful awareness.
Diaphragmatic breathing	Bring awareness to the breath as a point of concentration, deepening and steadying the breath.
Systematic relaxation	From the crown of your head to your fingers and toes, bring relaxation to each area of the body using awareness and breath.
Dharana: one-pointed concentration	Bring awareness to the breath, another object of concentration, or a mantra.
Dhyana	Cultivate the noticing of unification with the true self as the mantra fades. Practice meditative contemplation on the oneness of self and object.
Samadhi	Complete unification with the present moment, bare awareness, and truth.

Source: Anderson and Sovik, 2000; Simpkins and Simpkins, 2011; Sovik, 2005; Stephens, 2010.

crown of the head (Anderson & Sovik, 2000). At each area at which attention is focused, maintain deep, diaphragmatic breath while bringing release and relaxation to the muscle (Anderson & Sovik, 2000). Systematic relaxation is like the body scan (see Chapter 5). However, in the body scan, awareness is brought to each area of the body and in systematic relaxation deep relaxation is brought to each area of the body. Once awareness, breath, and relaxation have been brought through the body, focus is returned to the breath for 10 breath cycles (Anderson & Sovik, 2000). Associated embodied practices (see Chapter 3) include: (1) be mindfully aware, (2) honor your breath and physical experience, and (8) prioritize self-care.

PRACTICE SCRIPT 8.4: Systematic Relaxation

(Approximate Timing: 20 Minutes for Practice)

Lie down or get in a very comfortable, supported seated position. Bring your awareness to your breath, becoming aware of its qualities. Is it smooth and even? Are you moving from inhalation to exhalation without pause? Slowly deepen your breath to diaphragmatic breathing. Feel your belly expand with each inhalation and release with each exhalation. Breathe here for three deep cycles of breath.

Now, bring your awareness to the crown of your head. Breathe as if you could breathe into the crown of your head. Notice if you feel any tension in the muscles. Breathe into the tension and bring a softness, a letting go into the muscles. With each inhalation bring awareness and with exhalation bring relaxation and softness. As you relax the crown of the head and muscles of your scalp, be aware of your breathing and bring attention back to deep diaphragmatic breathing when necessary. Breathe here and relax. (Pause.)

[Continue this same process through the rest of your body, pausing to relax at each of these points: crown of the head, forehead, temples, eye area, nose, cheeks, jaw, mouth, chin, throat, neck, shoulders, arms, hands, fingers, palms of the hands, back of the arms, shoulders, chest, rib cage, spine, heart, belly, sides, lower back, hips, gluteus region, thighs, knees, calves, feet, toes, and the soles of the feet. Pause at the feet and reverse the order, going all the way back through the body to the crown of the head.]

Bring your awareness to your whole body. Breathe as if you can breathe into your whole body for three cycles of deep, diaphragmatic breath. Allow your breath to return to normal. Continue with 10 breath cycles. Slowly bring your awareness back to the room; bend your elbows and your knees. Roll to your right side, the softest side for your heart. Slowly come to a seated position. Cross your ankles and bring your hands to touch in front of your heart. Slowly open your eyes.

Source: Anderson and Sovik, 2000; Sovik, 2005.

Mantra and Mala Beads

Mantra yoga is a path to self-realization that utilizes sound and words as a means of growth (Anderson & Sovik, 2000; see Chapter 7). In mantra meditation, the breath is united with the sound of a word (Anderson & Sovik, 2000; Sovik, 2005; Weintraub, 2012). The first syllable, *man*, means "to think," and *tra* means "to guide or lead" (Anderson & Sovik, 2000). In this way, a mantra is a guiding or leading sound upon which we can organize our thoughts. When practicing with a mantra, you can say it out loud or internally in your mind (Anderson & Sovik, 2000). The mantra can be coordinated with your breathing during your practice (see Practice Script 8.5; Anderson & Sovik, 2000).

Mala beads can be a helpful tool in mantra meditation (Tigunait, 1996). A mala is a set of beads (traditionally 108) for keeping count of mantras while reciting, chanting, or mentally repeating the mantra (Stephens, 2010). The material used to make the beads can vary according to the purpose of the mantras used. Yogis sometimes set a gradual course of increasing *japa* (i.e., a specific number of repetitions of a mantra over a certain period of time; Tigunait, 1996). To use the mala beads, make a circle by touching the tip of your thumb to the tip of your ring finger (Tigunait, 1996). Next, hold the mala bead with your thumb and your third finger, gently supporting the string of beads with your ring finger and using any of your second through fourth fingers to turn the beads. According to tradition, using our first finger is discouraged (Tigunait, 1996).

The mantra *soham* is a good beginning mantra (Stephens, 2010). With two syllables it is easy to remember and lies naturally on the inhalations and exhalations of the breath. The word *soham* comes from the roots *sah*, which means "that referring to the true, uppercase 's' Self" (Anderson & Sovik, 2000), and the word *aham*, which refers to the word "I," reflecting all that comprises our individual personality, the ego self. Together they translate to "I am that" (Anderson & Sovik, 2000, p. 214). In this mantra education, you are reciting the connection between the ego self and the soul Self. In some lineages of yoga, mantras are given to an individual student through a process of initiation (Tigunait, 1996). The mantra given to a student becomes his or her personal mantra, which is intended to guide and protect the student (Anderson & Sovik, 2000). Associated embodied practices (see Chapter 3) include: (1) be mindfully aware, (2) honor your breath and physical experience, (6) discern what is not-self, and (7) allow what is with nonjudgment.

PRACTICE SCRIPT 8.5: Mantra Meditation Soham
With Mala Beads

(Approximate Timing: 20 Minutes for Practice)

Sit in a comfortable position. Be sure your sitting bones are grounded, your lower back is supported, and your core is engaged. Bring your awareness to your breath and close your eyes. Relax and allow your thoughts to come and go. Begin to become aware of the sounds that your breath makes as you inhale and exhale. As you inhale, begin to create the sound "so. . . ." for the entirety of the inhalation. As you exhale, begin to create the sound "hum. . . ." for the entirety of the exhalation. Each of the sounds should continue through the entirety of the inhalation or exhalation. It is important to allow the breath to be smooth, steady, and regular and then to imprint the sound on the breath. Continue for one round of the mala beads or 108 breaths.

Source: Anderson and Sovik, 2000; McCall, 2007; Sovik, 2005; Stephens, 2010.

Meditation on Chakras

As described in Chapter 7, the chakras are energy centers in the body. Meditation can be done on the chakras (see Practice Script 8.6), helping draw awareness inward and integrate energy within the body. For a step-by-step guide to meditation in yoga, see *Moving Inward: The Journey of Meditation* by Rolf Sovik (2005) and Amy Weintraub's (2012) *Yoga Skills for Therapists: Effective Practices for Mood Management*. Associated embodied practices (see Chapter 3) include: (1) be mindfully aware, (2) honor your breath and physical experience, (6) discern what is not-self, and (7) allow what is with nonjudgment.

PRACTICE SCRIPT 8.6: Meditation on Chakras

(Approximate Timing: 20 Minutes for Practice)

Sit in a comfortable position, being sure you are grounded and your spine is erect. Bring your awareness to your breath. Notice the natural inhalations and exhalations of the breath. Consciously pressing down into your sitting bones, breathe deeply into your experience of feeling grounded, stable, and rooted. As you breathe in, consider the concepts of earth and belonging. The mantra of the first chakra is "lam" (Stephens, 2010, p. 271). Press your sitting bones into your

seat and exhale saying "lam." Repeat this five times as you maintain your aware-
ness of the root chakra (pause and breathe).

Next, bring your awareness to the very center of your pelvis. From the
rooted connection with the mat, feel the openness and space in your pelvic area.
Breathe into a sense of openness, creativity, and water. As you exhale, say the
mantra "vam" (Stephens, 2010, p. 271). Breathe into creativity and possibility
and breathe out the sound "vam." Repeat this five times as you maintain your
awareness of the sacral chakra (pause and breathe). Now, move your awareness
to the center of your belly. As you inhale, consider empowerment, a sense of self,
and fire. As you exhale, say the mantra "ram" (Stephens, 2010, p. 271). Repeat
this five times as you maintain your awareness of the solar plexus chakra (pause
and breathe).

Next, bring your awareness to your heart. Breathe into a sense of love,
trust, acceptance, and the openness of air. As you exhale, say the mantra "ham"
(Stephens, 2010, p. 271). Repeat this five times as you maintain your aware-
ness of the heart chakra (pause and breathe). Next, bring your awareness to
your throat. Know that this is a place of action and voice. Bring awareness to
the power you have in effective communication and the expression of yourself.
Honor the power of sound. As you inhale, consider the power of your voice, and
as you exhale, say "vam" (Stephens, 2010, p. 272). Repeat this five times as you
maintain your awareness of the throat chakra (pause and breathe). Bring your
awareness through your grounded root, the pelvis, the belly, the heart, and the
throat, and into the area above your eyes in the center of your forehead. Cultivate
a sense of intelligence, intuition, and inner wisdom. Sense light as you inhale.
As you exhale, say "ke-sham" (Stephens, 2010, p. 272). Repeat this five times as
you maintain your awareness of the third eye chakra.

Finally, bring your awareness to your whole body. Breathe, ultimately cen-
tering your awareness on the crown of your head. Maintain a deep and steady
breath. As you inhale, cultivate a sense of pure consciousness and spaciousness.
As you exhale, say "om." Cultivate a sense of being connected with all things, all
beings, and the entire universe with each inhalation. Breathe out, saying "om."
Repeat this five times as you maintain your awareness of the crown chakra.

Source: Stephens, 2010; Weintraub, 2012.

SUMMARY

On-the-mat yoga practice is a pathway toward embodiment and the
promotion of well-being at the neurological and physiological levels in
these three ways: (a) it enhances neurological integration (i.e., neurological differentiation and linkage); (b) it reduces reactivity, increases reflective engagement, and improves access to restful and restorative states;

and (c) it improves emotional and behavioral regulation. Yoga can help your patients become present with and tolerate their feelings and ride the wave of being triggered or craving. The chapter reviewed specific techniques, including asana practice, breath work (pranayama), relaxation techniques, and meditation. Through yoga practice, your patients can learn through and with their bodies how to overcome triggers and cravings and move toward integration and well-being.

REFERENCES

Anderson, S., & Sovik, R. (2000). *Yoga: Mastering the basics.* Honesdale, PA: The Himalayan Institute.

Barwick, D. D. (1983). *A treasury of days: 365 thoughts on the art of living.* Florence, AL: CR Gibson.

Boudette, R. (2006). Yoga in the treatment of disordered eating and body image disturbance: How can the practice of yoga be helpful in the recovery from an eating disorder? *Eating Disorders, 14,* 167–170.

Bryant, E. F. (2009). *The Yoga Sutras of Patanjali.* New York, NY: North Point Press.

Carei, T. R., Fyfe-Johnson, A. L., Breuner, C. C., & Brown, M. A. (2010). Randomized controlled clinical trial of yoga in the treatment of eating disorders. *Journal of Adolescent Health, 46,* 346–351.

Damasio, A. (1999). *The feeling of what happens: Body and emotion in the making of consciousness.* New York, NY: Harcourt Brace.

Daubenmier, J. J. (2005). The relationship of yoga, body awareness, and body responsiveness to self-objectification and disordered eating. *Psychology of Women Quarterly, 29,* 207–219.

Douglass, L. (2011). Thinking through the body: The conceptualization of yoga as therapy for individuals with eating disorders. *Eating Disorders, 19,* 83–96.

Eisenstein, C. (2003). *The yoga of eating: Transcending diets and dogma to nourish the natural self.* Washington, DC: New Trends Publishing.

Eknath, E., & Nagler, M. N. (2007). *The Upanishads.* Tomales, CA: Nilgiri Press.

Field, T. (2011). Yoga clinical research review. *Complementary Therapies in Clinical Practice, 17,* 1–8.

Grabovac, A. D., Lau, M. A., & Willett, B. R. (2011). Mechanisms of mindfulness: A Buddhist Psychological Model. *Mindfulness.* doi: 10.1007/s12671-011-0054-5

Iyengar, B. K. S. (1966). *Light on yoga.* New York, NY: Schocken Books.

Jackson, E. (2013, November). *Resilience from trauma: Examination of a gender-responsive trauma-informed mind–body program in Haiti.* Presentation at 141st APHA Annual Meeting, November 2–November 6, 2013.

Koole, S. L., van Dillen, L. F., & Sheppes, G. (2011). The self-regulation of emotion. In K. D. Vohs & R. F. Baumeister (Eds.), *Handbook of self-regulation: Research, theory and applications* (2nd ed.) (pp. 22–40). New York, NY: Guilford Press.

Kraftsow, G. (1999). *Yoga for wellness: Healing with the timeless teachings of Viniyoga.* New York, NY: Penguin Putnam.

Levine, P. L. (2010). *In an unspoken voice: How the body releases trauma and restores goodness.* Berkeley, CA: North Atlantic Books.

Marlatt, G. A., Bowen, S. W., & Lustyk, K. (2012). Substance abuse and relapse prevention. In C. K. Germer & R. D. Siegel (Eds.), *Wisdom and compassion in psychotherapy: Deepening mindfulness in clinical practice* (pp. 221–233). New York, NY: Guilford Press.

McCall, T. (2007). *Yoga as medicine: The yogic prescription for health and healing.* New York, NY: Bantam Dell, Random House.

McIver, S., McGartland, M., & O'Halloran, P. (2009). Overeating is not about the food: Women describe their experience of a yoga treatment program for binge eating. *Qualitative Health Research, 19,* 1234–1245.

Nummenmaa, L., Glerean, E., Hari, R., & Hietanen, J. K. (2014). Bodily maps of emotions. *Proceedings of the National Academy of Sciences, 111,* 646–651.

Oosterwijk, S., Lindquist, K. A., Anderson, E., Dautoff, R., Moriguchi, Y., & Barrett, L. F. (2012). States of mind: Emotions, body feelings, and thoughts share distributed neural networks. *NeuroImage, 62,* 2110–2128.

Porges, S. W. (2011). *The polyvagal theory: Neurophysiological foundations of emotions, attachment, communication, and self-regulation.* New York, NY: W. W. Norton.

Prabhavananda, S., & Isherwood, C. (2007). *How to know God: The yoga aphorisms of Patanjali.* Hollywood, CA: Vedanta Press.

Reindl, S. M. (2001). *Sensing the self: Women's recovery from bulimia.* Cambridge, MA: Harvard University Press.

Rybak, C., & Deuskar, M. (2010). Enriching group counseling through integrating yoga concepts and practices. *Journal of Creativity in Mental Health, 5,* 3–14.

Siegel, D. (2012). *Pocket guide to interpersonal neurobiology: An integrative handbook of the mind.* New York, NY: W. W. Norton.

Siegel, D. J. (2010). *The mindful therapist: A clinician's guide to mindsight and neurological integration.* New York, NY: W. W. Norton.

Simpkins, A. M., & Simpkins, C. A. (2011). *Meditation and yoga in psychotherapy: Techniques for clinical practice.* Hoboken, NJ: John Wiley & Sons.

Sovik, R. (2005). *Moving inward: The journey to meditation.* Honesdale, PA: The Himalayan Institute Press.

Stephens, M. (2010). *Teaching yoga: Essential foundations and techniques.* Berkeley, CA: North Atlantic Books.

Tigunait, P. R. (1996). *The power of mantra and the mystery of initiation.* Honesdale, PA: The Himalayan International Institute of Yoga.

Weintraub, A. (2012). *Yoga skills for therapists: Effective practices for mood management.* New York, NY: W. W. Norton.

YogaHOPE. (2015). *TIMBo program.* Retrieved from http://yogahope.org/timbo-program/

Creating a Regulating Practice
Yoga Teachers, Styles, Risks, and Tools

*What I know now is that having the idea of change
isn't enough.*—BARON BAPTISTE (2013, p. xii)

FROM IDEA TO PRACTICE

When I first began my work researching yoga as a tool for preventing eating disorders among early adolescent girls, I either worked with or hired experienced yoga teachers to implement the yoga practice aspect of the program (Cook-Cottone, Kane, Keddie, & Haugli, 2013). Although I had a strong conceptual belief that yoga worked, my own practice and training lagged behind. I practiced in stops and starts, lost in the stress of pretenure academic life. I was not using the tools that I knew worked. In 2009, I was accepted into the Himalayan Institute's 200-hour yoga teacher training. It was then that my practice moved into what I now call a *therapeutic dose*. I was learning the yoga texts and the health benefits of postures, and, perhaps most important, I began practicing three or more times a week. I was going to studios and practicing with effective teachers. Critically, I moved from thinking about yoga to practicing, embodying yoga. As time passed, my yoga progressed into yet another level. I now had a conceptual understanding of yoga, a solid home practice, and the determination to embody my practice in my world. Today, my yoga is the integration of conceptual knowing, embodied practice, and daily living.

The process was a bit like an uncharted hike through a forest with few well-worn paths and many heart-opening learning experiences. Although this makes sense for therapists and academics with goals such as curiosity, stress reduction, spiritual growth, and physical health, guiding a client in the midst of struggle needs to be more specific. Guidance must detail clearer instruction and note risks and contraindications. Accordingly, this chapter provides a broad guide for supporting the creation of a regulating yoga practice. The process of finding a teacher and style is offered. Also, risks and contraindications are reviewed. Finally, tools for setting up a home practice are detailed.

This text does not provide detailed pose-by-pose instructions. This is intentional. As a tradition, yoga is a practice taught teacher to student. It is embodied in your own practice as well as within the relationship between student and teacher. An effective yoga teacher brings the technique to students in a personal and highly specific manner, giving each student what he or she needs. Further, there are, currently, no generally accepted, empirically based sets of guidance detailing particular poses for specific mental health challenges. The research simply isn't at that level of specificity at this time. As noted in Chapter 1 and Chapter 8, there are many guides for instruction in asana practice. These include texts and videos (see Anderson & Sovik, 2000; Iyengar, 1966: Kraftsow, 1999; McCall, 2007; Stephens, 2010). There are also many online resources. Several established yoga teachers have online video channels (see Christina Sell at www.livethelightofyoga.com/ and search Christina Sell on YouTube). *Yoga Journal* (www.yogajournal.com) and the Himalayan Institute's *Yoga International* (yogainternational.com) offer free access to asana, yoga, classes, and boundless information on yoga. As excellent resources, each offers descriptions of asana, including step-by-step instructions, tips, and contraindications for each pose.

CHOOSING A YOGA TEACHER AND YOGA STYLE

There are many styles of yoga practices and as many different types of teachers. Many types of yoga practices typically include stretching exercises or postures (i.e., asana), breath work, and meditation (Boudette, 2006; Field, 2011). Boudette (2006), who works with patients with eating disorders, refers patients to yoga classes that she knows will support their goals. She states that matching a student to the right kind of class is critical (Boudette, 2006). For example, a type A, perfectionistic individual might easily be drawn to a teacher who pushes students to and beyond their limits. A depressed individual might select only restorative classes, avoiding classes that might challenge or move him or her out of an habitual comfort zone (Boudette, 2006). A good fit is a class that aligns with an individual's general inclinations and desires, yet moves him or her toward integration and balance. The right yoga class will challenge habitual ways of being that might reinforce an individual's dysregulation. I have found that if I send a driven, intense person to a restorative class, the disconnect can be too great. The same can be true for a student who does not have a strong athletic drive, has been excessively using substances and his or her body is vulnerable, or has been avoiding physical experience altogether. Sending someone with these challenges to a power vinyasa or ashtanga class may be too big of a leap.

Get to know the teachers in your area, take classes, and have a sense of what being in each of the classes feels like in the body. In lived experience, how they teach? Do they push? Do they encourage the students to rest and take support or accommodate the pose? The Yoga Sutras guide students to a place between steadiness and comfort (e.g., Yoga Sutra II.46: *"sthira-sukkham asanam,"* which translates as "posture should be steady and comfortable"; Bryant, 2009, p. 283). See Figure 9.1.

Importantly, when a patient is struggling with self-regulation, the questions that he or she needs to ask about the best fit for a style and a teacher go beyond the matching of the need for structure and ease. The styles and the teacher must address the four areas described in earlier chapters: (a) neurologic integration; (b) reduction of reactivity, increased reflective engagement, and improved access to a restful state; (c) opportunities to feel feelings; and (d) a reduction in craving and symptom expression. To assess whether or not a practice is helpful, answer these questions:

- Do you have a sense of feeling more neurologically integrated? When you are increasing in neurologic integration you feel more emotionally and psychologically flexible, adaptive, coherent, and energized (Siegel, 2010). Can you go with the flow and adapt? Do your thoughts,

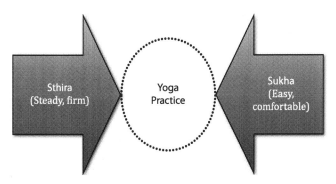

FIGURE 9.1 Finding balance and challenge.
Source: Boudette, 2006; Bryant, 2009; Simpkins and Simpkins, 2011.

feelings, and physical experiences feel more aligned? Do you have more energy?

- Are you less reactive?
- Are you more reflective when you interact with others? Can you pause before you act or talk?
- Do you feel you have improved access to restful and restorative states? Can you calm yourself down?
- Are you encouraged to feel what you are feeling in class (rather than pushing through or ignoring what you feel)?
- Have you experienced a sense of reduced craving or symptom reduction?

If a yoga practice is right for you or your patients the answer should be yes to many of these questions. If the style of practice feels like it triggers cravings and symptoms without support, then another style of yoga should be considered. Notably, what is right for one patient may not be right for another. For example, one patient in recovery from bulimia nervosa (BN) loved the Bikram yoga style because she felt very "rinsed out" after class and had immediate reductions in her drive to binge and purge. Another patient with BN felt very triggered in the Bikram classes by the sparse clothing the practitioners wore and the mirrors in the room. Sometimes assessing fit can go beyond the teacher's specific teaching techniques or the studio style, and rests in the clientele. For example, a patient might be triggered by the constant diet, cleansing, and body assessment talk shared by clients of the studio. By answering the questions just listed, you and your patients can have a better sense of whether the practice is supporting or triggering self-regulation challenges.

Choosing a Yoga Teacher

According to Anderson and Sovik (2000), "There is no substitute for a teacher" (p. 16). Choosing a yoga teacher takes time and should be done intentionally. The various styles of yoga are listed in the following section of this chapter, and this may influence your choice of yoga teacher. It may be helpful to experiment with different styles and then take classes from various teachers within that style. This, of course, is easier to do in larger cities or cities with many options. McCall (2007) lists six things to look for in a teacher: training, experience, reputation, flexibility of approach, whether or not he or she practices what he or she preaches, and the degree to which the teacher motivates you to practice.

Teachers often choose to become certified and registered. Certification as a yoga teacher is not as meaningful as you might think. Often confused with state certifications (e.g., New York State has a certification for school psychologists), registration as a yoga teacher (see Yoga Alliance), or licensure (by state as for medical doctors or psychologists, for example), yoga certification refers to the completion of a training program in yoga. Certification and registration can be offered by anyone—from a person with little training to an advanced group of yoga teachers associated with a reputable yoga school. That is, there are no universal standards for certification in yoga and quality can vary substantially.

The yoga teacher registry is not a certification program but a listing of teachers whose training and teaching experience meet minimum standards set by the Yoga Alliance (www.yogaalliance.org). Yoga teachers who completed training with registered yoga schools (which can be verified on the Yoga Alliance Web page) can receive varying levels of designation based on the amount of training and teaching experience they have. Graduates of registered yoga training programs can then individually register with the Yoga Alliance in order to become Registered Yoga Teachers (RYTs). Registration includes standard designations at the 200-, 300-, and 500-hour training levels, with the additional designation of "E" representing experience quantified as a certain number of hours teaching since the completion of teacher training.

As yoga grows in popularity, research support increases, and insurance companies reimburse for services, there is a push for universal standards of training. The field is in a time of substantial change and evolution. The role of state governments and the Yoga Alliance within the process is yet to be decided. Yoga teacher training is becoming increasingly sophisticated, with colleges and universities forming yoga teacher training programs. In 2012, the International Association of Yoga Therapists (www.iayt.org) published standards of training for becoming a yoga therapist (www.iayt.org/?page=AccredStds) and yoga therapist standards (www.iayt.org/?page=StandardsPartB). Universities such as Loyola Marymount University and Duke University now offer training in yoga therapy (academics.lmu.edu/extension/programs/yogatherapy) and yoga teacher training (www.dukeintegrativemedicine.org/professional-training/yoga-teacher-training).

Selecting a Style of Yoga

The following brief descriptions of yoga styles are offered as a short guide to what is available. It is important to note that there are so many different types of yoga that it is not feasible for all of them to be listed here. Several of the more popular styles of yoga are listed and described in alphabetic order. Note that there is no generally accepted source that delineates all types of yoga. Sources and discrepancies and similarities between and among sources are cited in the following discussion.

Anusara

Anusara yoga was developed by John Friend, a student of B. K. S. Iyengar (McCall, 2007). This style of yoga emphasizes limb alignment in asana, uses props to facilitate alignment, and integrates a positive philosophy. The main philosophical tenet is that an intrinsic energy of oneness underlies everyone and everything. It is known for free-flowing, vinyasa movements (Field, 2011). Each class is taught with a centering theme and includes asana and meditation. Learn more about anusara yoga at www.anusarayoga.com.

Ashtanga

Ashtanga yoga is based on the teachings of K. Pattabhi Jois (kpjayi.org; McCall, 2007). Taught by Krishnamacharya, Jois is the founder of the Ashtanga Yoga Research Institute in Mysore India (kpjayi.org/the-institute; Swenson, 1999). It is considered one of the more challenging and vigorous styles of yoga and is one of the foundational roots of power yoga (see discussion later in this chapter; McCall, 2007). The practice specialized in sequencing of postures, practiced in a continuous flow, and a set of breathing exercises (McCall, 2007; Swenson, 1999). Ujjayi breath (described in Chapter 8) is used during practice. Ashtanga teachers sometimes offer a Mysore class in which students practice at their own pace and can secure individual guidance from the teacher on the poses on which they are working (McCall, 2007). See Swenson (1999) for a detailed practice manual.

Bikram/Hot Yoga

Bikram yoga was created and founded by Choudhury Bikram (www.bikramyoga.com; McCall, 2007). Bikram yoga is practiced in higher temperatures (i.e., over 100°F; Field, 2011; McCall, 2007). It is a challenging practice that involves 26 postures done in a standard sequence (McCall, 2007). Postures are held for 30 seconds and nearly all of the asanas are repeated twice (McCall, 2007). People who like the Bikram style enjoy the heat, the sweating, the predicable sequence, and the standardization across studios. It is not recommended for those with high blood pressure, chronic illness such as multiple sclerosis or fibromyalgia, cardiovascular disease, or other medical illnesses that can be exacerbated by intense exercise in heat (Field, 2011; McCall, 2007).

Himalayan Institute

The Himalayan Institute was founded in 1971 by Swami Rama of the Himalayas. The asana practice emphasizes the therapeutic benefits of the poses, alignment, and physical and mental health. The Himalayan Institute offers teacher training that includes advanced studies in sequencing, verbal and hands-on assists, subtle body anatomy, pranayama, mantra meditation, therapeutic applications of yoga, and the study of sacred yoga texts. See the Himalayan Institute's Web page for more information (www.himalayaninstitute.org).

Integral

Integral yoga is considered to be a gentle style of yoga founded by Swami Satchidananda, who studied under Swami Sivananda (McCall, 2007). The practice includes asana, pranayama, chanting, meditation, and discussions of ancient yogic texts (McCall, 2007). The school reflects a commitment to selfless service encouraged in karma yoga, which is attributed to the lineage (McCall, 2007). Dean Ornish's early studies on yoga and cardiovascular health stylized this type of yoga (McCall, 2007). For more on integral yoga, see the Integral Yoga Institute's Web page (iyiny.org).

Iyengar

Iyengar yoga is known for longer holding of poses and inclusion of more strenuous poses (www.bksiyengar.com; Field, 2011). B. K. S. Iyengar is the founder of Iyengar yoga and the author of several books on yoga, including the seminal work *Light on Yoga* (Iyengar, 1966). Iyengar yoga focuses on alignment as the primary meditative focus of practice (McCall, 2007). Pranayama (i.e., breath work) is taught after a certain level of proficiency is attained in asana, a process that takes, on average, about 2 years of steady practice (i.e., postures; McCall, 2007). B. K. S. Iyengar is thought to be a pioneer in yoga in both use of props and in the development of restorative yoga. Props such as blocks, bolsters, straps, benches, and ropes mounted on the wall are used to enhance practice (McCall, 2007). Restorative yoga is useful for students who are in need of respite and recovery or have other physiological challenges (e.g., illness). Teacher training in Iyengar yoga is believed to be among the most rigorous (McCall, 2007).

Kripalu Yoga

Kripalu yoga was created by a group of yogis who followed yogi Amrit Desai in the 1970s (McCall, 2007). Kripalu yoga emphasizes emotional release, spiritual growth, and self-acceptance (Kripalu Center for Yoga and Health, 2015; McCall, 2007). There is a focus on creating a space for yoga students that is emotionally safe (McCall, 2007). The practice is presented in different levels of intensity ranging from gentle to more vigorous practices (McCall, 2007). Sequences stress coordination of movement and breath, awareness of energy in the body, and working to find your edge in postures (McCall, 2007). Sometimes teachers integrate breathing techniques and postures to elicit specific energy experiences (McCall, 2007). Kripalu yoga includes asana, chanting, pranayama, and meditation (McCall, 2007). Kripalu yoga is associated with the Kripalu Center for Yoga and Health in Lenox, Massachusetts (www.kripalu.org; McCall, 2007).

Mindful Yoga

Mindful yoga focuses on raising a practitioner's awareness of the patterns in his or her mind (Douglass, 2011). The methodologies include postures, breathing, deep relaxation, and concentration techniques (Douglass, 2011). Mindful yoga emphasizes embodied experience and mental responses, with teachers checking in with students as they move through poses and engage in breathing and relaxation techniques. Students are encouraged to bring awareness to thoughts, feelings, and physical postures and how they feel in the body, to discern thoughts and bodily sensations, and to notice that they can have multiple reactions to single sensations. Mindful yoga emphasizes awareness of sensations and the choice that follows (Douglass, 2011). Notably, it is not prescriptive but a form of inquiry in which negation and embracing of multiple meanings over experience, perceptions, sensations, and thoughts are encouraged (Douglass, 2011).

Power Yoga

Power yoga evolved during the 1980s as a physical practice with a focus on personal empowerment. Power yoga is often misunderstood as a practice that solely emphasizes an intense asana practice. Its roots are in vinyasa flow, ashtanga, and Bikram yoga. In Baptiste methodology, there is a standard sequence emphasizing different energetic foci, including integration, awakening, vitality, equanimity, grounding, igniting, stability, opening, release, rejuvenation, and deep rest (Baptiste, 2003). Physical and mental integration is reinforced via a central teaching tenet referred to as *true north alignment,* a continuous guidance to bring awareness and focus to the core of the physiological body and a grounded, mindful mental state. The power yoga emphasis on inquiry and personal growth is consistent with teachings in the Yoga Sutras and the Bhagavad Gita. Some power yoga classes use heat (i.e., around 90°F) and a standard sequence of poses (e.g., Baptiste, 2003). Others have more flexibility in the sequences and vary use of heat. Teachers typically encourage personal exploration and present inspiring physical classes. See the Baptiste Power Vinyasa Yoga Web page for more information (www .baronbaptiste.com).

Viniyoga

Viniyoga was disseminated by T. K. F Desikachar, the son of the guru Krishnamacharya (McCall, 2007). In the yoga culture, many find the lineage of teachers important—that is, who studied under whom. This helps people understand the emphasis, style, and general sense of the yoga culture a particular style might manifest. For example, B. K. S. Iyengar and Pattabhi Jois, two well-known yogis and founders of their own yoga methodologies, studied under the guru Krishnamacharya (McCall, 2007). Viniyoga focuses on breath, includes pranayama and chanting, and integrates pranayama techniques and chanting into asana practice (McCall, 2007). Consistent with the belief that yoga practice should be tailored to individual needs and challenges, yoga postures are typically practiced one-on-one, in a gentle, therapeutic manner (Kraftstow, 1999; McCall, 2007).

Vinyasa Yoga

The vinyasa style of yoga has its roots is ashtanga yoga. This style of yoga emphasizes flow, breath, and energy work. There are many different forms of vinyasa yoga. For example, Seane Corn, a modern vinyasa teacher who emphasizes self-acceptance, self-love, energy work, spirituality, and activism, exemplifies this type of practice (see www.seanecorn .com/about.php). As another example, Shiva Rea created Prana Flow, an energetic, creative, full-spectrum approach to embodying the flow of yoga. In Prana Flow yoga, practitioners learn classical and innovative approaches to vinyasa yoga and the state of flow drawn from Krishnamacharya's teachings, tantra, Ayurveda, bhakti, and somatics. For more information, see shivarea.com/about-prana-flow.

Yoga Nidra

Yoga nidra means "sleep" in Sanskrit (McCall, 2007). Yoga nidra is a guided meditation technique that involves a series of relaxation exercises beginning with the body, moving to the breath, then to the mind, and to total relaxation and meditation (Rybak & Deuskar, 2010). Yoga nidra is typically done while the practitioner lies in savasana (i.e., lying down on the floor or mat, face up, with the feet slightly more than hip distance apart and the palms a few inches from the sides of the body, palms facing up; the eyes are closed). The instructor guides the student through attentional focus to different areas of the body (McCall, 2007). For a step-by-step yoga nidra practice, see Weintraub (2012).

DOSAGE: HOW MUCH, HOW OFTEN, AND HOW LONG TO PRACTICE

Dosage refers to how often, how long of a session, and for how many years an individual practices yoga (Cook-Cottone, 2013). It also refers to the components or limbs of yoga practiced during sessions (Cook-Cottone, 2013). Researchers have yet to quantify exactly how much and what limb of yoga practice show positive benefits for which disorders or challenges (Cook-Cottone, 2013). As the field of yoga research evolves, researchers are getting closer to answering these questions. What research suggests at this time is that there may be a threshold below which activities such as yoga may not produce significant effects (Cook-Cottone, 2013). That means that in order to have positive outcomes or benefits from your yoga practices, you need to practice it often enough and for long enough.

The most effective practice is regular and systematic (Anderson & Sovik, 2000). The Yoga Sutras tell us this: "Practice becomes firmly grounded when well attended to for a long time without break and in all earnestness" (Chapter I: 14; Satchidananda, 2012). According to the current body of research and experienced yogis, this looks like three sessions per week for at least 1 hour per session, or two sessions per week with 75 to 90 minutes per session (Anderson & Sovik, 2000; Cook-Cottone, 2013). Also, positive outcomes are typically seen after 8 to 12 weeks of practice (Cook-Cottone, 2013; Sherman, 2012). It is important to think of yoga as an ongoing practice, rather than a short intervention that helps patients improve and can then be discontinued. Studies suggest that maintenance of practice may be important.

When establishing initial practice routines, it can be very helpful to join a studio. Many studios offer drop-in sessions as well as weekly, monthly, and yearly packages in which students self-select into the classes that they would like to take. Drop-in classes are often taught in isolation and do not have a thread of instruction over days, weeks, or months. Studios also offer workshops and multisession packages, which do have a longer instructional thread. For example, a studio may offer a 4- to 8-week beginners' yoga program that begins with diaphragmatic breathing, teaches basic postures, and reviews shorter sequences. Advanced workshops might include lessons on nutrition, yoga for kids, or how to do challenging poses such as arm balances.

CONTRAINDICATIONS IN YOGA PRACTICE

Contraindications are warnings in regard to areas in which the practice of yoga can potentially do harm. McCall (2007) reminds of ahimsa, a foundational yama of yoga that directs yogis to do no harm. McCall (2007) notes that as with any physical exercise, the practice of yoga postures involves some risk. It is important to remain aware of your body, pursue good instruction, and follow basic precautions in your practice (McCall, 2007). If you have doubts or concerns about any particular asana or breathing technique, consult with your doctor (McCall, 2007). Use your common sense. If a posture hurts, don't do it (McCall, 2007). Also, be sure you and your clients let the yoga teacher know if there are any medications, injuries, or past medical conditions that might affect practice (e.g., surgeries, chronic conditions, pregnancy; McCall, 2007). Ask for accommodations and support. Be wary of a teacher who will not readily provide accommodations, alterations of postures, and support for your needs.

Another Expression of Your Struggle?

One aspect that is frequently seen in yoga studios is when someone uses the practices as another form of expression of his or her disorder. For example, Mark is a 24-year-old engineer who is struggling with gaming. He has a serious girlfriend who is about to leave him. He has been late for work and even neglected taking showers and getting food when he is lost in a video game. He has acknowledged that there are times when he clearly cannot stop playing. He decided to go to yoga class after work before going home to take the edge off and help him avoid the gaming systems in his den. However, in yoga class, his compulsive drive has simply shape-shifted into a compulsively driven yoga practice. He has always been strong and flexible and the poses have come easy. In class, he takes every pose to the highest level, often ignoring the teacher and engaging in what is practically an independent practice in the front corner of the room. He makes few friends, having little awareness of how the pressured aspects of his practice make people nervous and distract the teachers. When he comes home, he tells his girlfriend about his achievements and the next advanced poses he'd like to try. His misses every opportunity in class to be present, become breath aware, and notice the processes of his mind and body as they work together in asana. Mark is not really doing yoga.

Pushing Too Hard

A close cousin to shape shifting your struggle into your yoga practice is pushing too hard. McCall (2007) suggests that yoga students can focus too intently on the outward appearance, or form, of an asana and not on the experience that is occurring on the inside during asana practice. When completing an asana practice, a yogi's breath should be steady and easy, the face should present as light and calm, and the mind and body should be integrated in service of both (McCall, 2007). Further, some poses are not meant for every body shape and type. Other poses may take many years of steady practice to achieve. Pushing too hard, moving too fast, and ignoring the realities of the physical aspects of the body can lead to injury (McCall, 2007). The pose should be done from the inside out with respect for the natural limitations of the body and the current level of ability achieved by the student.

Mathew Sanford (2006), author of the deeply moving and inspiring book *Waking: A Memoir of Trauma and Transcendence,* articulately described the moment he had taken his self-destructive struggle into his yoga practice. Sanford's book details the story of his recovery from a traumatic car accident, which killed members of his family and left him with a severe spinal cord injury. Yoga was his pathway to healing and, for a while, he used this healing tool against himself. He notes, "I know the moment my yoga practice passed over into the threshold into violence" (Sanford, 2006, p. 203). Mathew describes pushing and straining so hard in a pose that he broke his own leg. The injury was complicated, as was his recovery from it. Sanford (2006) states, "Breaking my leg was the harshest lesson that I have ever experienced in yoga. For me, nonviolence is no longer an intellectual platitude within my practice. It is an energetic fact" (p. 213).

Finding the Just Right Edge

McCall (2007) speaks about the edge in physical terms. When you are holding an asana, move into the shape of the pose until you feel a resistance to further movement (McCall, 2007). That is the physical edge. At this point, bring your awareness to your breath and gently move into and out of the edge. You will want to look for a deep stretching or strength building in the belly of the muscles (i.e., located in the middle, bulkiest part of the muscle). This is the place to gently explore the edge. You do not want to feel sharp pain, sudden pain, or any pain at the joints (McCall, 2007). This is a sign that you could be pushing toward an injury. Also, muscles tighten to prevent injuries (McCall, 2007). Forceful, quick movements can result in defensive tightening. Conversely, gentle, deep, slow movement supported by breath and awareness can encourage growth (McCall, 2007).

Baptiste talks about finding the edge in a slightly different way. Baptiste (2003) suggests that it is at the edge where opportunities for physical and emotional transformation lie. He states that the edge is where we come up against our conceptualization of self—"the boundary between where we are and where we grow" (p. 30). For each pose, there is a physical edge and an emotional edge. Careful discerning of which one you are approaching is critical for safe practice. For example, I am working on doing a handstand in the middle of the room. I have carefully built up strength and competency doing a handstand against the wall. With the wall right there, I can easily hold the pose for 60 seconds or more, never touching the wall. I have learned how to cartwheel out of the pose so that if I try it away from the wall I am safe. Currently, I am facing my emotional edge. I am working on the anxiety I feel when doing the pose without the wall. I am physically safe, yet outside of my comfort zone. When I practice, I feel the same feelings I felt when I challenged myself to apply for my first teaching job, when I gave my first lecture at the university, and when I taught my first yoga class. These are good feelings for me to face and playing the edge with my handstand is just what I need. This is the edge that Baptiste (2003) is talking about. Risk comes from erroneously thinking that you are pushing through an emotional or psychological edge when, in fact, you are not physically prepared or your body is sending you strong physical warnings that you are injuring yourself. Playing the edge should be done carefully and with full awareness of exactly what edge you are pushing.

Hands-On Adjustments

Many yoga teachers offer hands-on adjustments. Provide clear feedback to the instructor about what does and does not feel good in your body. Some teachers can be overly aggressive in their adjustments and create risk for injury (McCall, 2007). Some studios provide a chip, or a cue, for the yoga teacher to indicate that you do not want a physical assist during your class. If you are unsure or have an injury, let the teacher know so that adjustments can be sensitive to your area of concern.

Use of Supports

For beginners and individuals with chronic illnesses or other physical challenges, it can be important to use supports during asana. For example, beginners and those with physical challenges or issues with balance can be susceptible to falling out of a pose (McCall, 2007). Practice with a chair or the wall for support can be very helpful (McCall, 2007).

Risk in Breath Work and Meditation

When I first began doing yoga with patients with eating disorders, I quickly realized the challenges that presented when individuals have experienced trauma or have depression or anxiety (Cook-Cottone, Beck, & Kane, 2008). What many of us take for granted (e.g., lying peacefully in savasana) can be very scary or disconcerting for someone struggling with traumatic memories and fears. As with postures, it is important to provide support and offer alternatives for individuals with mental and emotional struggles. For example, if a patient is feeling too vulnerable in savansana, rather than lying on her back with her eyes closed, provide the option of sitting against the wall, supported, with the eyes open and a gentle gaze toward the floor. McCall (2007) warns that yoga, meditation, and breath work can be triggers for emotional experiences that have not yet been negotiated. Practitioners should be supported and encouraged to work at their own pace. When working with patients with these backgrounds in therapy, I discuss the practice or pose first, address concerns and challenges, provide accommodations and options, and then practice watching carefully and supporting as needed. For those with problems with self-regulation, we want the practice to be supportive, challenging, and ultimately down-regulating. Challenges should be approached with intention and calming; breath work should be done to bring the patient down to baseline before the session ends.

ESTABLISHING A HOME PRACTICE

Studio practice and individual instruction can be wonderful learning and practicing supports for you and your patients. However, initiation of a home practice may be an important step in internalizing yoga techniques and improved emotional and behavioral outcomes (Cook-Cottone, 2013). In a study by Ross, Friedmann, Bevans, and Thomas (2012), home practice was more strongly correlated with mindfulness, subjective well-being, healthy eating, and sleep than number of years of yoga practice.

Anderson and Sovik (2000) offer an excellent guide for a beginning home practice. They suggest starting each session with a brief relaxation (e.g., body scan, about 1–3 minutes). Next, bring awareness to the breath, maintaining this awareness throughout the practice. Keep your eyes soft and open (Anderson & Sovik, 2000). Begin with a basic sequence, gently warming up the body. Move into more vigorous poses, balance poses, and grounded poses, and end with inversions, resting poses, and restorative poses. See Anderson and Sovik (2000) and McCall (2007) for suggested sequences. Throughout practice, nurture feelings of lightness as you work toward elongating through poses and building strength and endurance (Anderson & Sovik, 2000). Maintain mindful awareness, noticing when you have found the edge. Breathe here as you deepen poses and challenge yourself (Anderson & Sovik, 2000). Notice the arising and passing away of thoughts, feelings, triggers, and desires to leave a pose. It is in these peaks that the greatest lessons are learned. At the end of practice, take time to rest in savasana, allowing your practice to integrate in your mind and body. Associated embodied practices (see Chapter 3) include: (1) be mindfully aware, (2) honor your breath and your physical experience, (3) live in inquiry, (4) accept impermanence, (5) cultivate nonattachment, (6) discern what is not-self, and (7) allow what is with nonjudgment.

Setting Up a Yoga Space at Home

Setting up a yoga space at home is relatively easy. You need a floor space, free of breakables, that is about 2 feet longer than you are tall and about 2 feet wider than the span of your arms. When I first started practicing at home, I practiced in our television room, scooting back the coffee table and two large chairs. As my husband and I established a regular home practice, we changed our upstairs office into a yoga and meditation room. This provided more privacy during meditation and allowed us to keep our yoga mats, meditation candles, blocks, straps, and pillows ready for use.

Generally, yoga requires little equipment. The props you need often depend on the type of yoga you will be practicing, with some requiring more props than others (McCall, 2007). In the West, most yoga practitioners use a yoga mat. These range in texture, including rough, smooth, and sticky. It is good to try out a few before you purchase one, as mats can range from as low as $15 to as high as $90. For those who practice yoga in a warm or hot room, a hand towel and a mat towel can be helpful. Yoga supply companies sell towels that have nonslip material on one side specifically designed for hotter yoga classes.

One or two yoga blocks can be very helpful. Most studios supply blocks for your use. Yoga blocks can help support postures such as triangle, extended side angle, and half moon, in which supporting your hand on the block allows the yogi to feel stable and stretch through the sides of the body. Blocks can help with restorative poses, too. For example, placing a block under the sacrum while lying on the floor and then lifting the feet toward the ceiling is a wonderful restorative inversion. Heavy blankets or bolsters can also help with restorative poses and support (McCall, 2007). Some like a small pillow for savasana (the final resting pose).

A yoga strap is essential for support with stretches such as a seated forward fold. For some, lengthening through the hamstrings and attempting to reach the toes encourages rounding in the lower back. A yoga strap can be very helpful with these types of hamstring-stretching poses. By placing the strap around the feet and holding onto the strap with both hands, the practitioner can lengthen through the back while drawing the chest toward the toes, deepening into a hamstring stretch. Other poses, such as standing extended-toe pose and poses that open the chest, can be enhanced by using the strap. Straps can also be used to stabilize the arms when working on arm balances (e.g., loop and tighten the strap around the upper arms so that they are stabilized at shoulder distance apart for forearm balance). Props are not required. Ultimately, yoga can be done without any props.

CONCLUSIONS

Yoga is an active, embodied practice. There are many potential benefits. However, the practice must be used to bring equanimity and regulation to current struggles and not misused as another way to express pathological tendencies. Finding the right teacher and the best-fit style is critical. There is an old quote for which I can find no source, "There is no right or wrong, but what is right is right and what is wrong is wrong." I often use this quote in private practice. Ultimately, across yoga styles and techniques, there are few styles and practices that are universally accepted as wrong. When they are, the community has highlighted their risks and contraindications. Similarly, there is no right style or practice for all yogis. Each patient, therapist, and yogi must find the practice that is effective for him or her given current challenges, risk, and goals. Over time, for each person what is right may change and evolve. Practice, styles, and teachers may change. That is the practice—finding the right fit, right now.

REFERENCES

Anderson, S., & Sovik, R. (2000). *Yoga: Mastering the basics.* Honesdale, PA: The Himalayan Institute.

Baptiste, B. (2003). *Journey into power: How to sculpt your ideal body, free your true self, and transform your life with yoga.* New York, NY: A Fireside Book by Simon and Schuster.

Baptiste, B. (2013). *Being of power: The 9 practices to ignite an empowered life.* Carlsbad, CA: Hay House.

Boudette, R. (2006). Yoga in the treatment of disordered eating and body image disturbance: How can the practice of yoga be helpful in the recovery from an eating disorder? *Eating Disorders, 14,* 167–170.

Bryant, E. F. (2009). *The Yoga Sutras of Patanjali.* New York, NY: North Point Press.

Cook-Cottone, C., Beck, M., & Kane, L. (2008). Manualized-group treatment of eating disorders: Attunement in mind, body, and relationship (AMBR). *The Journal for Specialists in Group Work, 33*(1), 61–83.

Cook-Cottone, C. P. (2013). Dosage as a critical variable in yoga therapy research. *International Journal of Yoga Therapy, 23,* 11.

Cook-Cottone, C. P., Kane, L., Keddie, E., & Haugli, S. (2013). *Girls growing in wellness and balance: Yoga and life skills to empower.* Stoddard, WI: Schoolhouse Educational Services.

Douglass, L. (2011). Thinking through the body: The conceptualization of yoga as therapy for individuals with eating disorders. *Eating Disorders, 19,* 83–96.

Field, T. (2011). Yoga clinical research review. *Complementary Therapies in Clinical Practice, 17,* 1–8.

Iyengar, B. K. S. (1966). *Light on yoga.* New York, NY: Schocken Books.

Kraftsow, G. (1999). *Yoga for wellness: Healing with the timeless teachings of Viniyoga.* New York, NY: Penguin Putnam.

Kripalu Center for Yoga and Health. (2015). Retrieved from http://www.kripalu.org

McCall, T. (2007). *Yoga as medicine: The yogic prescription for health and healing.* New York, NY: Bantam Dell, Random House.

Ross, A., Friedmann, E., Bevans, M., & Thomas, S. (2012). Frequency of yoga practice predicts health: Results of a national survey of yoga practitioners. *Evidence-Based Complementary and Alternative Medicine, 2012,* Article ID 983258.

Rybak, C., & Deuskar, M. (2010). Enriching group counseling through integrating yoga concepts and practices. *Journal of Creativity in Mental Health, 5,* 3–14.

Sanford, M. (2006). *Waking: a memoir of trauma and transcendence.* Emmaus, PA: Rodale.

Satchidananda, S. (2012). *The Yoga Sutras of Patanjali.* Buckingham, VA: Integral Publications.

Sherman, K. J. (2012). Guidelines for developing yoga interventions for randomized trials. *Evidence-Based Complementary and Alternative Medicine, 16.*

Siegel, D. J. (2010). *Mindsight: The new science of personal transformation.* New York, NY: Bantam Dell.

Simpkins, A. M., & Simpkins, C. A. (2011). *Meditation and yoga in psychotherapy: Techniques for clinical practice.* Hoboken, NJ: John Wiley & Sons.

Stephens, M. (2010). *Teaching yoga: Essential foundations and techniques.* Berkeley, CA: North Atlantic Books.

Swenson, D. (1999). *Ashtanga yoga: The practice manual: An illustrated guide to personal practice, the primary and intermediate series, plus three short forms.* Austin, TX: Ashtanga Yoga Productions.

Weintraub, A. (2012). *Yoga skills for therapists: Effective practices for mood management.* New York, NY: W. W. Norton.

Off the Mat
Informal Yoga Practices

We are what we repeatedly do.—ARISTOTLE

Love, compassion, joy, and equanimity are the very nature of an enlightened person. They are the four aspects of true love within ourselves and within everyone and everything.—THICH NHAT HANH (1999, p. 170)

THE BUILDING BLOCKS OF OFF-THE-MAT PRACTICE

Off-the-mat yoga practices are the informal practices in which your clients can engage throughout the day (Stahl & Goldstein, 2010) and do not require a mat or a scheduled practice time. They include basic physiological foundational practices that develop a steady experience of the body (e.g., breathing exercises, nutrition, physical activity), behavioral practices (i.e., the yamas and niyamas) that help organize individual behavior and behavior within relationships, cultivation of positive emotions, and, finally, spiritual practices that help create a life with meaning. These areas of practice support each other (Figure 10.1). The daily practice of healthy physical and emotional behaviors is critical to securing and maintaining recovery. This is well understood in recovery circles. Those in recovery often use the word HALT, which stands for times when relapse or symptom expression is at high risk (i.e., [H] hungry, [A] angry, [L] lonely, and [T] tired). In this manner, utilizing the off-the-mat practices supports a nourished, steady, self-validated and rested self—a self better prepared to negotiate triggers and challenges.

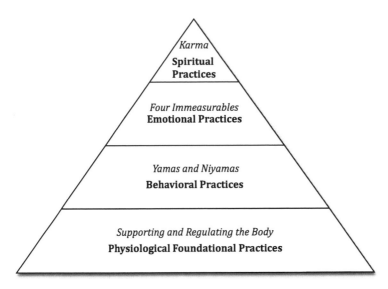

FIGURE 10.1 The building blocks of off-the-mat yoga practice.

BUILDING WELL-BEING FROM THE BODY UP: PHYSIOLOGICAL FOUNDATIONAL PRACTICES

Western psychology has focused on changing individual behavior from the top down for many years. These top-down approaches have taken many forms ideologically. For example, there is the notion that one must understand his or her trauma or past history before he or she can change (e.g., psychoanalysis), or that reframing a way of thinking about something can shift behavior (e.g., cognitive behavioral approaches). For some patients these approaches are very effective. However, for others a focus on actionable methodologies moves them more effectively toward positive self-regulating behaviors and away from self-destructive inclinations.

In a memoir documenting his journey from trauma, spinal cord injury, and transformation through yoga, Mathew Sanford (2006) speaks clearly of the mind–body disconnect that can manifest. He says of his body, "I judge it rather than connect to it. I leave it rather than feel it. This only deepens my sense of separation. It also gives me better access to anger and disgust. Both are effective ways 'out' of body. Ask [someone with] Anorexi[a]" (p. 69). Sanford's (2006) story of transformation is a moving and instructive piece about what is possible in yoga, given seemingly overwhelming obstacles. Describing his first yoga session, Sanford recounts the embodiment experienced as he takes his paralyzed legs into an extended V on the floor for the first time since a car accident many years before. Sanford captures the powerful role of the body in well-being. A bright, gifted writer, a man capable of fully understanding and processing his trauma and challenges, ultimately felt the authentic movement toward healing when he was able to reconnect with his body.

Linehan (1993), whose work focuses on behavioral self-regulation among patients with borderline personality disorder, was among the first to suggest focus must begin in the provision of skills to negotiate experiences prior to digging deeper into more complex issues. There are two main conceptual components of the physiological foundations: (a) a calm and relaxed body fosters a calm and relaxed mind, and (b) taking reliable, steady care of your body fosters a reliable, steady state of mind.

Calm Body, Calm Mind

My patients and yoga students are often fairly well versed in positive affirmations, the power of positive thinking, and the ability to look at the positive side of things. However, I have noticed that they rarely consider the body as a potential source of soothing. Citing the effectiveness of progressive muscle relaxation and breathing techniques, Bourne (2010), in his top-selling anxiety workbook, suggests that it is quite difficult for one to have an anxious mind within a relaxed body. In both private practice and in yoga classes, I provide guidance and support in ways to access the body as a source of soothing, groundedness, and calm during stressful situations. Of course, going for a walk, attending a relaxation-based yoga class (i.e., a yin class), or attending a traditional yoga class can all be ways to calm down the body and relax the mind. However, it is often in daily life, when there is no yoga mat to be found, that we need access to calming tools. Effective strategies include diaphragmatic breathing (see Chapter 8), sensate focus, and the stop–refocus–breathe (SRB) technique. See Bourne's (2010) *The Anxiety and Phobia Workbook, Fifth Edition* for a variety of breathing, relaxation, and meditation techniques for calming the mind. Two effective techniques are explicated here.

Sensate Focus

In Linehan's (1993) manual for dialectic behavioral therapy (DBT), self-soothing, as a bottom-up approach, takes the form of sensate focus (Siegel, 2010). Sensate focus refers to bringing mindful awareness of the sensory input from each of the senses. For example, sensate focus using the eyes refers to the intentional awareness of what you are seeing. Perhaps you bring your attention to each and every detail of a rose. You study the curve of the petal, the sturdiness of the stem, each leaf, and how all the different parts of the flower come together, creating the whole flower. You notice the shadows and places where the light reflects. This can be done with each of the senses—vision, hearing, smell, taste, and touch. By bringing your awareness back to your sensations, you allow your mental processes to clear, becoming immersed in sensations rather than thoughts (Siegel, 2010). This can lead to a new way of considering things, free from confining or habit-reinforcing conceptualizations. Associated embodied practices (see Chapter 3) include: (1) be mindfully aware, (2) honor your breath and your physical experience, and (3) live in inquiry.

Stop–Refocus–Breathe (SRB)

Mindful breathing techniques are helpful in recovery (e.g., Garland, Schwarz, Kelly, Whitt, & Howard, 2012; Stahl & Goldstein, 2010). SRB is a simple breathing technique that can be applied as needed or used prophylactically to down-regulate the physical and emotional systems (see Practice Script 10.1, Stop–Refocus–Breathe). I explain to patients that the brain can be like a toddler fascinated with an electrical outlet. The toddler, curious and persistent, will continually return to the outlet, unless you give him or her something else upon which to focus. More effectively, you tell the toddler, "No!" and then you say to the toddler, "Look over here," as you point to something that will catch the toddler's interest. Patients use SRB in this same way to refocus the brain. The *outlet* is a metaphor for anything that might be triggering or anxiety provoking and the *toddler* is a metaphor for the easily guided brain. In the SRB, the brain is redirected to the breath as a point of concentration. In order to maintain focus, a breath in three parts can be practiced (i.e., inhale for a count of four, hold for a count of four, and exhale for a count of four). Repeat the breath cycle four times. Associated embodied practices (see Chapter 3) include: (1) be mindfully aware, (2) honor your breath and your physical experience, and (3) live in inquiry.

PRACTICE SCRIPT 10.1: Stop–Refocus–Breathe

(Approximate Timing: 3 Minutes for Practice)

Stop:	*Either in response to an internal or external stressor or as a systematic practice scheduled throughout the day, tell your brain to "STOP" thinking. This might be a gentle reminder or a firm directive.*
Refocus:	*Tell your brain, "Refocus" as a gentle reminder or a firm directive. Direct your brain to your breath.*
Breathe:	*Complete a mindful breath in three parts. Hold your attention on the breath. Breathe in and count to four—one, two, three, and four.*

Now hold the breath for a count of four—one, two, three, and four. Next, exhale for a count of four—one, two, three, and four. Repeat this cycle three more times.

The Six Pillars of Emotional Regulation

Emotional regulation is inextricably connected to physical stability and homeostasis (Cook-Cottone, Tribole, & Tylka, 2013). The more regulated the body, the more regulated and steady the mind. Daily maintenance of the body provides a physiological steadiness, reducing cravings and sensitivity to triggers and supporting healthful, positive behavioral choices (Anderson & Sovik, 2000). In Linehan's (1993) manual for DBT, sleep, nutrition, avoidance of mood-altering drugs, and exercise are key components of the emotional regulation facet of treatment. See Figure 10.2 for the six pillars of self-regulation.

During early sessions with clients, I review their nutritional patterns in terms of what a typical day of eating looks like, including hydration practices. Nutrition is known to play a role in mood, sleep, cognitive efficiency, and emotional stability (e.g., Anderson & Sovik, 2000; Kennedy, Jones, Haskell, & Benton, 2011). Further, even mild dehydration has been linked to alterations in mood (e.g., Armstrong et al., 2012). Often patients with substance use and eating disorders struggles have compromised nutritional status (e.g., Zahr, Kaufman, & Harper, 2011). I partner with a nutritionist with nearly all of the patients I see who have eating disorder struggles and/or substance use issues. The nutritionist helps patients develop a meal plan that is aligned with their treatment goals and can help stabilize their physiological experience. Patients frequently do not understand the link between adequate protein, fat, and micronutrient intake and the dips and peaks in energy, fatigue, and coping throughout the day. When not understood and minded, nutrition- and hydration-based drops in energy can quickly become triggers for symptoms.

Although more research is needed, there is some evidence suggesting that daily exercise plays a role in preventing, delaying the onset of, and enhancing treatment outcomes in mental disorder (e.g., Zschucke,

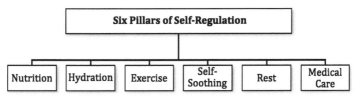

FIGURE 10.2 The six pillars of self-regulation.

Gaudlitz, & Ströhle, 2013). Linehan (1993) encourages at least 20 minutes of vigorous exercise every day. I encourage patients to target 30 to 60 minutes a day depending on the exercise. This would translate to a yoga class, a hike, a walk with a friend, or a pick-up soccer game. Researchers suspect that the mechanisms of action include changes in neurotransmitters such as serotonin and endorphins, which relate to mood and positive effects on stress reactivity (e.g., the hypothalamus–pituitary–adrenal axis; Zschucke et al., 2013). Potential psychological mechanisms of action may include changes in body-related and health-based attitudes and behaviors, social reinforcement, experience of mastery, shift of external to more internal locus of control, and improved coping strategies (Zschucke et al., 2013).

Getting adequate rest matters (Anderson & Sovik, 2000). Sleep deprivation can place patients at risk for symptoms. For example, in their review of research Gujar, Yoo, Hu, and Walker (2011) concluded that sleep deprivation is associated with enhanced reactivity toward negative stimuli, amplified reward-relevant reactivity toward pleasure-evoking stimuli, and increased emotional reactivity. Simple rest, the allowing of yourself to do nothing, is also an important aspect of creating a stable base for self-regulation (Stahl & Goldstein, 2010). Doing nothing and resting can take many forms: lying on a hammock, sitting on the deck, sitting by the lake, and putting the cell phone and the computer away (Stahl & Goldstein, 2010).

The final two pillars of self-regulation are self-soothing and engagement in consistent medical care. Chapter 12 reviews each of these, along with the other pillars, as critical to a stable experience of recovery and symptom prevention. Each pillar, and other aspects of self-care, is assessed by the Mindful Self-Care Scale in Chapter 12. This scale can be used to help patients explore their current self-care practices and set goals in areas that need improvement. Associated embodied practices (see Chapter 3) include: (1) be mindfully aware, (2) honor your breath and your physical experience, and (8) prioritize self-care.

YAMAS AND NIYAMAS

The yamas and the niyamas are described by Anderson and Sovik (2000) as "the ten principles of self-regulation" (p. 224). Recall (see Chapter 7) that the yamas are the five restraints, the guidelines of conduct for the self within the context of others (i.e., nonharming, truthfulness, nonstealing, moderation of the senses, and nonpossessiveness; Adele, 2009; Simpkins & Simpkins, 2011). The niyamas are the five observances, or guidelines for the conduct of the self (i.e., purity, contentment, self-discipline, self-study, and self-surrender; Adele, 2009; Simpkins & Simpkins, 2011). Accordingly, Simpkins and Simpkins (2011) describe the yamas and niyamas as "a rudder to help people steer through difficult times" (p. 121). The daily study and practice of both the restraints and the observances complement the physiological building blocks reviewed earlier (i.e., calm body, calm mind, and the pillars of self-regulation). The yamas and niyamas are also a suitable way to provide a structure for the decision-making process as they provide guidelines for behavior within relationships and toward the self (Simpkins & Simpkins, 2011).

For example, the yamas and niyamas can be wonderful ways of enhancing motivational interviewing (MI; Rubak, Sandbæk, Lauritzen, & Christensen, 2005). The yamas and the niyamas can be integrated into MI in order to elicit clients' statements of desire, ability, and reasons and need for change as the therapist keeps an eye toward evoking increasingly strong commitment to change (Miller & Rose, 2009). In MI, it is believed that as commitment language emerges, behavior change is more likely to occur (Miller & Rose, 2009). In MI, patients are asked to look at their behaviors within the context of the benefits and the costs of the behaviors in their lives (e.g., compulsive shopping, eating disorders, gaming, gambling, self-injury, and substance use). These are often explored in terms of implications such as finances, relationships, careers, and so forth. Adding the yamas and niyamas can help patients explore the costs and benefits in greater depth (Simpkins & Simpkins, 2011).

To illustrate, using Table 10.1, I asked a patient, Jeannette, to consider her bulimia nervosa (BN) and whether or not it allowed her these lived experiences in life. I explained that in yoga philosophy, these practices are believed to help you remove obstacles to well-being and finding your own true nature, your authentic self, something Jeannette had told me she wanted for herself. I suggested that we consider the BN through the lens of yama and niyama and see if the BN could be an obstacle. In each

TABLE 10.1   The Yamas and the Niyamas

Yamas	Niyamas
• Nonharming	• Purity
• Truthfulness	• Contentment
• Nonstealing	• Self-discipline
• Moderation of the senses	• Self-study
• Nonpossessiveness	• Self-surrender

of the areas, she saw cost and no benefit. For example, she identified how the BN was harming her body and her relationship with her mother. She shared about how she had to lie to everyone, almost every day. She was stealing food out of the kitchen and having to spend time and money to replace it before anyone noticed. There was no moderation and she craved food constantly. She felt physically horrible, dehydrated and bloated a lot of the time. She had no sense of contentment—ever—and felt as if she completely lacked discipline. She saw self-study as something that was coming from her work in therapy and self-surrender as something that might be possible as she acknowledged the impact of the BN in her life. Associated embodied practices (see Chapter 3) include: (1) be mindfully aware, (3) live in inquiry, and (9) be of your values.

FOUR IMMEASURABLES

The four immeasurables are addressed both in mindful and yogic traditions, reflecting the intertwining of the roots of these practices. The four immeasureables are equanimity, joy, loving-kindness, and compassion (Hanh, 1999). They are understood to be parallel to a set of negative states (McCown, Reibel, & Micozzi, 2010). It is believed that cultivating equanimity makes it more difficult for anxiety, attachment, and aversion to grow; loving-kindness can be developed to soften anger; joy for others combats jealously; and compassion is a counterbalance for cruelty to self and others (McCown et al., 2010).

Equanimity

Equanimity is the quality of balance within the context of challenge or change (Stahl & Goldstein, 2010). In yoga, true balance in a posture happens when the body has become neurologically integrated. That is, the various areas of the brain involved in maintaining a posture are working together. In life, equanimity is quite similar. Being truly steady and in equanimity involves integration of the feeling and thinking aspects of the self (Linehan, 1993). In Linehan's DBT, she refers to joining of the emotional and cognitive aspects of self as *wise mind* (p. 109). The goal is to be present and process the experience fully, including the physical, emotional, and cognitive aspects, without falling into reaction (Linehan, 1993). In private practice, I find it effective to draw a picture of the brain and explain that there are parts of the brain generally responsible for thinking and other parts of the brain that are primarily responsible for feeling (Cook-Cottone, Tribole, et al., 2013). When we defer to either thoughts or emotions, we run the risk of missing critical information that we need for making a decision. We run the risk of losing our emotional balance. McCown et al. (2010) describe equanimity as the most difficult of all of the immeasurables, as it means to embrace all that arises—the feeling, thinking, good, bad, pleasant, and unpleasant. Despite the inherent challenge, I explain to my patients that we make the best decisions when we process all of the information available, integrating the thinking and the feeling brain (Cook-Cottone, Kane, Keddie, & Haugli, 2013; Figure 10.3).

This way of conceptualizing the brain has been very helpful for Katie. She is 17 years old and struggles with obsessive-compulsive tendencies and anorexia nervosa. Since as long as she can remember she has been trying to handle her life with the thinking part of her brain. She actively avoids feeling her feelings and focuses on food restriction, counting calories, and adding up the calories she has burned working out whenever she is faced with challenge, stress, or anything emotional. Without actively processing the emotional content of her life, she overrelies on the cognitive functions of her brain that are not working effectively. She makes things meaningful that are not (such as calories, and how many miles she ran). She is afraid to get too involved in relationships for fear of

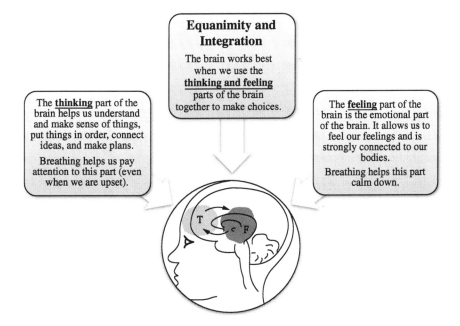

FIGURE 10.3 Equanimity and integration—the thinking and feeling brain.
Source: Cook-Cottone et al., 2013; Cook-Cottone, Tribole, et al., 2013.

getting hurt. She spends a lot of time making judgments, making evalua-tions, and being in reaction. Katie is rarely present in the current moment. She is always two or three thoughts away.

Sometimes patients are concerned that equanimity, or balance in reactions, is like dissociation or not connecting. Equanimity is not the same as dissociating, not caring, or completely disconnecting. It is a process of staying centered during times of seemingly great fortune and times of seemingly great challenge. There is an old story of a farmer and a horse. His horse was lost and then returned. The next day, his son rode the horse, fell, and broke his leg. This accident ultimately saved the farmer's son from being recruited for active duty in the war. Throughout the story, the farmer stayed steady as his neighbor watched in reaction to the tragedy and fortune as it moved in and out like the tide. Instruc-tional Story 10.1 is like this. It is the story of Sophie, a waitress, who works through her day experiencing both good fortune and challenges. Throughout she stays in equanimity.

INSTRUCTIONAL STORY 10.1: Sophie the Waitress

There was a young woman who grew up very poor. Her name was Sophie. She worked hard as a waitress every day. Thoughtful and reliable, she was kind and compassionate to all she served. One day a very old woman came into the res-taurant and sat in Sophie's section. Her friend said, "Oh no! Sophie! That old woman is sitting in your section. She never leaves a tip. This is very bad!" Sophie said to her friend, "I don't know if it is very bad. I just know that there is a cus-tomer sitting in my section." Then, Sophie went to serve the woman lunch. The woman left her a very large tip, $50, for her cup of tea and toast. Sophie's friend said, "Sophie, that is very wonderful! What a great day! She left you a $50 tip!" Sophie said, "I don't know if it is very wonderful. I do know that the woman was kind and I now have $50."

Some teenagers sat down in Sophie's section. She served them hamburgers, fries, and soda. They ate and made quite a mess. While Sophie was in the kitchen, the teenagers ran out of the restaurant without paying their bill. Sophie's friend said, "Sophie, this is truly horrible! You know the policy. We have to cover the costs when people leave and do not pay! Oh! This is the worst day ever!" Sophie said, "I don't know if this is very horrible. I do know that most people are good and some struggle. I also know that I need to clean the table and pay $50 for this meal."

Later, the other regular costumers had heard what happened to Sophie and chipped in to help her out. They gave her over $500. Her friend said, "Oh, Sophie, this is wonderful! You now have more money than before. Perhaps this is the *best day ever!" Sophie said, "I don't know if this is the best day ever. I do know that I am surrounded by generous people and that I have $500." And, like this, Sophie's day continued.*

In practice, I like to explain the thinking and feeling brain, equanimity, and integration. Sophie's story can be very helpful in exploring these issues. Ask your client:

- Is anything gained or lost in Sophie's reactions?
- What was different about Sophie and her friend?
- What are the benefits of an approach like Sophie's? The downside?
- How would the story have been different if Sophie became very upset about the old woman in her section or the teenagers leaving?
- Do our emotions need to swing to extremes based on what fortune or misfortune is happening in our lives?
- What do you imagine is steady in Sophie's day-to-day life that helps her to feel steady like this?

Cultivating equanimity can bring a sense of peace and contentment into the lives of our patients (Hanson & Mendius, 2009). Stahl and Goldstein (2010) suggest that equanimity allows for a deep understanding of the nature of change and how to be with change. As the practice of equanimity dampens the stress-response system, we need not overthink or get lost in our emotional reaction (Hanson & Mendius, 2009). Linehan (1993) asks clients to focus on controlling their attention and move away from trying to control what is being said or what is happening. Next, simply put words onto the experience as we saw Sophie do. Finally, as Sophie did, Linehan (1993) asks patients to participate as needed. Work with Figure 10.4 as you walk your patients through a life event. Ask them

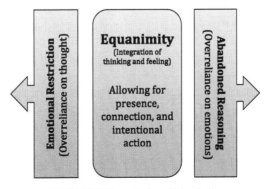

FIGURE 10.4 Equanimity within challenge.

to identify times when they abandoned reason and let emotions take over and times when they shut down the emotional self and allowed reason to run the show. Ask them to consider what could happen if they used both sources of wisdom to guide action during times of change.

The process of cultivating equanimity in daily life involves acceptance, nonjudgment, and a focus on speaking and behaving in service of effectiveness and *not* in service of reaction (Linehan, 1993). When experiencing the integration and presence that can be found in the center (Figure 10.4), Siegel (2010) suggests that these five qualities present: flexibility, adaptability, coherence, energy, and stability (i.e., FACES). That is, as we saw with Sophie, your patients will be able to show more (F) flexibility in response to challenge, they will be (A) adaptive to new situations, their response will reflect a central (C) coherence and organization, they will have (E) energy, and they will show more (S) stability over time (Siegel, 2010). Associated embodied practices (see Chapter 3) include: (1) be mindfully aware, (4) accept impermanence, (5) cultivate nonattachment, (6) discern what is not-self, (7) allow what is with nonjudgment, and (11) maintain equanimity.

Joy and Loving-Kindness

Joy and loving-kindness are positive emotional states associated with our feelings toward ourselves and others. Cultivation of positive feelings states has been found to be an important component in programs that effectively address self-regulation (e.g., Hanson & Mendius, 2009; Linehan, 1993; Shapiro & Carlson, 2009). Hanson and Mendius (2009) remind us that the brain preferentially scans for negative and potentially threatening information. Our negative implicit memory system grows faster than our positive implicit memory system (Hanson & Mendius, 2009). It is critical to purposely cultivate positive emotions such as joy and loving-kindness. In the emotional regulation module of DBT, patients are taught to build positive emotions, joyfulness, by scheduling and engaging in pleasant events each day (Linehan, 1993). By accumulating positive events and corresponding positive emotional states, patients begin to experience a life within which they want to be present (Linehan, 1993). Linehan (1993) and Stahl and Goldstein (2010) both provide lists of over 100 activities that can help cultivate positive experiences.

In the mindful and yogic teaching, sympathetic joy goes a step beyond simply cultivating joy. Sympathetic joy involves the cultivation of joyful feelings when we see others doing well. The practice of sympathetic joy pairs well with loving-kindness practices. Consistent with these teachings, Linehan (1993) instructs patients to change current emotions by active opposition to the current emotion. Loving-kindness meditation (see Chapter 5 for a practice script) is useful for cultivating feelings of loving-kindness and warmth toward yourself, people whom you care about in your life, as well as people with whom you struggle (Stahl & Goldstein, 2010). It is important to encourage patients to be self-validating. That is, help them acknowledge the struggle they are experiencing within the context of their relationship with another individual. Then, move toward addressing how this struggle gets in their way and the use of loving-kindness practices as a method for removing this resistance as an obstacle. Siegel (2010) believes that practice of loving-kindness meditation helps activate the social and self-engagement systems of the brain. Stahl and Goldstein (2010) recommend that you practice loving-kindness meditation in the face of resistance: "Perhaps there is no greater healing than to learn to love yourself and others with an open heart" (p. 150). Associated embodied practices (see Chapter 3) include: (1) be mindfully aware, (5) cultivate nonattachment, (6) discern what is not-self, (7) allow what is with nonjudgment, and (12) cultivate loving-kindness and joy.

Compassion for Self and Others

Compassion means to wish for the suffering in others to be removed (McCown et al., 2010). The roots of the word *compassion* are shared with those of the word *kindness* (Wallace, 2010). When you experience compassion, you are fully present with the struggle within the other or yourself. There is no avoidance, denial, or dissociation. Compassion for self and others also includes the awareness that struggling is part of being human. In private practice and in yoga class I remind patients and yoga students that it is not about the winning, getting it right, or being perfect. It is about the trying. Further, in the trying there will be some instances of getting right, landing the play, and nailing the test, performance, maybe even the pose. However, there will also be times when they get it wrong, fall, lose a sense of purpose, and experience what the world sees as failure. Self-compassion is loving yourself through all of it. Compassion is the kindness you show to others as they succeed, fail, try, and forget how to try. To assess compassion, see Pommier (2011), which is accessible at www.self-compassion.org/CompassionScale.pdf.

Research suggests that self-compassion may promote the successful self-regulation of health-related behaviors (Terry & Leary, 2011). It is believed that the mechanisms of change are the promotion of self-regulation via a lowering defensiveness, reduction of emotional states and self-blame that interfere with self-regulation, and increase in compliance with medical recommendations (Terry & Leary, 2011). Additionally, it is theorized that as people high in self-compassion are less depleted, they cope better, with greater self-regulatory resources to devote to self-care (Terry & Leary, 2011). To assess self-compassion see Raes, Pommier, Neff, and Van Gucht (2011). The scale is accessible at www.self-compassion .org/ShortSCS.pdf. Associated embodied practices (see Chapter 3) include: (1) be mindfully aware, (5) cultivate nonattachment, (6) discern what is not-self, (7) allow what is with nonjudgment, and (10) observe compassion for self and others.

KARMA: PLANTING SEEDS

According to the Yoga Sutras as interpreted by Prabhavananda and Isherwood (2007), there are three kids of karma: (1) karma that has already been created, stored, and may bear fruit in the future; (2) karma that was created in the past that is bearing fruit in this present moment; and (3) karma that we are in the process of creating right now in our current thoughts and actions. Only one of these types of karma is in our control. That is the karma we are creating right now. The Yoga Sutras explain that the already-existing karmas are beyond our control and one can only wait until they have worked themselves out. However, right now, we can make the changes, be in the present moment, and create the karma that we want in our lives (Prabhavananda & Isherwood, 2007).

Karma-yoga is a technique for performance of actions such that the soul (i.e., the uppercase "S" Self) is not bound by the results of the actions (Mulla & Krishnan, 2009). According to Mulla and Krishnan (2009), Karma-yoga has three dimensions: duty-orientation, indifference to rewards, and equanimity. Illustrative of the expression of karma service in yoga is the Off the Mat and into the World (OTM; www .offthematintotheworld.org) service organization. Founded in 2007, OTM is led by Seane Corn, Kerri Kelly, Marianne Manilov, and Taj Jame and uses the power of yoga to inspire conscious, sustainable activism and ignite grassroots social change. The OTM organization does this by facilitating personal empowerment through leadership trainings, fostering community collaboration, and initiating local and global service projects. Service foci include a global seva (i.e., service) challenge, the empowered youth initiative, and yoga votes, an initiative to support yogis in political engagement.

It is a continuous process. Karma holds that you are now, and have always been, planting seeds. Each thought, word, and action is a seed that is planted with a potential to yield a bountiful, soulful harvest or to create suffering. Acknowledging that we can't control seeds that we have already planted is challenging for those who have been struggling with self-regulation. If you have been lying, stealing, and evading people you love to support your eating disorder, shopping addiction, self-injury, gaming, or gambling problems, there are many seeds that have been planted. It is frightening to think about them. Still, thought about or not—they are there. For example, Sean, a 32-year-old in recovery from alcohol abuse and gambling addiction, hurt many people in service of his struggles. He stole from his mother, his boyfriends, and his sisters. He lied about where he was. He actively ignored their pleas for him to stop and avoided their company. Before he was willing to face his behaviors and the impact it had on others, his avoidance fueled his drinking and addiction.

Facing what he had done and acknowledging the *karma debt* that already exists has been a powerful motivator in Sean's sobriety and abstinence from gambling. To stay on track, he ends each of his morning meditations with a commitment to planting positive karma seeds each day. He has a goal to be a sponsor in Alcoholics Anonymous and currently supports others in recovery at daily meetings. Every day, he intentionally seeks ways to support his mom and his sisters. Sean also assists at the free yoga classes at his studio. His conscious planting of karma seeds is not done for reward or acknowledgment. He does this in right action and to remind himself that he is part of something bigger than himself. He does this to be in service, and this is giving his life meaning. Finally, the meaning is giving him a reason to stay sober.

To plant good karma seeds, engage in acts of service for something bigger than yourself (i.e., your ego self). Do this with no concern about reward or acknowledgment, while cultivating a sense of equanimity. It does not matter how bad things have gotten or how far you have traveled down a difficult path. At any point you can begin to plant positive seeds. I have had patients tell me that they feel like they are too far gone, too lost to ever get it right. I often tell them the story of the Vietnam veteran Clause Thomas (2004). Thomas (2004) explains, "At the age of seventeen I enlisted in the US Army and volunteered for service in Vietnam. By taking up arms, I was directly responsible for killing several hundred people, and the killing didn't stop until I was honorably discharged and sent home with numerous medals . . ." (p. xi). Troubled by war and all he had seen and done, Thomas actively avoided his memories, dissociated from his feelings, and struggled with addiction. It was through the teaching of Thich Nhat Hanh that he was able to turn his life around into one of service. By taking all that he had learned through his experiences of war and turning it into motivation to do good, be good, and support good, Thomas began to create a life in which he could be present. Finding this type of meaning, a reason for being that is bigger than the ego self and serves the true, soul Self, can be critical to long-term negotiation of symptoms. Associated embodied practices (see Chapter 3) include: (1) be mindfully aware, (3) live in inquiry, (5) cultivate nonattachment, (6) discern what is not self, (7) allow what is with nonjudgment, (9) be of your values, (10) observe compassion for self and others, (11) maintain equanimity, and (12) cultivate loving-kindness and joy.

SUMMARY

This chapter reviews off-the-mat practices from the physiological foundation up. The off-the-mat practices serve self-regulation by providing a steady physical, body-based stability cultivated from daily health and down-regulating practices. The yamas and niyamas provide a structure for organizing behavioral choices for the self and for the self within relationships. Next, the four immeasurables provide guidance for cultivating emotional well-being in daily living. Finally, karma practice encourages pursuit

TABLE 10.2   Off-the-Mat Yoga Practice Assessment

Off-the-Mat Practice	Current Daily Practices (Practices I'd Like to Start)
Karma practices	
In what ways do you provide service for others?	
What gives you a sense of greater purpose in your life?	
Emotional practices	
Review the ways you cultivate equanimity in your daily life.	
List ways you foster joy and loving-kindness as you manage your relationships.	
Explain how you currently integrate compassion into your understanding of the people in your life and your own self-understanding.	
Behavioral practices	
What are the guidelines that you use to make daily decisions about your behavior?	
Do your self-regulation problems interfere with your ability to be the kind of person that you want to be (see yamas and niyamas)?	
Physiological foundational practices	
In what ways do you support and regulate the body?	

of service and meaning as a pathway to long-term recovery. In practice, it can be helpful to review the off-the-mat yoga practice assessment from the bottom up. Work with your patients, discussing the daily practices they currently integrate into their day-to-day lives and which ones they would like to cultivate (Table 10.2). It can be helpful to review each of the sections in this chapter with your patients, using guiding questions, figures, and assessments. Next, Chapter 11 reviews comprehensive treatment protocol and Chapter 12 details the maintenance of self-care throughout the process of recovery and service.

REFERENCES

Adele, D. (2009). *The yamas and the niyamas: Exploring yoga's ethical practice.* Duluth, MN: On-Word Bound Books.

Anderson, S., & Sovik, R. (2000). *Yoga: Mastering the basics.* Honsedale, PA: The Himalayan Institute.

Armstrong, L. E., Ganio, M. S., Casa, D. J., Lee, E. C., McDermott, B. P., Klau, J. F., . . . Lieberman, H. R. (2012). Mild dehydration affects mood in healthy young women. *The Journal of Nutrition, 142*(2), 382–388.

Bourne, E. J. (2010). *The anxiety and phobia workbook* (5th ed.). Oakland, CA: New Harbinger Publications.

Cook-Cottone, C. P., Kane, L. S., Keddie, E., & Haugli, S. (2013). *Girls growing in wellness and balance: Yoga and life skills to empower.* Stoddard, WI: Schoolhouse Educational Services.

Cook-Cottone, C. P., Tribole, E., & Tylka, T. L. (2013). *Healthy eating in schools: Evidence-based interventions to help kids thrive.* Washington, DC: American Psychological Association.

Garland, E. L., Schwarz, N. R., Kelly, A., Whitt, A., & Howard, M. O. (2012). Mindfulness-oriented recovery enhancement for alcohol dependence: Therapeutic mechanisms and intervention acceptability. *Journal of Social Work Practice in the Addictions, 12*(3), 242–263.

Gujar, N., Yoo, S. S., Hu, P., & Walker, M. P. (2011). Sleep deprivation amplifies reactivity of brain reward networks, biasing the appraisal of positive emotional experiences. *The Journal of Neuroscience, 31,* 4466–4474.

Hanh, T. N. (1999). *The heart of Buddha's teachings: Transforming suffering into peace, joy, and liberation.* New York, NY: Broadway Books.

Hanson, R., & Mendius, R. (2009). *Buddha's brain: The practical neuroscience of happiness, love, and wisdom.* Oakland, CA: New Harbinger Publications.

Kennedy, D., Jones, E., & Haskell, C. (2011). Vitamin status, cognition and mood in cognitively intact adults. In D. Benton (Ed.), *Lifetime nutritional influences on cognition, behaviour and psychiatric illness* (pp. 194-250). Cambridge, UK: Woodhead.

Linehan, M. (1993). *Cognitive-behavioral treatment of borderline personality disorder.* New York, NY: Guilford Press.

McCown, D., Reibel, D., & Micozzi, M. S. (2010). *Teaching mindfulness: A practical guide for clinicians and educators.* New York, NY: Springer.

Miller, W. R., & Rose, G. S. (2009). Toward a theory of motivational interviewing. *American Psychologist, 64,* 527–537.

Mulla, Z. R., & Krishnan, V. R. (2009). Do Karma-yogis make better leaders? Exploring the relationship between the leader's Karma-yoga and transformational leadership. *Journal of Human Values, 15*(2), 167–183.

Pommier, E. A. (2011). The Compassion Scale. *Dissertation Abstracts International Section A: Humanities and Social Sciences, 72,* 1174.

Prabhavananda, S., & Isherwood, C. (2007). *How to know God: The yoga aphorisms of Patanjali.* Hollywood, CA: Vedanta Press.

Raes, F., Pommier, E., Neff, K. D., & Van Gucht, D. (2011). Construction and factorial validation of a short form of the Self-Compassion Scale. *Clinical Psychology & Psychotherapy, 18,* 250–255.

Rubak, S., Sandbaek, A., Lauritzen, T., & Christensen, B. (2005). Motivational interviewing: A systematic review and meta-analysis. *British Journal of General Practice, 55,* 305–312.

Sanford, M. (2006). *Waking: A memoir of trauma and transcendence.* Emmaus, PA: Rodale.

Shapiro, S. L., & Carlson, L. E. (2009). *The art and science of mindfulness: Integrating mindful into psychology and the helping professions.* Washington, DC: American Psychological Association.

Siegel, D. J. (2010). *The mindful therapist: A clinician's guide to mindsight and neural integration.* New York, NY: W. W. Norton.

Simpkins, A. M., & Simpkins, C. A. (2011). *Meditation and yoga in psychotherapy: Techniques for clinical practice.* New York, NY: John Wiley & Sons.

Stahl, B., & Goldstein, E. (2010). *A mindfulness-based stress reduction workbook.* Oakland, CA: New Harbinger Publications.

Terry, M. L., & Leary, M. R. (2011). Self-compassion, self-regulation, and health. *Self and Identity, 10,* 352–362.

Thomas, C. A. (2004). *At hell's gate.* Boston, MA: Shambhala Publications.

Wallace, B. A. (2010). *The four immeasurables: Practices to open the heart.* Ithaca, NY: Snow Lion Productions.

Zahr, N. M., Kaufman, K. L., & Harper, C. G. (2011). Clinical and pathological features of alcohol-related brain damage. *Nature Reviews Neurology, 7*(5), 284–294.

Zschucke, E., Gaudlitz, K., & Ströhle, A. (2013). Exercise and physical activity in mental disorders: Clinical and experimental evidence. *Journal of Preventive Medicine and Public Health, 46*(Suppl. 1), S12–S21.

ೞ IV ೞ

Evolving Mindful and Yogic Approaches

Comprehensive Treatment Protocols and Empirical Support

*. . . if you hope to mobilize your inner capacities for growth and for healing
and to take charge in your life on a new level,
a certain kind of energy on your part will be required . . .
there are times when you have to light one fire to put out another.*
—JON KABAT-ZINN (2013, p. xlix)

THE RESEARCH PERSPECTIVE

To be accepted as viable treatments and complements to current treatments, mindful and yogic approaches must be scientifically validated. In order to adhere to the standards of the scientific method, the intervention (in this case, mindful and yogic approaches) must be detailed in a manner that allows for treatment integrity and replication. Issues such as intervention content, process, dosage, method of delivery, control groups, and group assignment can be critical variables affecting whether or not the outcomes are due to the intervention or some other variable. For example, in mindfulness and yoga interventions it has yet to be determined if interventions can be delivered effectively by a trained teacher, therapist under supervision, researcher, experienced mentor, or guru. Other specific questions have yet to be answered, such as the following: Can a therapist effectively deliver a mindfulness intervention in therapy when coached by a trained facilitator? Does he or she need additional training or will a manual with instructions be sufficient? Are interventions effective in a group format or one-on-one? Which mindfulness techniques are most effective for depression, anxiety, eating disorders, gambling addiction, self-harm, or alcohol abuse? As you can see, there are many questions yet to be answered. Groups of researchers have made progress in standardizing mindful and yogic techniques with various degrees of success. This has resulted in bodies of research ranging from emergent to reliable levels of maturity. This chapter briefly reviews mindfulness-based and yoga protocols, recommends texts and handbooks, and provides preliminary evidence in support of mindful and yoga techniques. Cautions and contraindications are noted. Finally, the conclusion details weaknesses and future directions in research.

A THIRD WAVE OR NEW PARADIGM?

The emergence of mindful approaches to mental illness is seen by some as a new wave, a third wave, and even a paradigm shift in psychology (Cook-Cottone, Tribole, & Tylka, 2013; Greco & Hayes, 2008). Others argue that comprehensive treatment protocols such as dialectic behavioral therapy (DBT; Linehan, 1993) and acceptance and commitment therapy (ACT) are an extension of traditional cognitive behavioral therapy (CBT) and not a new wave of interventions (Hofmann, Sawyer, & Fang, 2010). Notably, yoga has yet to be acknowledged as part of the third wave of therapies. It is true that both mindful and yogic approaches address cognitive interpretations of events and encourage active, behavioral change (Young, DeLorenzi, & Cunningham, 2011). Researchers posit that the deviations from CBT are specific to the theoretical explanations of the role of cognitions (Hofmann et al., 2010). Like many others, Hofmann and colleagues (2010) argue that these distinctions from CBT are not irreconcilable in requiring a separate classification of *new wave* treatments. They contend that although subtle and important differences on the theoretical and procedural levels exist, research findings to date do not favor one treatment over another. Further, they argue that there are no differential mechanisms of action that warrant a dramatic separation from the CBT family of approaches. Yes, some of the mindfulness-based and informed protocols that are currently being researched are essentially CBT packaged with mindfulness and/or yoga practice add-ons. In this way, they are an extension of previous methodologies. Mindfulness and yoga, from their traditions, as described in this text and not as an add-on to CBT, are something different. When used in practice honoring core, traditional features, they are a new wave of being with patients.

Arguably, traditional mindfulness and yoga offer conceptually distinct ways to negotiate thoughts and feelings; are a set of daily, life-long practices rather than a remedy for disordered functioning; are preventive and proactive in nature; and enhance neurologic integration. First, unlike CBT, within mindful and yogic approaches, thoughts, sense impressions, and feelings are not the target of change (e.g., the Buddhist Psychological Model [BPM]; Grabovac, Lau, & Willett, 2011). Rather, these experiences are felt and accepted as they are (e.g., Cook-Cottone, Tribole, et al., 2013; Grabovac et al., 2011).

Experiencing, accepting, and allowing thoughts, sense impressions, and feelings is more than another form of CBT. It is a form of self-validation and external validation. Years ago, I realized that when I told a client that the thought she was expressing was irrational, I was acting in ways that were completely invalidating. When a patient with a seemingly out-of-control struggle with bulimia nervosa (BN) tells you that she feels she can no longer face another meal, she does not want to restructure this thought and consider a more rational way of being around food. She wants to be heard and understood. She feels this way and has likely struggled alone with these difficult feelings. During a session much like this back in the 1990s, I realized the invaliding nature of a standard CBT methodology. Although traditional CBT seemed to work well with patients with anxiety-based struggles, it was not a good fit for those with substantial emotional and self-regulation issues. I decided to change my approach. Connecting to Rogerian roots, I began validating patients' feelings and working with their sense of overwhelm. The core mechanisms of change here are acceptance and relaxation with what is (Young et al., 2011). In a validating manner, I worked with my patients to make a distinction between *what is*, what something feels like (i.e., sense impressions and feelings), and how they could come to be with *what is* differently.

Shortly after, I began reading about dialectic behavior therapy. I realized that I was one of many psychologists who was looking for a deeper, more complex way of being with my patients. I began studying DBT and integrating these techniques into my sessions with patients. Inspired by the efficacy, my own study of mindfulness and yoga commenced. I discovered that mindful and yogic approaches not only validate the notion that thoughts, sense impressions, and feelings can be uncomfortable, in their traditional forms they refer to daily, human experience as *painful*. In fact, one of the main tenets of both approaches is learning to not add *suffering* to that which is already painful (Black, 2014). Yes! The things we think and feel on a daily basis can be painful, and often this *not* irrational. Distinct from CBT, at their core these approaches begin with validation of the human experience.

Second, unlike CBT, both mindful and yogic approaches include sets of daily practices that continually challenge and sculpt ways of thinking, being, and acting within the context of our lives. In this way, mindful and yogic approaches are embodied in daily life. Despite 6-, 8-, and 12-week protocols designed to explore research outcomes and efficacy, mindful and yogic approaches are meant to be integrated into a person's life for the long term. Seeing them as interventions is, perhaps, a necessity within the context of Western empirical methodologies. However as traditions, these practices were not considered to be short-term interventions that once completed shift your patient forever. They are daily, life-long practices.

Third, unlike CBT, mindful and yogic practices such as meditation and asana generate daily opportunities for growth. Addiction researchers have referred to this as exposure (Young et al., 2011). Specifically, rather than waiting for an urge, trigger, or stimulating context to manifest, mindful and yogic practices bring forth opportunity for and awareness of challenging thoughts, sense impressions, and feelings (Young et al., 2011). In this way, the patient creates his or her own challenges while seated in meditation or moving on the yoga mat. Thoughts, feelings, and sense impressions manifest, as they always do, while the patient is *on the cushion* or *on the mat*, providing a safe and low-consequence arena for facing uncomfortable and unpleasant thoughts, sense impressions, and feelings. Within the practice sessions, the patient gains a sense of self-efficacy from the doing of it, the managing of it—the embodiment of it.

Finally, there is evidence that embodied practices that bring together the cognitive, emotional, and physical aspects of self increase neurologic integration, thus increasing self-regulation and a sense of well-being, and decrease cravings (see Chapters 4 [on mindfulness] and 7 [on yoga]; Forfylow, 2011; Froeliger, Garland, Modlin, & McClemon, 2012; Witkiewitz, Bowen, Douglas, & Hsu, 2013; Young et al., 2011). Researchers believe that mindfulness practice may, in fact, disrupt the craving cycle, serving as a counter-conditioning alternative to addiction (Witkiewitz et al., 2013; Witkiewitz, Marlatt, & Walker, 2005).

A full explanation is beyond the scope of this text. However, to illustrate, Marlatt, Bowen, and Lustyk (2012) describe how mindfulness-based activities such as meditation can thicken the prefrontal cortical tissues critical to self-regulation and the inhibition required for sobriety and reductions in substance use. Further, they describe how approaches that enhance self-compassion are able to modify emotional cues, thereby improving emotional regulation. Further, in a study of yoga practitioners and a control group, researchers found that yoga practitioners exhibited less reactivity in areas of the brain associated with negative affect (Froeliger et al., 2012). Yoga practitioners may learn and practice strategies that help reduce reactions to negative stimuli. Finally, reviews of research on yoga consistently document regulation of the autonomic nervous system and improvement in neurotransmitter and hormonal functioning (e.g., Forfylow, 2011). Siegel (2010) writes at length about the neurologic integration possible with mindfulness practice. See *The Mindful Therapist: A Clinician's Guide to Mindsight and Neural Integration*.

Here is what this might look like in therapy. In CBT, a therapist might ask a client to complete a worksheet upon which the client records thoughts and feelings, behavioral choices that come to mind, the behavioral choice made, and associated consequences of the behavioral choice. This can happen in mindful and yogic approaches as well. In fact, you have seen some worksheets in this book. A key difference is that in yogic and mindful approaches, the client is asked to (a) address (not necessarily change) symptomatic thinking and feeling through behavioral homework; and is also asked to (b) do something (or several things) daily to practice new ways of being with routine thoughts and behaviors. In this way, yogic and mindful approaches address both symptom reduction and the cultivation of a new framework for approaching life. For example, recall Danny, the young law clerk who was struggling with drinking, shopping, and eating behaviors. Her life was quite chaotic and she was unable to stay present with any uncomfortable thoughts or feelings. Fed up with her life and ready for change, Danny went to a psychologist who was well versed in both mindful and yogic techniques.

Early in treatment, the psychologist encouraged Danny to give an embodied practice, such as yoga, a try. She also encouraged Danny to: (a) sit for meditation for 2 to 5 minutes a day; (b) begin a daily log of her eating, sleep, and hydration behaviors; and (c) log her two most troubling symptoms. Danny chose drinking and purging. Initially, the psychologist helped Danny work with her symptoms by becoming aware of and journaling her triggers; discerning the nature of the triggers and the feelings that accompanied them, coding them as pleasant, neutral, or unpleasant; and then recording whether or not symptoms followed. She also taught Danny how to meditate and explained the Buddhist Psychological Model (see Chapter 4). Session by session, they discussed the lessons that Danny learned *on the cushion* and *on the mat* and how those lessons translated into Danny's way of being in her daily life. Danny was truly overwhelmed by her tendency to avoid uncomfortable thoughts and feelings as well her tendency to label nearly every thought and feeling as bad. Following 2 weeks of observing and documenting baseline thoughts, feelings, and behaviors, she was ready to integrate her work in yoga and meditation into her work on her symptoms. Within several weeks of solid practice, Danny was able to negotiate her uncomfortable thoughts and feelings that often trigger symptoms. Her competency on the cushion and on the yoga mat had increased her sense of self-efficacy, empowering her efforts when she was exceptionally triggered. Ultimately, Danny was able to consider herself recovered and continues to practice yoga to date.

MINDFULNESS

Mindfulness interventions typically include psychoeducation and active practices that help clients develop mindful awareness, acceptance, and nonjudgment, as well as competency in various forms of meditation and relaxation methods (see Chapters 4, 5, and 6 for a review of mindfulness and formal and informal practices). Central to mindfulness-based and informed therapies is the treatment of internal events (see earlier discussion; Greco & Hayes, 2008). Mindfulness to the present moment involves consciously and actively attending to and relating with experiences (Levin & Hayes, 2012; Linehan, 1993; van Goethem, Mulders, Muris, Arntz, & Egger, 2012). Protocols typically employ a variety of techniques to allow patients practice in noticing and allowing thoughts, sense impressions, and feelings; exploring the context of events; and practicing mindful awareness.

Specific to embodied self-regulation, mindfulness interventions help patients cultivate a willingness to experience and tolerate thoughts and cravings with self-compassion (Levin & Hayes, 2012). In this way, the urge to escape that drives many addictive and compulsive behaviors is reduced (Levin & Hayes, 2012). For example, Levin and Hayes (2012) describe a common strategy that clients use when attempting abstinent- suppression of cravings and urges. Mindfulness interventions help break the old patterns of use. These interventions interrupt the process by facilitating a flexible and nonreactive awareness of triggers. In this way, there is a space cultivated, from which clients can notice triggers, accept them, and actively choose how to respond to them (Levin & Hayes, 2012). When patients have a more accepting approach to the automatic urges and cravings for substance use, they have been less likely to engage them, even when motivations are strong (Levin & Hayes, 2012; Witkiewitz et al., 2013). In DBT clients are encouraged to see urges like waves and imagine that they are surfing the wave, riding it to its peak and then down the other side (Levin & Hayes, 2012; Young et al., 2011). In this way, awareness is used like a surfboard, riding the wave of the urge without wiping out (Young et al., 2011).

Mindfulness-Informed and Mindfulness-Based Interventions

There are several mindfulness-informed and mindfulness-based approaches. These include mindfulness-based stress reduction, DBT, mindfulness-based cognitive therapy, and acceptance and commitment therapy. Research has found positive outcomes in self-regulation (e.g., van Goethem et al., 2012; Wanden-Berghe, Sanz-Valero, & Wanden-Berghe, 2010). Across studies the main outcomes include increased subjective well-being, reduced psychological symptoms and emotional reactivity, and improved behavioral regulation (Keng, Smoski, & Robins, 2011). Mechanisms of change include increased mindfulness, metacognitive awareness, exposure, attentional control, memory functioning, and values clarification (Keng et al., 2011).

Mindfulness-Based Stress Reduction

Mindfulness-based stress reduction (MBSR) was the first mindfulness-based protocol (Black, 2014; Shapiro & Carlson, 2009). It was developed by John Kabat-Zinn in 1979 in a behavioral medicine setting for patients with chronic pain and stress (Baer & Krietemeyer, 2006; Black, 2014; Shapiro & Carlson, 2009). It is a standardized protocol with a duration of 8 weeks with weekly sessions from 2.5 to 3.0 hours and an all-day intensive session occurring on the 6th week (Baer & Krietemeyer, 2006; Black, 2014; Shapiro & Carlson, 2009). There are often individual and small-group intake sessions with preprogram assessment. Participants are asked to complete extensive home practice of at least 45 minutes a day at least 6 days a week (Baer & Krietemeyer, 2006). Program content is didactic, covering education on stress and its effects, as well as experiential, devoting time to mindfulness exercises and processing these experiences in a group format (Baer & Krietemeyer, 2006). Experiential activities include formal and informal mindfulness practices such as the body scan, mindful eating, sitting meditation, Hatha yoga, walking meditation, and incorporating mindfulness into daily life (Baer & Krietemeyer, 2006; Shapiro & Carlson, 2009). For training, courses, and further information on MBSR, see the Center for Mindfulness in Medicine, Health-Care and Society at the University at Massachusetts Medical School (www .umassmed.edu/cfm/stress-reduction). For an easy-to-read and easy-to-use resource on specific techniques, see *The Relaxation and Stress Reduction Workbook*, 6th edition, by Davis, Eshelman, and McKay (2008).

Mindfulness-Based Cognitive Therapy

Emerging in the late 1990s, mindfulness-based cognitive therapy (MBCT) is based on MBSR and utilizes many of its components (i.e., mindful eating, body scan, sitting meditation, yoga, walking meditation, and informal daily mindful practices; Baer & Krietemeyer, 2006; Shapiro & Carlson, 2009). Like MBSR, MBCT includes the observing of pleasant and unpleasant events (Baer & Krietemeyer, 2006). Developed specifically to address the prevention of relapse of a major depressive episode, the didactic component of MBCT addresses depression rather than stress (Baer & Krietemeyer, 2006).

As in MBSR, homework and group discussions are critical factors in implementation. The format is a group-based, 8-week intervention delivered in 2-hour weekly sessions (Shapiro & Carlson, 2009).

The MBCT protocol also includes additional exercises: 3-minute breathing space, triggering meditations, cognitive therapy exercises, pleasure and mastery exercises, and relapse prevention action plans (Baer & Krietemeyer, 2006; Shapiro & Carlson, 2009). First, the 3-minute breathing space is taught as a mini-meditation in which patients learn to take a moment to step back, breathe, and establish awareness of the present moment (Baer & Krietemeyer, 2006). Specifically, they are taught to ask themselves, "What is my experience right now?" (Baer & Krietemeyer, 2006, p. 14). They are encouraged to scan their bodies and minds for thoughts, sense impressions, and feelings and to experience and accept without judgment (Baer & Krietemeyer, 2006; Shapiro & Carlson, 2009). Next, patients are asked to move their awareness to the breath and then to the whole body. The breathing space is designed to increase awareness and give space for new behavioral choices rather than default to maladaptive, automatic responses (Baer & Krietemeyer, 2006). Challenging meditations are also included in MBCT. The technique extends the instructions for meditation in order to deliberately bring to mind a difficult issue and bring awareness to the associated body sensations (Baer & Krietemeyer, 2006). Patients are asked to notice any attempts to resist or avoid the feelings that arise and to acknowledge the feelings and the tendencies to avoid them with open awareness and acceptance. Patients are encouraged to imagine "breathing with" difficult sensations and feelings (Baer & Krietemeyer, 2006, p. 15). Of note, there is no formal loving-kindness instruction (Shapiro & Carlson, 2009).

Addressing cognitive aspects of the treatment, the MBCT protocol includes a thoughts and feelings exercise, discussion of automatic thoughts, and an exercise that focuses on mood, thoughts, and alternative viewpoints (Baer & Krietemeyer, 2006). The thoughts and feelings exercise involves guided imagery in which patients see someone they know, stop and wave, and that individual walks on without seeming to notice the patient's kind gestures (Baer & Krietemeyer, 2006). Patients are asked to notice the thoughts, sense impressions, and feelings that accompany this imagery (Baer & Krietemeyer, 2006). They are taught the ABC model (A = triggering situation, B = associated thoughts, and C = associated feeling or emotions; Baer & Krietemeyer, 2006). The activity is designed to bring awareness to each component and the chain of events that occurs following a triggering situation.

The protocol also includes exploration of automatic negative thoughts, a critical depressive symptom. Patients complete an automatic thoughts questionnaire and then discuss these thoughts as symptoms of depression rather than statements of truth (Baer & Krietemeyer, 2006). In another exercise, patients explore how a negative mood or experience and a positive mood or experience might affect their interpretation of an event, such as someone not having time to listen or talk. Each of these activities is designed to help patients gain insight into how depressive symptoms and thought patterns are affecting their life experiences (Baer & Krietemeyer, 2006).

Pleasure and mastery activities are included in the protocol to help combat depressive symptoms. Pleasure activities include pleasant activities that are fun and enjoyable to do (Baer & Krietemeyer, 2006). Mastery activities are those activities that leave a patient with a sense of accomplishment (e.g., complete a household task; Baer & Krietemeyer, 2006). Patients generate lists of these activities so that they have the lists as a go-to when they are struggling. Finally, the MBCT protocols include sessions in which patients develop a relapse prevention plan that brings together the lessons and insights learned (Baer & Krietemeyer, 2006). They record a list of the symptoms that manifest as they begin relapse. When a symptom is noticed, they are encouraged to take a breathing space, notice how they are feeling, and choose an exercise they have learned, a mastery activity, or a pleasure activity. For more on MBCT, see Ruth Baer's (2006) *Mindfulness-Based Treatment Approaches: A Clinician's Guide to Evidence Base and Applications.* For more on MBCT, including resources and training, go to mbct.com.

Dialectic Behavioral Therapy

DBT was developed by Marsha Linehan for patients with borderline personality disorders (BPDs; Linehan, 1993). More recently, it has been adapted for use with other populations, including those who struggle with self-regulation. The term *dialectic* refers to the central tenet of the therapy: an emphasis on balance and integration of opposing ideas such as acceptance and change (Baer & Krietemeyer, 2006). Specifically, DBT provides psychosocial skills training in four modules: core mindfulness skills, interpersonal effectiveness skills, emotional regulation skills, and distress tolerance skills (Linehan, 1993). Given the substantial struggles with self-regulation among those with BPD, the mindfulness practices as presented in MBSR and MBCT were seen as too lengthy and formal to be accepted by BPD patients (Baer & Krietemeyer, 2006). Accordingly, a set of shorter and less formal mindfulness exercises was utilized (Baer & Krietemeyer, 2006). Outpatient DBT involves a 1-year commitment with weekly individual therapy and group-based skills training sessions.

The core mindfulness skills module includes didactic information that provides a rationale for practicing mindfulness and controlling attention (Baer & Krietemeyer, 2006). Further, it serves to help patients integrate thoughts and feelings in the service of behavioral choice. Linehan (1993) refers to the integration of the cognitive (i.e., reasonable) mind and the emotional mind as *wise mind*. The specific skills include teaching patients what to do when being mindful (i.e., observe, describe, and participate [attend to activity in the present moment]; Linehan, 1993). Patients are taught how to be mindful (i.e., nonjudgmentally, one-mindfully, and effectively; Linehan, 1993). The emotional regulation and distress tolerance modules of DBT also integrate mindfulness skills (Baer & Krietemeyer, 2006). For example, identifying and labeling emotions is a central component of the emotional regulation model (Baer & Krietemeyer, 2006). Further, within the distress tolerance module, patients are taught to notice the rising and passing away of distressful or uncomfortable feelings or urges (Linehan, 1993). Patients are taught other skills such as distraction and breath work to assist in tolerating distress. Currently, there are many studies documenting the positive outcomes associated with DBT in the reduction of symptoms such as self-injury (e.g., van Goethem et al., 2012).

There are many adapted manuals for DBT. For a detailed description of DBT, see *Skills Training Manual for Treating Borderline Personality Disorder* (Linehan, 1993) and *The Dialectic Behavioral Therapy Skills Workbook for Bulimia: Using DBT to Break the Cycle and Regain Control of Your Life* (Astrachan-Fletcher & Maslar, 2009). For more on DBT, including training and resources, go to the Linehan Institute at behavioraltech.org/index.cfm.

Acceptance and Commitment Therapy

Acceptance and commitment therapy (ACT) is viewed as a general approach to psychotherapy designed to increase psychological flexibility (Baer & Krietemeyer, 2006; Wilson, Schnetzer, Flynn, & Kurz, 2012). Psychological flexibility has been defined as "the willingness to accept all aspects of one's experience without engaging in unnecessary avoidance behaviors, when doing so serves the development of patterns of values-congruent activity" (Wilson et al., 2012, p. 27). Specifically, ACT addresses mindfulness and acceptance skills and behavioral changes needed to help patients engage in a life that is vital and meaningful (Baer & Krietemeyer, 2006).

Central to ACT is the negotiation of experiential avoidance of feelings, sensations, cognitions, or urges (Baer & Krietemeyer, 2006). Experiential avoidance is seen as a root cause of many forms of psychopathology (e.g., substance abuse, binge eating; Baer & Krietemeyer, 2006). This model of treatment is based on six functional processes believed to underlie human suffering and adaptability: acceptance, diffusion (i.e., the decoupling of words and their cognitive and emotional referents), present-moment awareness, self-processes (i.e., de-emphasizing the self-definition and emphasizing the things we experience and do, our processes), value-based living (i.e., a focus on what is important), and committed action (i.e., action in areas of value; Wilson et al., 2012). Acceptance work involves openness to and nonjudgmental awareness of thoughts, sensations, and emotions as they occur (Baer & Krietemeyer, 2006). There is a specific focus on abandonment of efforts to control the uncontrollable and an acknowledgment that attempts to control the uncontrollable can exacerbate circumstances (Baer & Krietemeyer, 2006). Exposure to previously avoided experiences, such as anxiety, are promoted (Baer & Krietemeyer, 2006).

Cognitive diffusion involves considering thoughts and feelings as something to be noticed, yet not necessarily to be believed (Baer & Krietemeyer, 2006). Thoughts can be offensive and aversive in content and yet not harmful if we do not accept them or acknowledge them as true (Baer & Krietemeyer, 2006; Young et al., 2011). Diffusion is addressed through several approaches, such as nonjudgmental and nonreactive observation, thought labeling, and guided meditation. For example, in one activity, thoughts are viewed as leaves that fall from a tree and are allowed to float down the river (Baer & Krietemeyer, 2006).

Present-moment awareness in ACT is consistent with present-moment awareness activities described throughout this text. It involves a series of mindfulness activities that encourage observation of present-moment experience, accompanying internal and external sensations, labeling experiences without judgment or evaluation, and acceptance (Baer & Krietemeyer, 2006). Self-as-context expands present-moment awareness by seeing the self as the context within which these experiences are occurring (Baer & Krietemeyer, 2006). For example, rather than thinking, "I can't control myself; I have no power here," a patient is encouraged to say, "I am having the thoughts: 'I can't control myself' and 'I have no power'" (Baer & Krietemeyer, 2006). Internal experiences are not viewed as indicators of qualities of the self. Rather, they are experiences that can be reacted to or not.

Values and committed action is a feature unique to ACT (Baer & Krietemeyer, 2006). The ACT protocol includes activities that help patients address goals and values related to specific areas of their lives (e.g., career, relationships, personal growth, and health; Baer & Krietemeyer, 2006). Goals and values are used to organize intentions and behaviors around meaning (Baer & Krietemeyer, 2006).

For a text on ACT and substance use and addictions, see Steven C. Hayes and Michael E. Levin's (2012) *Mindfulness and Acceptance for Addictive Behaviors: Applying Contextual CBT to Substance Abuse and Behavioral Addictions.* Also, see the Association for Contextual Behavioral Science (ACBS; www.contextualpscyhology.org) for ACT protocols and texts. For a text on ACT for children and adolescents, see Greco and Hayes's (2008) *Acceptance and Mindfulness Treatments for Children and Adolescents: A Practitioner's Guide.*

Mindfulness-Based Relapse Prevention

Mindfulness-based relapse prevention (MBRP) involves the stepping out of the cycle of addiction by bringing awareness to the series of smaller daily choices that potentiate enduring self-destructive patterns of behavior (Khanna & Greeson, 2013; Marlatt et al., 2012; Witkiewitz et al., 2013). Where substance abuse and addiction are involved, low threat, easy-entry protocols are needed. Mindfulness provides a less threatening entryway into the process of making better choices (Marlatt et al., 2012). Step by step, the patient can slowly create a path that leads to less destructive behavior, thereby accruing a sense of self-efficacy, a baseline of positive growth, and confidence (Marlatt et al., 2012). The 8-week, group-based sessions within the MBRP protocol begin with cultivating wisdom and compassion. Wisdom is viewed as coming from observation of one's own experience (Marlatt et al., 2012). Your patient asks, "What is actually happening?" and "What does my mind do with what is happening?" (Marlatt et al., 2012, p. 227). Over time, the patient begins to differentiate between what is arising (e.g., thought, sense impression, or feeling) and how he or she is relating to it (e.g., judgment, aversion, clinging; Khanna & Greeson, 2013; Marlatt et al., 2012). The patient works to create flexibility in choosing a response, and this is freedom from addiction. This awareness is gleaned through a series of activities that helps the client see the pattern of reaction and to use compassion (Marlatt et al., 2012).

Urge surfing is a practice that is used as an alternative to willpower when facing urges to use a substance. In urge surfing, patients are guided to bring awareness to the situation that is triggering an urge to use. They are asked to imagine the scenario and pause at the point during which they would typically react. Here, they are encouraged to notice the sensation, emotions, and thoughts that are arising. They are encouraged to be present right to the edge of almost reacting and soften into the experience rather than resist it. They are asked to notice the wave of sensations, emotions, and thoughts as the surge swells in intensity. Rather than fight the wave, they are encouraged to ride the urge to the other side, where it slowly drops in intensity (Marlatt et al., 2012).

The MBRP protocol also includes several other mindful activities described in this text (e.g., loving-kindness meditation). The protocol is delivered in a group setting, allowing for patients to validate and support each other. The goal is to generalize skills learned in sessions to daily life (Marlatt et al., 2012). For more on MBRP, see Marlatt et al.'s chapter on substance abuse and relapse prevention in Germer and Siegel's (2012) *Wisdom and Compassion in Psychotherapy: Deepening Mindfulness in Clinical Practice*. For more on MBRP, including training and resources, go to www.mindfulrp.com.

Mindfulness-Based Eating Awareness Training

Mindfulness-based eating awareness training (MB-EAT) is a modification of the MBSR curriculum for individuals with binge-eating disorder and obesity (Kristeller & Wolever, 2010; Shapiro & Carlson, 2009). The methodology was informed by models of food intake regulation that emphasize psychological and physiological control mechanisms and their interplay, self-regulation theory, and neurocognitive models of mindfulness meditation (Kristeller & Wolever, 2010). The protocol integrates elements of MBSR with CBT and guided eating meditations (Shapiro & Carlson, 2009). The conceptual underpinning of this intervention holds that overeating is a symptom of a larger problem with self-regulation of affect, cognition, and behaviors (Shapiro & Carlson, 2009). Mindfulness is utilized to help patients increase awareness of patterns, become less reactive, and make healthier behavioral choices (Shapiro & Carlson, 2009).

The four main components are: (a) cultivating mindfulness, (b) cultivating mindful eating, (c) cultivating emotional balance, and (d) cultivating self-acceptance (Kristeller & Wolever, 2010). There is some work with the body, although comparatively less than with the traditional MBSR protocol (Shapiro & Carlson, 2009). Evidence to date indicates that the intervention decreases binge episodes, improves sense of self-control regarding eating, and reduces depressive symptoms (Kristeller & Wolever, 2010). Further, in a recent randomized controlled trial, researchers found that the reductions in binge eating were associated with continued mindfulness practice (Kristeller, Wolever, & Sheets, 2014). For a more detailed review of the protocol, see Kristeller and Wolever (2010), and for more on mindful eating, go to www.thecenterformindfuleating.org.

YOGA

As detailed in Chapters 7, 8, 9, and 10 of this text, the term *yoga* reflects a set of practices intended to integrate the mind and body in harmonious relaxation (Forfylow, 2011; Khanna & Greeson, 2013). Western practice of yoga typically entails emphasis on physical postures (i.e., asana), breathing techniques (i.e., pranayama), and meditation (see Chapter 8; Forfylow, 2011; Khanna & Greeson, 2013). Although there has been a dramatic increase in number and quality of yoga-related research publications since 2000 (McCall, 2014), research in the area of yoga lags behind mindfulness research. In part, this is due to the lack of manualization of the methodology, the variety of types of yoga, and the variability in interpretations and practices of the eight limbs of yoga. It is also important to note that there has been some resistance to standardizing and manualizing yoga to conform to empirical methodologies and comprising its authenticity. There are core scientific requirements that have not been addressed in much of the research. For example, basics such as dosage (e.g., frequency and duration) have not been adequately addressed in research (Cook-Cottone, 2013). Currently, researchers believe that yoga is helpful for several reasons, including simultaneous relaxation and activation; improved neurologic integration, self-regulation, and sense of well-being and quality of life; and increased awareness and tolerance of bodily sensations, feelings, and physical experience (Simpkins & Simpkins, 2011; van der Kolk et al., 2014; Woodyard, 2011).

Self-regulation, the focus of this text, has also been identified as one of the key mechanism of change associated with yoga as an intervention (Simpkins & Simpkins, 2011). In yoga, self-regulation effects appear to be, in part, related to the effects on the sympathetic and parasympathetic aspects of the autonomic nervous system. As individuals practice yoga, they become increasingly competent in regulating these systems intentionally. Yoga is believed to foster executive control, allow patients to move from activation to deactivation, and promote neurologic integration (Simpkins & Simpkins, 2011). Relatedly, those who practice yoga appear to be able to produce deep relaxation while remaining activated and alert. Staying alert and relaxed at the same time has many performance-improving benefits (Simpkins & Simpkins, 2011). What follows is termed absorption, "the ability to fully engage in the emotional process as an object of attention" (Simpkins & Simpkins, 2011, p. 18). Essentially, you become absorbed in the moment and all else slips to the background. Siegel (2010) refers to two aspects of absorption, openness and focused attention.

Yoga appears to improve mood, which enhances a sense of well-being, increases quality of life, and supports treatment outcomes across a variety of self-regulatory disorders (Woodyard, 2011). Further, yoga may help practitioners learn to tolerate uncomfortable physical and sensory experiences while increasing emotional awareness and affect tolerance (van der Kolk et al., 2014). For example, in an randomized controlled trial (RCT) exploring mood and quality of life among women undergoing heroin detoxification, a 6-month yoga intervention was found to significantly improve mood and quality of life as compared to controls (Zhuang, An, & Zhao, 2013). Chapters 7, 8, 9, and 10 detail some of the benefits of yoga as well as philosophical foundations and formal and informal practices.

Yoga Interventions

There are few manualized yoga interventions. Research to date presents a relatively diverse array of interventions using various forms, aspects, and dosages of yoga (e.g., Klein & Cook-Cottone, 2013). Given the substantial variability from study to study, it is difficult to compare outcomes across studies or to meaningfully aggregate outcomes using systematic reviews or meta-analyses. Much of the work has been focused on physical and health outcomes. Given the current body of research on yoga and mental health outcomes, we can be cautiously informed. To date, yoga has been found to have positive effects on correlates of difficulties with behavioral self-regulation (e.g., anxiety, depression, post-traumatic stress disorder [PTSD], and traumatic symptomatology) and on specific behaviors and disorders (e.g., binge eating, eating disorder symptoms and correlates, addiction, and substance use; Khalsa, 2004; Klein & Cook-Cottone, 2013; McIver, O'Halloran, & McGartland, 2009; Simpkins & Simpkins, 2011; van der Kolk et al., 2014; Woodyard, 2011). In light of the known mechanisms of action, yoga has the potential for positive effects on pathological gambling, compulsive gaming, compulsive Internet use, and shopping addictions, although research is needed to explore these possibilities.

It is important to note that not all studies have shown significant effects. For example, in a small RCT study of the effects of yoga on alcohol dependence ($n = 18$), the yoga-plus-treatment-as-usual group reduced daily alcohol intake comparatively more than the treatment-as-usual-only group. However, outcomes were not statistically significant (Hallgren, Romberg, Bakish, & Andreasson, 2014). Similarly, in a review of the effects of yoga on eating disorder symptoms and correlates, nearly all studies reviewed showed positive outcomes, with the exception of one study, which utilized a comparatively low dosage of yoga (Klein & Cook-Cottone, 2013). Accordingly, a better understanding of the conditions under which yoga can be an effective intervention for disorders (e.g., as an adjunct therapy, sufficient statistical power, and dosage) should be the target of future research. Next, research in the area of trauma and eating disorders is described in order to illustrate the work that is being done.

Trauma-informed yoga has implications for addressing issues with self-regulation. It is thought that if those who have been traumatized learn to negotiate emotional, cognitive, and physical symptoms, they will be less likely to adopt or continue dysregulated behaviors in efforts to cope (e.g., substance use; compulsive shopping, gambling, and gaming; self-harm; and disordered eating). Trauma-informed yoga is a 10-week, hour-long yoga class that incorporates breathing, postures, and meditation (Emerson & Hopper, 2011). Certified yoga professionals, with advanced degrees in psychology, created the program. The program emphasizes exploration of body sensations, self-inquiry, and subtle directional language encouraging participants to move and act when they are ready. Self-directed bodily control is emphasized as participants are asked to modify, stay in, or release a posture as they choose (Emerson & Hopper, 2011).

A recent RCT using an active control group found trauma-informed yoga to significantly reduce PTSD symptomatology, showing effect sizes comparable to those of other forms of accepted therapy (van der Kolk et al., 2014). Researchers hypothesize that yoga may improve the functioning of individuals who have been traumatized by helping them to tolerate physical and sensory experiences associated with fear and helplessness while increasing emotional awareness and affect tolerance (van der Kolk et al., 2014). There have been other yoga-based interventions addressing the dysregulating symptoms of trauma, such as the Trauma Informed Mind-Body (TIMBo) program (yogahope.org). Early research on TIMBo suggests efficacy for those struggling with trauma symptoms (Jackson, 2013). See Chapter 8 for a brief overview of TIMBo.

There is emerging evidence on the use of yoga for treatment of eating disorders (EDs; Klein & Cook-Cottone, 2013). In 2013, a systematic review was conducted exploring the current body of research (Klein & Cook-Cottone, 2013). Of the 14 articles reviewed, 40% used cross-sectional designs to examine risk and protective factors for EDs among yoga practitioners, and 60% used longitudinal designs to assess the effectiveness of yoga interventions for preventing and treating EDs. Significant effects were found in the reduction of eating-disorder-symptom correlates such as drive for thinness and body dissatisfaction. Less convincing data were found for the reduction of ED symptoms.

Notably, nearly all studies utilized dosage levels at or below two sessions per week. There is growing evidence that there may be a minimal therapeutic dosage (Cook-Cottone, 2013). Consistent with exercise science research (Martin, Church, Thompson, Earnest, & Blair, 2009) and research on traditional interventions for mental illnesses such as depression (Uebelacker et al., 2010), there may be a dosage of yoga practice below which yoga will not have a significant, measurable effect. The review suggests that dosage levels at or above two sessions per week of a duration of at least 1 hour per week were most likely to be effective (e.g., Carei, Fyfe-Johnson, Breuner, & Brown, 2010).

To illustrate, Carei et al. (2010) conducted the first RCT exploring the effectiveness of yoga in the treatment of eating disorders, finding decreases in eating disorder symptoms at week 12 and a reduction of food preoccupation immediately after yoga sessions. The treatment-as-usual group showed an initial decline in symptoms with a return to baseline at week 12. Dosage levels appear to have been sufficient. Participants in the yoga group received 1 hour of yoga twice a week for 8 consecutive weeks along with their typical treatment. Although the program did not utilize a manual, the yoga protocol was detailed, including specific statements and postures to administer to participants.

Dale and colleagues (2009) studied the effect of a 6-day yoga workshop for women with a history of eating disorders. The workshop was developed by experienced yoga instructors to help women with eating disorders develop a healthier relationship with food and their bodies. The intervention focused on three strategies: (a) yoga practice, (b) healthy eating, and (c) self-reflection and interpersonal interactions (Dale et al., 2009). Specifically, yoga practice was implemented to address the participants' physical and emotional needs through breath work, addressing of physical and emotional injuries, and development of effective tools for managing fear and struggle. Healthy eating was addressed through the provision of an interactive cooking class emphasizing organic foods and elimination of highly processed food and food with low nutritional value. Mindful eating was also practiced. Finally, self-reflection and interpersonal skills were addressed via process work such as journaling and sharing in small groups.

Following the workshop, a repeated-measures design was used to analyze the data from the small group of women ($n = 5$). Results indicated that participants showed improvements in emotional regulation and the ability to recognize and respond to emotional states, along with decreases in mood instability, anger, self-destructive behaviors, and eating disorder symptoms (Dale et al., 2009). Methodological problems include failure to utilize a control group, no randomization, and small sample size. However, findings suggest that intensive workshops may be a viable delivery and dosage option when implementing yoga as a treatment for eating disorders. More research is needed.

The attunement in mind, body, and relationships (AMBR) treatment program integrates CBT, DBT, cognitive dissonance, positive psychology, and yoga in a manualized program for the treatment of eating disorders (Cook-Cottone, Beck, & Kane, 2008). Specifically, each of the eight sessions begins with a yoga practice aligned with the content to be covered for that day. For example, in the first session breath work as a calming practice is a key aspect of the didactic lesson and group discussion. Accordingly, the yoga practice that opens the session integrates a strong focus and instruction on the breath.

Didactic sessions cover key factors associated with risk and recovery in eating disorders (Cook-Cottone et al., 2008). A CBT framework is used to deconstruct patterns of eating-disordered behavior into antecedents and triggers, behavioral response, and associated consequences. Training in distress tolerance, emotional regulation, and interpersonal effectiveness is integrated into didactic, psychoeducational sessions (see Cook-Cottone et al. [2008] and Linehan [1993] for descriptions of modules). A positive psychology framework is used to reframe conceptualizations of self as human, vulnerable, and capable. Symptoms are viewed as opportunities to learn about the self. Further, symptoms are not described within group discussions; rather, the antecedents and consequences are explored. Finally, the body is reviewed in terms of its potential to serve as a tangible representation of the self. When seen this way, the body offers a seemingly accessible, measurable object of conflict (Cook-Cottone, 2006; Cook-Cottone et al., 2008). It can be measured, weighted, judged, and controlled. The body, as object, is juxtaposed alongside life's more abstract, elusive challenges (e.g., relationships, careers, security, love, and identity). Through a combination of group discussions and activities, these concepts are explored. Alternative coping and self-care skills are taught and practiced. Each didactic and discussion session is followed by a journaling activity and systematic relaxation or a guided meditation.

In a repeated measures design, the group was found to significantly reduce drive for thinness and body dissatisfaction (two central symptoms of anorexia nervosa and bulimia nervosa), as well as show a nonsignificant reduction in bulimic symptomatology (Cook-Cottone et al., 2008). This intervention illustrates a lower dosage of yoga (i.e., one 45-minute session per week for 8 weeks) resulting in only partial impact on eating disorder symptoms. Methodological problems include failure to utilize a control group, no randomization, and low dosage of yoga. More research is needed.

The *Girls Growing in Wellness and Balance: Yoga and Life Skills to Empower* (Cook-Cottone, Kane, Keddie, & Haugli, 2013) program is the first eating disorder prevention program to use yoga as the central feature of the intervention. The protocol is experiential and didactic in nature and includes constructivist activities in which the participants create their own understanding of concepts such as assertiveness, cultural and media pressures to be thin, and intrapersonal self-regulation. Based on the Attuned Representational Model of Self (ARMS; Cook-Cottone, 2006), the program teaches self-regulation skills such as breath work and yoga asana, integration of thoughts and feelings to make choices, and self-care. Each session begins with an asana practice, includes journaling, and transitions into group sessions that explore key conceptual issues. The 14-session program concludes with the participants creating their own magazine that reflects their personal values of self-development. Each session runs 90 to 120 minutes and ends with guided relaxation or meditation.

Studies of this program show reduction in risk and eating disorder symptoms (Scime & Cook-Cottone, 2008; Scime, Cook-Cottone, Kane, & Watson, 2006). Matched controlled analysis shows that the program was equally effective for girls identified as minorities and those who were not (Cook-Cottone, Jones, & Haugli, 2010). Further, a recent study found that the group format may be most effective with girls who are more externally oriented (Norman, Sodano, & Cook-Cottone, 2014). This program was designed for middle school females. The manual provides adaptation and extension for high school females and adults. Methodical issues include lack of randomization and lower dosage of yoga (i.e., one 45-minute session per week for 12 to 14 weeks). Please see the manual for a more comprehensive review of the program (Cook-Cottone, Kane, et al., 2013).

CAUTIONS AND CONTRAINDICATIONS

"Do no harm" is the guiding principle for health care experts (Dobkin, Irving, & Amar, 2012, p. 45). However, in the field of mindful and yogic interventions guidance is limited. The current body of research lacks sufficient data on cautions and contraindications (Forfylow, 2011). It is good to start with what is known. Cohen and Schouten (2007) wisely encourage therapists to utilize interventions with research evidence in support of use. Further, when treating a mental disorder it is critical to begin treatment with conventional treatments known to effectively remediate symptoms associated with a disorder (Cohen & Schouten, 2007). The following known cautions and contraindications should be noted.

Gain informed consent and be sure the mindful and/or yogic approach that you intend to implement is acceptable to the patient. As a therapist, it is your ethical responsibility to gain informed consent before integrating any treatments with clients (Forfylow, 2011). Clients should be fully informed regarding the maturity of the specific field of research, intervention content, risk, and known benefits associated with treatments (Forfylow, 2011). This includes honesty about your own competency and training associated with implementation of the intervention (Forfylow, 2011). Secure training and supervision when needed and inform your clients of the supervision structure.

Researchers have reviewed the extant literature associated with mindfulness interventions, and some risks have been identified (e.g., Dobkin et al., 2012). As you introduce techniques to your clients, explain that on some occasions patients have experienced the side effects in the following list. Review the side effects and ask if they have any questions or concerns. As you proceed with the mindful or yogic intervention, check in with your clients intermittently to ensure that they are not experiencing side effects. If they report side effects, stop the intervention, seek consultation if needed, and return to traditional treatments known to address the patient's primary disorder as well as the side effect. For example, if a patient is working to reduce binge eating and experiences substantial anxiety with panic attacks during meditation, return to CBT and address anxiety and panic attacks through standard protocol. Known risks that should be shared with your clients include: relaxation-induced anxiety and panic, a feeling of the need to escape, paradoxical increases in tension, decreased motivation, boredom, pain and discomfort, impaired reality testing, confusion, disorientation, spaced-out feelings, depressed mood, increase in feelings of negativity, and feelings of being addicted to meditation and/or yoga (Dobkin et al., 2012). Dobkin et al. (2012) describe case reports of meditation triggering onset of bipolar disorder, mania, and meditation-induced psychosis. Many cases of substantial decompensation were associated with preexisting mental health concerns.

As you review techniques and procedures with clients, assess acceptability. Young et al. (2011) warn that counselors should seek to understand a client's cultural identity and worldview before using practices such as mindfulness and yoga with a client. Boudette (2006) suggests that clients must be accurately matched as suitable for interventions such as yoga and mindfulness. For example, patients with certain religious backgrounds simply do not see mindfulness and yoga as compatible with their beliefs. Suitability can also be related to particular symptoms (i.e., attention problems, a tendency to dissociate or depersonalize) or disorder-specific challenges. To illustrate, individuals who are severely clinically depressed can find it nearly impossible to concentrate (Dobkin et al., 2012). Young et al. (2011) state that it is essential to match the implementation of techniques to stage of recovery. For example, meditation tends to work best in the middle stages of recovery from addiction (Young et al., 2011). In early recovery, patients often experience physical withdrawal symptoms that can hinder the ability to focus and sit still, potentially hindering their initial experiences at meditation (Young et al., 2011).

Review patients' medical histories for potential physical contraindications. There is some evidence that individuals with certain preexisting medical conditions (e.g., pregnancy, high blood pressure, a tendency to hyperventilate and/or faint) should use caution when practicing yoga and should avoid certain breathing techniques that may exacerbate these conditions (Cohen & Schouten, 2007; Forfylow, 2011; Sharma, 2007). Cohen and Schouten (2007) recommend requiring patients to have a full physical exam prior to the practice of any complementary mind–body practice.

When referring your patient to mindfulness and yoga teachers who are not trained mental health professionals, do so cautiously. Verify that the individuals teaching meditation and yoga have sufficient training in mental health to handle the challenges presented by individuals struggling with self-regulation, addiction, and mood problems. Address any gaps in competency by having patients sign a release of information and co-manage clients (Forfylow, 2011). Further, Douglass (2009) recommends working with yoga teachers with advanced training. She suggests that the yoga teacher should have considerable experience in working with typical populations prior to engaging in specialization with clinical populations. Also, the agency, clinic, or therapist should provide specialized training for the yoga teacher as needed, as well as supervision relevant to the disorder being addressed. Finally, the yoga teacher should be capable of working as part of a team providing yoga as a complement to the other prescribed healing modalities used (Douglass, 2009).

Prior to engaging in or referring for mindful or yogic techniques, therapists should assess the following:

- Can the patient generally manage affect, listen and respond in the present moment, follow instructions, remain in a classroom or office during an intervention, physically practice yoga and breath work, organize thoughts and logistics, and adhere to a commitment (Dobkin et al., 2012)?
- Does the patient decompensate when his or her cognitive controls are loosened (Germer, 2005)?

- Does the patient have a history of trauma, traumatic stress, or PTSD? If so, does the patient have a tendency to dissociate, experience body arousal, or display avoidance, or have tools for negotiating these tendencies (Dobkin et al., 2012)?
- If a patient presents as cognitively reactive, can you effectively prime the patient for the challenges of initial practices, encourage short practices to build competency, and teach skills for addressing uncomfortable or disconcerting emotions as they arise (Dobkin et al., 2012)?
- Can the patient maintain sobriety for periods of sufficient length to practice the mindful or yogic techniques when sober (Dobkin et al., 2012)?
- If you are referring a patient, is the patient willing to sign a release so that you can work with the mindful or yogic practitioner as a treatment team member who is supervised?

CONCLUSIONS AND FUTURE DIRECTIONS

Overall, the current state of research in areas of mindful and yogic interventions is in its early stages, with some specific areas (e.g., MBSR, self-injury, substance use) having well-developed bodies of research and others being only in their infancy (e.g., gaming, compulsive shopping, compulsive/addictive Internet use, and gambling). Notably, particular disorders have insufficient research in both mindfulness and yoga. For example, although patients who struggle with problematic gambling find mindfulness-based approaches acceptable, and cross-sectional and case studies suggest that interventions may be helpful, there is a dearth of controlled trials and RCTs (de Lisle, Dowling, & Allen, 2011; Shonin, Van Gordon, & Griffiths, 2013; Toneatto, Vettese, & Nguyen, 2007). Much more research is needed, and continued funding and initiatives from the National Center for Complementary and Alternative Medicine (NCCAM; nccam.nih.gov) is necessary for the field to continue to move forward. Overall, integration of mindful and yogic interventions into clinical practice can be cautiously informed by the current body of research. As the rate of publications in this area is rapidly increasing, therapists are encouraged to stay informed. Research concerns and limitations as well as recommendations for future research are detailed here.

More rigorous research, particularly on yoga interventions (i.e., RCTs), needs to be conducted (Forfylow, 2011). Other standard quality-of-research issues are not yet addressed in much of the mindful and yoga research. For example, more research is needed with extended follow-up assessments (McIver et al., 2009). Many studies use self-report measures, with little use of performance measures (Keng et al., 2011). Moreover, research in mindfulness and yoga needs to expand across ethnicity, age, sex, levels of experience, and ranges of disorder-specific symptoms in order to provide a sufficient body of evidence that can be generalized to particular groups of individuals (Forfylow, 2011). Further, studies with larger sample sizes are needed (Hallgren et al., 2014).

Dosage is a key variable that has not been effectively addressed in mindful or yoga research (e.g., Cook-Cottone, 2013). Strongly considered in other fields (e.g., pharmacology), standardized dosages are essentially missing from mindful and yogic research. Specifically, frequency, duration, session length, and content of sessions should be detailed and accounted for (Cook-Cottone, 2013). Relatedly, few studies measure whether or not the treatment or control group members practice meditation, yoga, or breath work at home or outside of the scope of the study intervention (Cook-Cottone, 2013). Few studies report a content-specific treatment integrity percentage (e.g., Were all the breath work activities completed during the session? Were all of the prescribed yoga postures implemented?; Cook-Cottone, 2013). Further, few studies assess engagement in other confounding physical activities, an important potentially confounding variable (Cook-Cottone, 2013). For example, did the control participants engage in mindful walking or attend a Tai Kwon Do class?

Finally, the content of interventions must be better detailed. This is especially salient within the context of yogic interventions. Specifically, the type of yoga, aspect of yoga, and amount of each type and aspect of yoga should be detailed and evaluated for efficacy (Cook-Cottone, 2013; Forfylow, 2011). There is some evidence that the type of yoga utilized may matter (Delaney & Anthis, 2010). Researchers should study the use of mindful and yogic approaches as complementary to therapy and when integrated into traditional therapy (Forfylow, 2011). Outside of standardized protocols and manualized methods, how are mindful and yogic approaches being integrated?

As our popular culture embraces alternative approaches such as yoga and mindfulness, it is critical for the scientific community to continue to carefully evaluate effectiveness, honoring both the scientific method as well as the roots and authenticity of these ancient practices. The deconstruction of mindfulness and yoga in service of empirical exploration must be addressed (Forfylow, 2011). There is adequate space within the field of mindfulness and yoga interventions for the practice of traditions, as well as the modification, standardization, and application of these powerful methods for use in the field of mental health. Further, it is in the innovation that we may find efficacy, such as the integration of compassion into work with self-injury (i.e., compassion-focused approaches to self-injury; Van Vliet & Kalnins, 2011). There are at least two truths at play. First, using tools such as the scientific method is necessary within the current cultural zeitgeist. Second, use of qualitative methods and other tools that allow for practices such as mindfulness and yoga to be explored exactly as they are occurring naturalistically is also critical. It is a dialectic. Perhaps it is in the simultaneous embracing of tradition and change that we will find the effectiveness we seek.

REFERENCES

Astrachan-Fletcher, E., & Maslar, M. (2009). *The dialectic behavioral therapy skills workbook for bulimia: Using DBT to break control of the cycle and regain control of your life.* Oakland, CA: New Harbinger Press.

Baer, R. A. (2006). *Mindfulness-based treatment approaches: A clinician's guide to evidence base and applications.* New York, NY: Academic Press.

Baer, R. A., & Krietemeyer, J. (2006). Overview of mindfulness- and acceptance-based treatment approaches. In R. A. Baer (Ed.), *Mindfulness-based treatment approaches: A clinician's guide to evidence base and applications* (pp. 3–30). New York, NY: Academic Press.

Black, D. S. (2014). Mindfulness-based interventions: An antidote to suffering in the context of substance use, misuse, and addiction. *Substance Use & Misuse, 49,* 487–491.

Boudette, R. (2006). Question & answer: Yoga in the treatment of disordered eating and body image disturbance: How can the practice of yoga be helpful in recovery from an eating disorder? *Eating Disorders, 14,* 167–170.

Carei, T., Fyfe-Johnson, A. L., Breuner, C. C., & Brown, M. A. (2010). Randomized controlled clinical trial of yoga in the treatment of eating disorders. *Journal of Adolescent Health, 46,* 346–351.

Cohen, M. H., & Schouten, R. (2007). Legal, regulatory, and ethic issues. In J. Lake & D. Spiegel (Eds.), *Complementary and alternative treatments in mental health care* (pp. 21–33). Arlington, VA: American Psychiatric Association.

Cook-Cottone, C. (2006). The attuned representation model for the primary prevention of eating disorders: An overview for school psychologists. *Psychology in the Schools, 43,* 223–230.

Cook-Cottone, C. (2013). Dosage as a critical variable in yoga therapy research. *International Journal of Yoga Therapy, 2,* 11–12.

Cook-Cottone, C., Beck, M., & Kane, L. (2008). Manualized-group treatment of eating disorders: Attunement in mind, body, and relationship (AMBR). *The Journal for Specialists in Group Work, 33*(1), 61–83.

Cook-Cottone, C., Jones, L. A., & Haugli, S. (2010). Prevention of eating disorders among minority youth: A matched-sample repeated measures study. *Eating Disorders, 18,* 361–376.

Cook-Cottone, C. P., Kane, L., Keddie, E., & Haugli, S. (2013). *Girls growing in wellness and balance: Yoga and life skills to empower.* Stoddard, WI: Schoolhouse Educational Services.

Cook-Cottone, C. P., Tribole, E., & Tylka, T. L. (2013). *Healthy eating in schools: Evidence-based interventions to help kids thrive.* Washington, DC: American Psychological Association.

Dale, L. P., Mattison, A. M., Greening, K., Galen, G., Neace, W. P., & Matacin, M. L. (2009). Yoga workshop impacts psychological functioning and mood of women with self-reported history of eating disorders. *Eating Disorders, 17,* 422–434.

Davis, M., Eschelman, E. R., & McKay, M. (2008). *The relaxation and stress reduction workbook* (6th ed.). Oakland, CA: New Harbinger Publications.

de Lisle, S. M., Dowling, N. A., & Allen, J. S. (2011). Mindfulness-based cognitive therapy for problem gambling. *Clinical Case Studies.* doi: 1534650111401016

Delaney, K., & Anthis, K. (2010). Is women's participation in different types of yoga classes associated with different levels of body awareness satisfaction? *International Journal of Yoga Therapy, 1*, 62–71.

Dobkin, P. L., Irving, J. A., & Amar, S. (2012). For whom may participation in a mindfulness-based stress reduction program be contraindicated? *Mindfulness, 3*, 44–50.

Douglass, L. (2009). Yoga as an intervention in the treatment of eating disorders: Does it help? *Eating Disorders, 17*, 126–139.

Emerson, D., & Hopper, E. (2011). *Overcoming trauma through yoga.* Berkeley, CA: North Atlantic Press.

Forfylow, A. L. (2011). Integrating yoga with psychotherapy: A complementary treatment for anxiety and depression. *Canadian Journal of Counseling and Psychotherapy, 45*, 132–150.

Froeliger, B. E., Garland, E. L., Modlin, L. A., & McClemon, J. (2012). Neurocognitive correlates of the effects of yoga meditation practice on emotion and cognition: A pilot study. *Frontiers in Integrative Neuroscience, 6*, 1–11.

Germer, C. K. (2005). Teaching mindfulness in therapy. In C. K. Germer, R. D. Siegel, & P. R. Fulton (Eds.), *Mindfulness and psychotherapy* (pp. 113–129). New York, NY: Guilford Press.

Germer, C. K., & Siegel, R. D. (Eds.). (2012). *Wisdom and compassion in psychotherapy: Deepening mindfulness in clinical practice.* New York, NY: Guilford Press.

Grabovac, A. D., Lau, M. A., & Willett, B. R. (2011). Mechanisms of mindfulness: A Buddhist Psychological Model. *Mindfulness, 2*, 154–166.

Greco, L., & Hayes, S. C. (2008). *Acceptance and mindfulness treatments for children and adolescents: A practitioner's guide.* Oakland, CA: New Harbinger Publications.

Hallgren, M., Romberg, K., Bakish, A., & Andreasson, S. (2014). Yoga as an adjunct treatment for alcohol dependence: A pilot study. *Complementary Therapies in Medicine, 22*, 441–445.

Hayes, S. C., & Levin M. (2012). *Mindfulness and acceptance for addictive behaviors: Applying contextual CBT to substance abuse and behavioral addictions.* Oakland, CA: New Harbinger Publications.

Hofmann, S. G., Sawyer, A. T., & Fang, A. (2010). The empirical status of the "new wave" of CBT. *The Psychiatric Clinics of North America, 33*, 701.

Jackson, E. (2013, November). *Resilience from trauma: Examination of a gender-responsive trauma-informed mind–body program in Haiti.* Presentation at 141st APHA Annual Meeting, November 2–November 6, 2013.

Kabat-Zinn, J. (2013). *Full catastrophe living: Using the wisdom of your body and mind to face stress, pain, and illness.* New York, NY: Bantam Books.

Keng, S. L., Smoski, M. J., & Robins, C. J. (2011). Effects of mindfulness on psychological health: A review of empirical studies. *Clinical Psychology Review, 31*, 1041–1056.

Khalsa, S. B. S. (2004). Yoga as a therapeutic intervention: A bibliometric analysis of published research studies. *Indian Journal of Physiology and Pharmacology, 48*, 269–285.

Khanna, S., & Greeson, J. M. (2013). A narrative review of yoga and mindfulness as complementary therapies. *Complementary Therapies in Medicine, 21*, 244–252.

Klein, J., & Cook-Cottone, C. (2013). The effects of yoga on eating disorder symptoms and correlates: A review. *International Journal of Yoga Therapy, 2*, 41–50.

Kristeller, J. L., & Wolever, R. Q. (2010). Mindfulness-based eating awareness training for treating binge eating disorder: The conceptual foundation. *Eating Disorders, 19,* 49–61.

Kristeller, J., Wolever, R. Q., & Sheets, V. (2014). Mindfulness-based eating awareness training (MB-EAT) for binge eating: A randomized clinical trial. *Mindfulness, 5,* 282–297.

Levin, M. E., & Hayes, S. C. (2012). Contextual cognitive behavioral therapies for addictive behaviors. In S. C. Hayes & M. E. Levin (Eds.), *Mindfulness and acceptance for addictive behaviors: Applying contextual CBT to substance abuse and behavioral addictions* (pp. 1–26). Oakland, CA: New Harbinger Publications.

Linehan, M. (1993). *Skills training manual for treating borderline personality disorder.* New York, NY: Guilford Press.

Marlatt, G. A., Bowen, S., & Lustyk, M. K. B. (2012) Substance abuse and relapse prevention. In C. K. Germer & R. D. Siegel (Eds.), *Wisdom and compassion in psychotherapy: Deepening mindfulness in clinical practice* (pp. 221–233). New York, NY: Guilford Press.

Martin, C. K., Church, T. S., Thompson, A. M., Earnest, C. P., & Blair, S. N. (2009). Exercise dose and quality of life. *Archives of Internal Medicine, 3,* 269–278.

McCall, M. C. (2014). In search of yoga: Research trends in a Western medical database. *International Journal of Yoga, 7,* 4–8.

McIver, S., O'Halloran, P., & McGartland, M. (2009). Yoga as a treatment for binge eating disorder: A preliminary study. *Complementary Therapies in Medicine, 17,* 196–202.

Norman, K., Sodano, S. M., & Cook-Cottone, C. (2014). An exploratory analysis of the role of interpersonal styles in eating disorder prevention outcomes. *The Journal for Specialists in Group Work, 39*(4), 301–315.

Scime, M., & Cook-Cottone, C. (2008). Primary prevention of eating disorders: A constructivist integration of mind and body strategies. *International Journal of Eating Disorders, 41,* 134–142.

Scime, M., Cook-Cottone, C., Kane, L., & Watson, T. (2006). Group prevention of eating disorders with fifth-grade females: Impact on body dissatisfaction, drive for thinness, and media influence. *Eating Disorders, 14,* 143–155.

Shapiro, S. L., & Carlson, L. E. (2009). *The art and science of mindfulness: Integrating mindfulness into psychology and the helping professions.* Washington, DC: American Psychological Association.

Sharma, V. P. (2007). Yoga therapy in practice: Pranayama can be practiced safely. *International Journal of Yoga Therapy, 17,* 75–79.

Shonin, E., Von Gordon, W., & Griffiths, M. D. (2013). Buddhist philosophy of the treatment of problem gambling. *Journal of Behavioral Addictions, 2,* 63–71.

Siegel, D. J. (2010). *The mindful therapist: A clinician's guide to mindsight and neural integration.* New York: NY: W. W. Norton.

Simpkins, A. M., & Simpkins, C. A. (2011). *Meditation and yoga in psychotherapy: Techniques for clinical practice.* New York, NY: John Wiley & Sons.

Toneatto, T., Vettese, L., & Nguyen, L. (2007). The role of mindfulness in the cognitive-behavioural treatment of problem gambling. *Journal of Gambling Issues,* Issue 19, 91–100.

Uebelacker, L., Epstein-Lubow, G., Gaudiano, B. A., Tremont, G., Battle, C. L., & Miller, I. W. (2010). Hatha yoga for depression: Critical review of the evidence for efficacy, plausible mechanism of action, and directions for future research. *Journal of Psychiatric Practice, 16,* 22–33.

van der Kolk, B. A., Stone, L., West, J., Rhodes, A., Emerson, D., Suvak, M., & Spinazzola, J. (2014). Yoga as an adjunctive treatment for posttraumatic stress disorder: A randomized controlled trial. *Journal of Clinical Psychiatry, 75*, e1–e7.

van Goethem, A., Mulders, D., Muris, M., Arntz, A., & Egger, J. (2012). Reduction of self-injury and improvement of coping behavior during dialectic behavioral therapy (DBT) of patients with borderline personality disorders. *International Journal of Psychology and Psychological Therapy, 12*, 21–34.

Van Vliet, J. K., & Kalnins, G. R. C. (2011). A compassion focused approach to self-injury. *Journal of Mental Health Counseling, 33*, 295–311.

Wanden-Berghe, R., G., Sanz-Valero, J., & Wanden-Berghe, C. (2010). The application of mindfulness to eating disorder treatment: A systematic review. *Eating Disorders: The Journal of Treatment Prevention, 19*, 24–48.

Wilson, K. G., Schnetzer, L., W., Flynn, M. K., & Kurz, A. S. (2012). Acceptance and commitment therapy for addiction. In S. C. Hayes & M. E. Leven (Eds.), *Mindfulness and acceptance for addictive behaviors: Applying contextual CBT to substance abuse and behavioral addictions* (pp. 27–68). Oakland, CA: New Harbinger Publications.

Witkiewitz, K., Bowen, S., Douglas, H., & Hsu, S. H. (2013). Mindfulness-based relapse prevention for substance craving. *Addictive Behaviors, 38*, 1563–1571.

Witkiewitz, K., Marlatt, G., & Walker, D. (2005). Mindfulness-based relapse prevention for alcohol and substance use disorders. *Journal of Cognitive Psychotherapy: An International Quarterly, 19*, 211–228.

Woodyard, C. (2011). Exploring the therapeutic effects of yoga and its ability to increase quality of life. *International Journal of Yoga, 4*, 49–54.

Young, M. E., DeLorenzi, L., & Cunningham, L. (2011). Using meditation in addiction counseling. *Journal of Addictions & Offender Counseling, 32*, 58–71.

Zhuang, S., An, S., & Zhao, Y. (2013). Yoga effects on mood and quality of life in Chinese women undergoing heroin detoxification. *Nursing Research, 62*, 260–268.

Mindful Self-Care

*Self-care is a personal challenge and professional imperative
that every psychotherapist—literally, everyone—must consciously
confront.*—NORCROSS AND GUY (2007, p. ix)

MINDFUL SELF-CARE AND SELF-REGULATION

At their core, mindfulness and yogic approaches are pathways to self-care. Self-care, as a contemporary practice, is defined as the daily process of being aware of and attending to one's basic physiological and emotional needs, including the shaping of one's daily routine, relationships, and environment as needed to promote self-care (Norcross & Guy, 2007). Self-care is seen as the foundational work required for physical and emotional well-being. Self-care is associated with positive physical health, emotional well-being, and mental health. Steady and intentional practice of mindful self-care is seen as protective by preventing the onset of mental health symptoms, preventing job/school burnout, and improving work and school productivity (Figure 12.1).

It is as important for the clinician to engage in self-care as it is for the patient (Norcross & Guy, 2007; Sayrs, 2012; Shapiro & Carlson, 2009; Siegel, 2010). Siegel (2010) emphasizes the significance of attending to the development of your own inner life in order to do your job well. He describes doing your job well as bringing a healthy and positive presence to your work in addition to bringing resilience to your life (Siegel, 2010). Consider that you cannot give what you do not have. As a therapist, presenting as overworked, exhausted, depleted, and overly self-sacrificing, even if not spoken, does not inspire. Siegel (2010) says it this way,

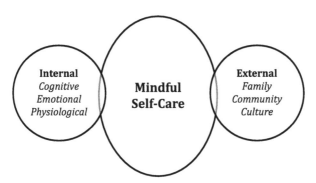

FIGURE 12.1 Mindful self-care.

"Caring for your self, bringing support and healing to your own efforts to help others and the larger world in which we live, is an essential daily practice—not a luxury, not some form of self-indulgence" (p. 3).

I first developed the self-care scale for use with a yoga-based eating disorder prevention program (Cook-Cottone, Kane, Keddie, & Haugli, 2013). The initial version of the scale addressed nutrition, hydration, exercise, soothing, rest, and medicines/vitamins. Appropriate for use with children of middle school age and above, the scale assesses children's self-care behaviors, including eating healthy foods in moderation, drinking enough water, exercising for at least 1 hour a day and not to excess, engaging in relaxation and rest behaviors throughout the day, and taking medicines prescribed and not taking those that are not (e.g., alcohol). Like the Mindful Self-Care Scale (MSCS), the children's self-care scale allows for an assessment of self-care behaviors across domains. As I worked with patients in private practice, the need for a psychometrically sound self-care scale aligned with mindful and yogic principles became increasingly clear.

Self-care practice is self-regulating (Figure 12.2; Cook-Cottone, Tribole, & Tylka, 2013). Self-care, mindful, and yogic practices can provide a foundation for self-regulation. Ironically, many people say that they will take better care of themselves and do healthy things like yoga and mindfulness once they feel better emotionally. I challenge patients to engage in self-care, yoga, and mindfulness practice as a foundation for feeling better (Cook-Cottone, Tribole, et al., 2013). I explain that emotional regulation is inextricably linked to physiological stability and homeostasis (Cook-Cottone, Tribole, et al., 2013). It can be helpful to remind patients that daily self-care practices can enhance physiological stability and support emotional regulation (Linehan, 1993).

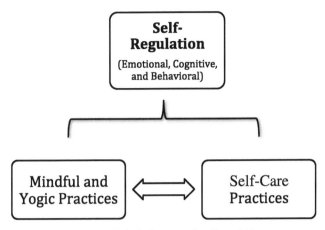

FIGURE 12.2 Self-care and self-regulation.

Mindful self-care goes beyond a basic assessment of and engagement in self-care behaviors. It is the integration of the practice of mindful awareness and self-care. Mindful self-care is a critical aspect of embodied self-regulation designed to help both patients and therapists negotiate personal needs and challenges and external demands (see Figure 12.1 and the discussion in Chapter 3 of embodied practice 8, prioritize self-care). Essentially, self-care practices are rooted in both mindfulness and yoga (e.g., yamas and niyamas; see Chapter 10). Mindful self-care begins with self-awareness and self-monitoring (Norcross & Guy, 2007).

The Mindful Self-Care Scale (MSCS) is an 84-item scale that measures the self-reported frequency of self-care behaviors. This scale is intended to help individuals identify areas of strength and weakness in self-care behavior as well as assess interventions that serve to improve self-care. The scale addresses 10 domains of self-care: nutrition/hydration, exercise, soothing strategies, self-awareness/mindfulness, rest, relationships, physical and medical practices, environmental factors, self-compassion, and spiritual practices (Figure 12.3). There are also three general items assessing the individual's general or more global practices of self-care. Research is currently being conducted on this specific self-care scale to evaluate psychometric properties and association of the scale with self-regulation. See gse.buffalo.edu/about/directory/faculty/cook-cottone for a version of the scale with formatting instructions and updates of research outcomes.

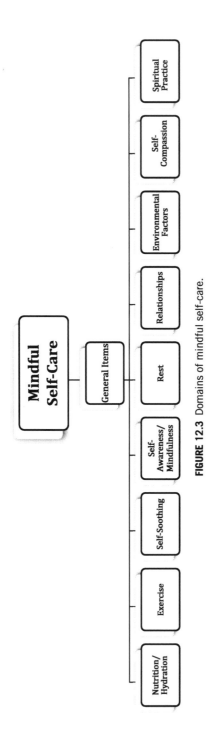

FIGURE 12.3 Domains of mindful self-care.

MINDFUL SELF-CARE: HOW TO USE THIS CHAPTER

Mindful self-care progress involves four steps: (a) mindful awareness of self-care as essential to well-being, (b) assessment of self-care domains, (c) assessment-driven self-care goal setting, and (d) engagement in self-care behaviors (Figure 12.4). The four steps are discrete phases of an ongoing process, a continuous mindful awareness of one's own self-care behaviors, continual assessment, and goal setting. As the Sanskrit term *smriti* (i.e., to recollect, to remember) conceptualizes, mindful self-care is a process of constant remembering. Both therapists and patients get pulled away from their own self-care by external contingencies and the needs of others (see Figure 12.1). Accordingly, mindful self-care involves a remembering of the self, a remembering to nurture the self.

This chapter is organized domain by domain in order to facilitate a mindful and intentional review of personal self-care. Each domain is defined and domain-specific questions follow. Whether you are working with a patient or exploring your own self-care, work through the chapter one domain at a time. Read the definition and then carefully answer the questions. The directions for scoring follow each set of questions. Please note that some questions are reversed scored. Once the domain is scored, average the scores across the domain. Averages of 0 to 2 in a domain suggest that this area of self-care is an area that can be targeted for improvement. The specific items are prescriptive in nature. For example, if your patient is not hydrating adequately, the item "I drank 6 to 8 glasses of water" can be easily translated to a goal, "I will drink 6 to 8 glasses of water each day."

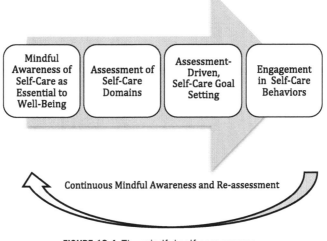

FIGURE 12.4 The mindful self-care process.

TABLE 12.1   Self-Care General Items*

- I engaged in a variety of self-care strategies (e.g., mindfulness, support, exercise, nutrition, spiritual practice).

- I planned my self-care.

- I explored new ways to bring self-care into my life.

---

*Ask yourself, "This past week, how many days did I do the following?" You can give yourself the following scores: 0 = *never* (0 days), 1 = *rarely* (1 day), 2 = *sometimes* (2 to 3 days), 3 = *often* (3 to 5) days, and 4 = *regularly* (6 to 7 days). Your score for this section can range from 0 to 12.

General (G)

The general (G) self-care items (Table 12.1) were designed to provide a broad sense of the variety of self-care strategies utilized, planning of self-care, and creativity and exploration of self-care. Norcross and Guy (2007) warn that there is no single self-care strategy that alone can help you or your patient manifest well-being. Further, for some individuals, one beloved hobby or leisure pursuit can be more effective than working to engage in a variety of self-care strategies (Norcross & Guy, 2007).

Nutrition and Hydration (NH)

Norcross and Guy (2007) identify nutrition and hydration as critical aspects of self-care. A healthy body responds to the unavoidable stress in life better than an unhealthy body (Davis, Eshelman, & McKay, 2008). Addressing basic nutritional needs can deeply affect self-regulation. This includes eating a healthy amount of healthy foods and engaging in the planning needed to make that happen. Issues such as drops in sugar levels, insufficient or excessive energy intake, and nutrient deficits (i.e., low iron intake, low vitamin D and B_{12} levels) have all been identified in variations in mood and sense of well-being and can be dysregulating. Stabilizing nutritional intake can reduce cravings and bolster resiliency in resisting triggers. For example, a careful analysis of when a patient was having anxiety issues and associated desire to use substances revealed that when she skipped meals or ate insufficient protein, she experienced anxiety. By stabilizing her nutritional intake across the day and adding higher-protein snacks, her anxiety issues completely abated, as did her associated urges to use. See *American Dietetic Association Complete Food and Nutrition Guide* (Duyff, 2011) and *The Relaxation and Stress Reduction Workbook,* 6th edition (Davis et al., 2008) for nutritional guidelines and tools for enhancing nutrition.

It is well accepted that water is essential for life, and maintaining recommended levels of hydration is critical to healthy functioning (i.e.,

TABLE 12.2 Self-Care Nutrition/Hydration Items*

- I drank at least 6 to 8 glasses of water.

- Even though my stomach felt full enough, I kept eating (reverse score).

- I adjusted my water intake when I needed to (e.g., for exercise, hot weather).

- I skipped a meal (reverse score).

- I ate breakfast, lunch, dinner, and, when needed, snacks.

- I ate a variety of nutritious foods (e.g., vegetables, protein, fruits, and grains).

- I planned my meals and snacks.

*Ask yourself, "This past week how many days did I do the following?" You can give yourself the following scores: 0 = *never* (0 days), 1 = *rarely* (1 day), 2 = *sometimes* (2 to 3 days), 3 = *often* (3 to 5) days, and 4 = *regularly* (6 to 7 days). For the items that state "reverse score" score as: 4 = *never* (0 days), 3 = *rarely* (1 day), 2 = *sometimes* (2 to 3 days), 1 = *often* (3 to 5) days, and 0 = *regularly* (6 to 7 days). Your score for this section can range from 0 to 28.

1.2 liters per day [about 6–8 glasses]; Benelam & Wyness, 2010). If water losses are not replaced, dehydration occurs (Benelam & Wyness, 2010). At extreme levels, dehydration is very serious and can be fatal. Mild dehydration (i.e., 2% loss of body weight) can result in headaches, fatigue, and reduced physical and mental performance, and too much water can result in hyponatremia (low levels of sodium in the blood; Benelam & Wyness, 2010). The items in Table 12.2 can give you and your patients a sense of basic nutrition and hydration self-care practices.

Exercise (E)

Review of the literature indicates that the association between exercise and well-being has been well documented (Norcross & Guy, 2007). Exercise reduces stress by releasing endorphins into the bloodstream, decreasing muscle tension and increasing alpha-wave activity; improves strength and flexibility; lessens fatigue; increases resting metabolism; rids your body of toxins; improves blood flow to the brain; and reduces risk for those with stress-related medical conditions (Davis et al., 2008). Further, you learn lessons on your mat, in your running shoes, and at the gym that you can apply to your life (e.g., persistence pays off; Davis et al., 2008). The beneficial effects of regular exercise include improvements in measures of cognition and psychological well-being in healthy individuals (Hopkins, Davis, VanTieghem, Whalen, & Bucci, 2012). The items in Table 12.3 address planning, duration, frequency, and quality of exercise as well as the amount of sedentary activity present. Assessment can aid in the development of specific physical activity goals.

TABLE 12.3 Self-Care Exercise Items*

- I exercised at least 30 to 60 minutes.

- I took part in sports, dance, or other scheduled physical activities (e.g., sports teams, dance classes).

- I did sedentary activities instead of exercising (e.g., watched TV, used the computer) (reverse score).

- I sat for periods of longer than 60 minutes at a time (reverse score).

- I did fun physical activities (e.g., danced, played active games, jumped in leaves).

- I exercised in excess (e.g., when I was tired, sleep deprived, or risking stress/injury) (reverse score).

- I planned/scheduled my exercise for the day.

*Ask yourself, "This past week how many days did I do the following?" You can give yourself the following scores: 0 = *never* (0 days), 1 = *rarely* (1 day), 2 = *sometimes* (2 to 3 days), 3 = *often* (3 to 5) days, and 4 = *regularly* (6 to 7 days). For the items that state "reverse score" score as: 4 = *never* (0 days), 3 = *rarely* (1 day), 2 = *sometimes* (2 to 3 days), 1 = *often* (3 to 5) days, and 0 = *regularly* (6 to 7 days). Your score for this section can range from 0 to 28.

Self-Soothing (S)

Self-soothing is an effective tool in emotional regulation (Linehan, 1993). Self-soothing is a positive, healthy response to feeling stress, distress, or an intense emotional reaction. Self-soothing includes relaxation techniques, deep breathing, and pursuit of stimuli or activities that are calming and relaxing. There are many other ways to self-sooth. For example, reading, writing, and cultivating sensory awareness are all effective forms of self-soothing (Davis et al., 2008; Norcross & Guy, 2007). Self-soothing can be in response to a trigger and planned as a preventive tool (Davis et al., 2008; Norcross & Guy, 2007). The items in Table 12.4 assess a wide range of self-soothing behaviors.

Self-Awareness/Mindfulness (SA)

Self-awareness and mindfulness are fundamental and unique features of mindful self-care. These self-care practices include formal and informal mindful and yogic practices (e.g., mindful awareness, yoga practice, and meditation). Well-reviewed and detailed throughout this text, self-awareness, one-mindedness, and active practices such as meditation and yoga are emphasized in several items in Table 12.5, as they are increasingly acknowledged for their effectiveness as self-care practices (Linehan, 1993; Norcross & Guy, 2007; Sayrs, 2012; Shapiro & Carlson, 2009).

TABLE 12.4 Self-Care Self-Soothing Items*

- I used deep breathing to relax.
- I did *not* know how to relax (reverse score).
- I thought about calming things (e.g., nature, happy memories).
- When I got stressed, I stayed stressed for hours (i.e., I couldn't calm down) (reverse score).
- I did something physical to help me relax (e.g., taking a bath, yoga, going for a walk).
- I did something intellectual (using my mind) to help me relax (e.g., read a book, wrote).
- I did something interpersonal to relax (e.g., connected with friends).
- I did something creative to relax (e.g., drew, played instrument, wrote creatively, sang, organized).
- I listened to relax (e.g., to music, a podcast, radio show, rainforest sounds).
- I sought out images to relax (e.g., art, film, window shopping, nature).
- I sought out smells to relax (e.g., lotions, nature, candles/incense, smells of baking).
- I sought out tactile or touch-based experiences to relax (e.g., pet an animal, cuddled a soft blanket, floated in a pool, put on comfy clothes).
- I prioritized activities that help me relax.

---

*Ask yourself, "This past week how many days did I do the following?" You can give yourself the following scores: 0 = *never* (0 days), 1 = *rarely* (1 day), 2 = *sometimes* (2 to 3 days), 3 = *often* (3 to 5) days, and 4 = *regularly* (6 to 7 days). For the items that state "reverse score" score as: 4 = *never* (0 days), 3 = *rarely* (1 day), 2 = *sometimes* (2 to 3 days), 1 = *often* (3 to 5) days, and 0 = *regularly* (6 to 7 days). Your score for this section can range from 0 to 52.

TABLE 12.5 Self-Care Self-Awareness/Mindfulness Items*

- I had a calm awareness of my thoughts.
- I had a calm awareness of my feelings.
- I had a calm awareness of my body.
- I carefully selected which of my thoughts and feelings I used to guide my actions.
- I meditated in some form (e.g., sitting meditation, walking meditation, prayer).
- I practiced mindful eating (i.e., paid attention to the taste and texture of the food, ate without distraction).
- I practiced yoga or another mind/body practice (e.g., Tae Kwon Do, Tai Chi).
- I tracked/recorded my self-care practices (e.g., journaling, used an app, kept a calendar).
- I planned/scheduled meditation and/or a mindful practice for the day (e.g., yoga, walking meditation, prayer).
- I took time to acknowledge the things for which I am grateful.

---

*Ask yourself, "This past week how many days did I do the following?" You can give yourself the following scores: 0 = *never* (0 days), 1 = *rarely* (1 day), 2 = *sometimes* (2 to 3 days), 3 = *often* (3 to 5) days, and 4 = *regularly* (6 to 7 days). Your score for this section can range from 0 to 40.

Rest (R)

The rest domain of self-care includes getting enough sleep, taking restful breaks, and planning time to rest and restore into your schedule. First, sleep is a critical aspect of self-care for both patients and mental health professionals. The National Sleep Foundation recommends 7 to 9 hours of sleep for adults per day (sleepfoundation.org). Lack of sleep and too much sleep are associated with negative outcomes. Both short and long duration of sleep are predictors, or markers, of cardiovascular outcomes (Cappuccio, Cooper, D'Elia, Strazzullo, & Miller, 2011). Researchers have noted cognitive effects of sleep deprivation (i.e., speed and accuracy; Lim & Dinges, 2010). Further, review of the literature suggests that insomnia impacts on diverse areas of health-related quality of life (Kyle, Morgan, & Espie, 2010). See the National Sleep Foundation for tips on addressing problems with sleep and ways to induce and maintain sleep (sleepfoundation.org).

Next, rest involves taking breaks from the current activity (Norcross & Guy, 2007). This can look very different depending on what you or your patients are doing. For example, rest for someone who is sitting all day might take the form of a brief walk throughout the building. Rest for someone who works on a computer all day would involve taking breaks from screen time. Rest for someone who is teaching yoga all day might be taking time to sit and have some green tea. Taking a break from electronics is relevant to nearly everyone. Sayrs (2012) highlights the importance of creating an enjoyable life outside of work.

Planned breaks and relaxation are vital (Norcross & Guy, 2007). Although seemingly counterproductive, breaks can actually create more time and energy (Norcross & Guy, 2007). Breaks and relaxation can be days off, lengthier vacations, as well as short 5- to 10-minute breaks away from work, the computer, or interpersonal interactions (Norcross & Guy, 2007). Taking breaks is consistent with the embodied practice 11, maintain equanimity (see Chapter 3). Sleep, rest, and taking breaks are all addressed in the items in Table 12.6.

Relationships (RR)

Supportive relationships enhance well-being (Norcross & Guy, 2007). Being mindful of the nature of the relationships that you are in is a critical aspect of mindful self-care. Norcross and Guy (2007) identify a range of potentially nurturing relationships: colleagues, staff, supervisors, peer support groups, clinical teams, community professionals, friends, spouse/partner, family, employee assistance professionals,

TABLE 12.6   Self-Care Rest Items*

- I got enough sleep to feel rested and restored when I woke up.
- I planned restful/rejuvenating breaks throughout the day.
- I rested when I needed to (e.g., when not feeling well, after a long workout or effort).
- I took planned breaks from school or work.
- I planned/scheduled pleasant activities that were not work or school related.
- I took time away from electronics (e.g., turned off phone and other devices).
- I made time in my schedule for enough sleep.

*Ask yourself, "This past week how many days did I do the following?" You can give yourself the following scores: 0 = *never* (0 days), 1 = *rarely* (1 day), 2 = *sometimes* (2 to 3 days), 3 = *often* (3 to 5) days, and 4 = *regularly* (6 to 7 days). Your score for this section can range from 0 to 28.

and consultants. The supportive aspects of relational self-care are operationalized in the following items in Table 12.7: "I felt supported by people in my life," "I made time for people who sustain and support me," and " I feel like I had someone who would listen to me if I became upset." For a therapist, this can include undergoing your own personal therapy and/or securing a mentor or supervision (Norcross & Guy, 2007).

An important aspect of healthy relationships is appropriate boundaries (Norcross & Guy, 2007; Sayrs, 2012). In relationships, a boundary "denotes maintenance of a distinction between self and other—what is within bounds and what is out of bounds" (Norcross & Guy, 2007, p. 93). In their review of the literature, Norcross and Guy (2007) concluded that setting boundaries was the most frequently used and highly effective self-care strategy among therapists. Norcross and Guy (2007) recommend that relationship boundaries (e.g., therapist and patient, spouse and spouse, partner and partner) be clear and flexible. The self-care process of setting boundaries is operationalized in the following items in Table 12.7: "I felt confident that people in my life would respect my choice if I said 'no,'" and "I knew that, if I needed to, I could stand up for myself in my relationships."

Physical and Medical (PM)

The physical and medical domain of self-care addresses the medical care and keeping of the body. The items in Table 12.8 speak to maintenance of medical and dental care, practicing daily hygiene, adherence to medical advice (e.g., taking prescribed medicines or vitamins and brushing teeth), and avoiding substance abuse. Despite cultural messages to the

TABLE 12.7   Self-Care Relationship Items*

- I spent time with people who are good to me (e.g., support, encourage, and believe in me).
- I scheduled/planned time to be with people who are special to me.
- I felt supported by people in my life.
- I felt confident that people in my life would respect my choice if I said "no."
- I knew that, if I needed to, I could stand up for myself in my relationships.
- I made time for people who sustain and support me.
- I felt that I had someone who would listen to me if I became upset (e.g., friend, counselor, group).

*Ask yourself, "This past week how many days did I do the following?" You can give yourself the following scores: 0 = *never* (0 days), 1 = *rarely* (1 day), 2 = *sometimes* (2 to 3 days), 3 = *often* (3 to 5) days, and 4 = *regularly* (6 to 7 days). Your score for this section can range from 0 to 28.

TABLE 12.8   Self-Care Physical and Medical Items*

- I engaged in medical care to prevent/treat illness and disease (e.g., attended doctor visits, took prescribed medications/vitamins, was up to date on screenings/immunizations, followed doctor recommendations).
- I engaged in dental care to prevent/treat illness and disease (e.g., dental visits, tooth brushing, flossing).
- I took/did recreational drugs (reverse score).
- I did *not* drink alcohol.
- I practiced overall cleanliness and hygiene.
- I accessed the medical/dental care I needed.
- I did not smoke.
- I did not drink alcohol in excess (i.e., more than 1 to 2 drinks [*1 drink = 12 ounces beer, 5 ounces wine, or 1.5 ounces liquor*]).

*Ask yourself, "This past week how many days did I do the following?" You can give yourself the following scores: 0 = *never* (0 days), 1 = *rarely* (1 day), 2 = *sometimes* (2 to 3 days), 3 = *often* (3 to 5) days, and 4 = *regularly* (6 to 7 days). For the items that state "reverse score" score as: 4 = *never* (0 days), 3 = *rarely* (1 day), 2 = *sometimes* (2 to 3 days), 1 = *often* (3 to 5) days, and 0 = *regularly* (6 to 7 days). Your score for this section can range from 0 to 32.

contrary, substance use should not be confused with self-care. Norcross and Guy (2007) refer to substance abuse as a form of unhealthy escape.

Environmental Factors (EF)

In their review of the literature, Norcross and Guy (2007) note that most approaches to self-care focus on changing the behaviors of the individual without adequately addressing environmental factors. The physical environment can affect well-being (Norcross & Guy, 2007). The comfort and appeal of lighting, furniture, decorations, flooring, and windows can make a difference in the overall tone of a space (Norcross & Guy, 2007). Barriers to daily functioning can play a large role in stress. Similar to the concept of micro-aggressions that can add up over time, *micro-stressors* can aggregate, chipping away at resiliency and the ability to cope.

For example, many years ago I worked for a small company that evaluated children and families. We used mini-cassettes to dictate our reports. Each day, we waited for tapes to become available from the typist. The delays could range from minutes to hours of work time lost. Despite our request, the administrators failed to provide a sufficient number of tapes. While at the electronics store, I decided to invest $50.00 in tapes. This small investment eliminated this daily annoyance and was surprisingly helpful in cultivating a more positive mood in the office. It is easy to underestimate the power of micro-stressors when left unaddressed. Self-care involves noticing and addressing these types of environmental issues. The environmental factors domain (Table 12.9) also addresses maintaining an organized workspace, balancing work for others and addressing your own initiatives, wearing suitable clothes, and doing small things to make each day a little bit better.

TABLE 12.9 Self-Care Environmental Factors Items*

- I maintained a manageable schedule.

- I avoided taking on too many requests or demands.

- I maintained a comforting and pleasing living environment.

- I kept my work/schoolwork area organized to support my work/school tasks.

- I maintained balance between the demands of others and what is important to me.

- Physical barriers to daily functioning were addressed (e.g., needed supplies for home and work were secured, light bulbs were replaced and functioning).

- I made sure I wore suitable clothing for the weather (e.g., umbrella in the rain, boots in the snow, warm coat in winter).

- I did things to make my everyday environment more pleasant (e.g., put a support on my chair, placed a meaningful photo on my desk).

- I did things to make my work setting more enjoyable (e.g., planned fun Fridays, partnered with a coworker on an assignment).

*Ask yourself, "This past week how many days did I do the following?" You can give yourself the following scores: 0 = *never* (0 days), 1 = *rarely* (1 day), 2 = *sometimes* (2 to 3 days), 3 = *often* (3 to 5) days, and 4 = *regularly* (6 to 7 days). Your score for this section can range from 0 to 36.

Self-Compassion (SC)

Self-compassion entails "treating oneself with kindness, recognizing one's shared humanity, and being mindful when considering negative aspects of oneself" (Neff, 2011, p. 1). Norcross and Guy (2007) address self-compassion throughout their text. However, it is most saliently addressed in their chapter on cognitive restructuring. In this chapter they cite several rigid, overarching beliefs that therapists hold that can lead to burnout. These include the belief that a therapist must be successful with all clients, that he or she must be one of the most outstanding therapists, and that he or she must be liked by all clients. Patients can have rigid beliefs as well. This is especially true among those with eating disorders (i.e., "I must look effortlessly perfect at all times"), although I have seen it across the array of self-regulation difficulties. Rigid beliefs often share a focus on perfectionism, a quality incompatible with self-compassion. Culturally, perfectionism is held as achievable and honorable. In practice, I actively discourage perfectionism by defining it as *romanticized rigidity*. Clients typically laugh and then get it. By dropping perfectionism and labeling it as just another way to be rigid, patients can more easily move toward more compassionate ways of thinking about behaviors, goals, and the self. Self-compassion is the focus of a very recent and growing body of research and appears to play a role in self-regulation. For example, self-compassion has been found to be negatively correlated with emotional regulation difficulties (Vettese, Dyer, Li, & Wekerle, 2011), negatively associated with Internet addiction (Iskender & Akin, 2011), and as a promising aspect of treatment for self-injury (Van Vliet & Kalnins, 2011). The items in Table 12.10 address self-compassion.

TABLE 12.10 Self-Care Self-Compassion Items*

- I noticed, *without judgment*, when I was struggling (e.g., feeling resistance, falling short of my goals, not completing as much as I'd like).

- I punitively/harshly judged my progress and effort (reverse score).

- I kindly acknowledged my own challenges and difficulties.

- I engaged in critical or harsh self-talk (reverse score).

- I engaged in supportive and comforting self-talk (e.g., "My effort is valuable and meaningful").

- I reminded myself that failure and challenge are part of the human experience.

- I gave myself permission to feel my feelings (e.g., allowed myself to cry).

---

*Ask yourself, "This past week how many days did I do the following?" You can give yourself the following scores: 0 = *never* (0 days), 1 = *rarely* (1 day), 2 = *sometimes* (2 to 3 days), 3 = *often* (3 to 5) days, and 4 = *regularly* (6 to 7 days). For the items that state "reverse score" score as: 4 = *never* (0 days), 3 = *rarely* (1 day), 2 = *sometimes* (2 to 3 days), 1 = *often* (3 to 5) days, and 0 = *regularly* (6 to 7 days). Your score for this section can range from 0 to 28.

TABLE 12.11 Self-Care Spiritual Practice Items*

- I experienced meaning and/or a larger purpose in my *work/school* life (e.g., for a cause).
- I experienced meaning and/or larger purpose in my *private/personal* life (e.g., for a cause).
- I spent time in a spiritual place (e.g., church, meditation room, nature).
- I read, watched, or listened to something inspirational (e.g., watched a video that gives me hope, read inspirational material, listened to spiritual music).
- I spent time with others who share my spiritual worldview (e.g., church community, volunteer group).
- I spent time doing something that I hope will make a positive difference in the world (e.g., volunteered at a soup kitchen, took time out for someone else).

*Ask yourself, "This past week how many days did I do the following?" You can give yourself the following scores: 0 = *never* (0 days), 1 = *rarely* (1 day), 2 = *sometimes* (2 to 3 days), 3 = *often* (3 to 5) days, and 4 = *regularly* (6 to 7 days). For the items that state "reverse score" score as: 4 = *never* (0 days), 3 = *rarely* (1 day), 2 = *sometimes* (2 to 3 days), 1 = *often* (3 to 5) days, and 0 = *regularly* (6 to 7 days). Your score for this section can range from 0 to 24.

Spiritual Practice (SP)

Spirituality involves inspiration from something greater than yourself (Norcross & Guy, 2007). Specifically, spirituality can be sourced from a sense of mission, purpose, and value as well as from religion (Norcross & Guy, 2007; Sayrs, 2012). Spirituality can be a source of strength and meaning (Norcross & Guy, 2007). The spirituality items (Table 12.11) address bringing meaning or purpose into work or school life as well as your personal life. The cultivation of spiritual moments, connections, and experiences is also addressed.

SUMMARY

Mindful self-care is a foundational self-regulating practice. It is a constant practice of bringing awareness to self-care, assessing self-care practices, setting self-care goals, and actively engaging in self-care practices. This chapter reviews self-care and mindful self-care and provides a domain-by-domain review, each with a set of questions to facilitate self-assessment. Based on the current body of research, the Mindful Self-Care Scale (MSCS) is currently undergoing psychometric evaluation and study. In its current form, it is a useful tool for reviewing and assessing self-care across the 10 domains for effective self-care goal setting. With the mindful and yogic tools provided in the text, as well as a steady practice of self-care, self-regulation can be achieved. The cultivation of healthy, integrating, embodied practices brings well-being, emotional stability, and physical health, while helping to remediate self-regulation difficulties.

Because no matter the challenges we confront. . . .
There is no escaping this reality, no matter what
others, or we, try to say about it.
If we don't care for ourselves, we'll be limited in how we can
care for others. It is that simple. And it is that important
—for you, for others, and for our planet.
DANIEL SIEGEL, THE MINDFUL THERAPIST (2010, p. 3)

REFERENCES

Benelam, B., & Wyness, L. (2010). Hydration and health: A review. *Nutrition Bulletin,* *35,* 3–25.

Cappuccio, F. P., Cooper, D., D'Elia, L., Strazzullo, P., & Miller, M. A. (2011). Sleep duration predicts cardiovascular outcomes: A systematic review and meta-analysis of prospective studies. *European Heart Journal, 32,* 1484–1492.

Cook-Cottone, C. P., Kane, L. S., Keddie, E., & Haugli, S. (2013). *Girls growing in wellness and balance: Yoga and life skills to empower.* Stoddard, WI: Schoolhouse Educational Services.

Cook-Cottone, C. P., Tribole, E., & Tylka, T. (2013). *Healthy eating in schools: Evidence-based interventions to help kids thrive.* Washington, DC: American Psychological Association.

Davis, M., Eshelman, E. R., & McKay, M. (2008). *The relaxation and stress reduction workbook* (6th ed.). Oakland, CA: New Harbinger Publications.

Duyff, R. L. (2011). *American Dietetic Association complete food and nutrition guide.* New York, NY: Houghton Mifflin Harcourt.

Hopkins, M. E., Davis, F. C., VanTieghem, M. R., Whalen, P. J., & Bucci, D. J. (2012). Differential effects of acute and regular physical exercise on cognition and affect. *Neuroscience, 215,* 59–68.

Iskender, M., & Akin, A. (2011). Self-compassion and Internet addiction. *Turkish Online Journal of Educational Technology—TOJET, 10,* 215–221.

Kyle, S. D., Morgan, K., & Espie, C. A. (2010). Insomnia and health-related quality of life. *Sleep Medicine Reviews, 14,* 69–82.

Lim, J., & Dinges, D. F. (2010). A meta-analysis of the impact of short-term sleep deprivation on cognitive variables. *Psychological Bulletin, 136,* 375.

Linehan, M. M. (1993). *Skills training manual for treating borderline personality disorder.* New York, NY: Guilford Press.

Neff, K. D. (2011). Self-compassion, self-esteem, and well-being. *Social and Personality Psychology Compass, 5,* 1–12.

Norcross, J. C., & Guy, J. D. (2007). *Leaving it at the office: A guide to psychotherapist self-care.* New York, NY: Guilford Press.

Sayrs, J. H. (2012). Mindfulness, acceptance, and values-based interventions for addiction counselors: The benefits of practicing what we preach. In S. C. Hayes & M. E. Levin (Eds.), *Mindfulness and acceptance for addictive behaviors: Applying contextual CBT to substance abuse and behavioral addictions* (pp. 187–215). Oakland, CA: New Harbinger Publications.

Shapiro, S. L., & Carlson, L. E. (2009). *The art and science of mindfulness: Integrating mindfulness into psychology and the helping professions.* Washington, DC: American Psychological Association.

Siegel, D. J. (2010). *The mindful therapist: A clinician's guide to mindsight and neural integration.* New York, NY: W. W. Norton.

Van Vliet, K. J., & Kalnins, G. R. (2011). A compassion-focused approach to nonsuicidal self-injury. *Journal of Mental Health Counseling, 33,* 295–311.

Vettese, L. C., Dyer, C. E., Li, W. L., & Wekerle, C. (2011). Does self-compassion mitigate the association between childhood maltreatment and later emotion regulation difficulties? A preliminary investigation. *International Journal of Mental Health and Addiction, 9,* 480–491.

Index